Davidson's Clinical Cases

Mark W.J. Strachan
BSc(Hons) MD FRCP Edin
Consultant Physician,
Western General Hospital, Edinburgh;
Part-time Senior Lecturer,
University of Edinburgh, UK

Surendra K. Sharma
MD PhD
Chief, Division of Pulmonary,
Critical Care and Sleep Medicine;
Professor and Head, Department of Medicine,
All India Institute of Medical Sciences,
New Delhi, India

John A.A. Hunter
OBE BA MD FRCP Edin
Professor Emeritus of Dermatology,
University of Edinburgh, UK

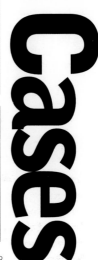

CHURCHILL
LIVINGSTONE

ELSEVIER

Edinburgh London New York Oxford Philadelphia St Louis Sydney Toronto 2008

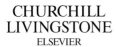

CHURCHILL
LIVINGSTONE
ELSEVIER

First published 2008

Main Edition ISBN: 978-0-443-06894-2
International Student Edition ISBN: 978-0-443-06893-5

British Library Cataloguing in Publication Data
A catalogue record for this book is available from the British Library

Library of Congress Cataloging in Publication Data
A catalog record for this book is available from the Library of Congress

Notice
Knowledge and best practice in this field are constantly changing. As new research and experience broaden our knowledge, changes in practice, treatment and drug therapy may become necessary or appropriate. Readers are advised to check the most current information provided (i) on procedures featured or (ii) by the manufacturer of each product to be administered, to verify the recommended dose or formula, the method and duration of administration, and contraindications. It is the responsibility of the practitioner, relying on their own experience and knowledge of the patient, to make diagnoses, to determine dosages and the best treatment for each individual patient, and to take all appropriate safety precautions. To the fullest extent of the law, neither the Publisher nor the Editors assume any liability for any injury and/or damage to persons or property arising out of or related to any use of the material contained in this book.

The Publisher

616/STK

Commissioning Editor: Laurence Hunter
Development Editor: Hannah Kenner
Project Manager: Frances Affleck
Designer: Stewart Larking
Illustrator: Chartwell Illustrators
Illustration Manager: Gillan Richards/Kirsteen Wright

Contents

Preface

Davidson's Principles and Practice of Medicine, now in its 20th edition, has stood the test of time because it continues to reflect Sir Stanley Davidson's determination to produce a book that was readable without ambiguity, uncertainty or wordiness. It is not a reference book and does not describe every rare disease or syndrome, but devotes most of its space to those disorders more commonly seen in practice. Inevitably, the content has changed considerably over the years, mirroring medical advances, and the approach over the last decade has become unashamedly problem-based, reflecting modern educational principles. *Davidson's Principles and Practice of Medicine* attempts to provide an international perspective on disease, to reflect the huge success that the book has had in many parts of the world, especially in the Indian subcontinent.

Davidson's Clinical Cases has been written in response to repeated suggestions from trainees that a companion case studies book would be well received. Patients do not appear in consulting rooms or hospitals with tags of 'Disease of such or such a system'; instead they come with problems that may cross many systems and which may even disguise the nature of the primary pathological culprit. This is the real world in which doctors practise; impressive physicians are those who accumulate knowledge gleaned from different cases and who can recall such experiences when faced with a similar new problem. We have made every effort to ensure that *Davidson's Clinical Cases* guides our reader, step by step, to follow the correct path in the maze between the presenting complaint of a patient and the final diagnosis. We emphasise the value of interpreting available clinical and investigative information in a logical way before considering a definitive diagnosis. Our selection of cases has not been arbitrary; it is based on the 'Presenting Problems' of the (20th) edition of *Davidson's Principles and Practice of Medicine* and illnesses that reflect an international outlook. We are more than aware that, for epidemiological, economic and other reasons, the practice of medicine in the developing world and in low-resource settings may be different from that in more privileged places, and the section on 'Global Issues' at the end of each case study addresses many of these important differences.

We chose our contributors carefully; they are all senior doctors, from different parts of the world, with considerable teaching experience. We tried to persuade them to take us through their cases in a personal way and to avoid regurgitating long and all-embracing lists from larger textbooks. We focus on the common disorders that are described in *Davidson's Principles and Practice of Medicine* and cross-references are included in every chapter. We have been strict in our editing in an effort to ensure uniformity in the layout and style of the many contributions. Inevitably, there is overlap between some of the cases and occasionally the approach of our contributors differs slightly from one to another. But this is medicine in diverse clinics.

Our editorial team works primarily in different specialties of medicine, though each of us has considerable experience of general internal medicine. In editing the text we have found it to be a most stimulating and effective method of learning about conditions of which we knew too little! We trust that our readers will also find that knowledge imparted in this manner is both easy and painless to digest. Welcome to *Davidson's Clinical Cases*!

M.W.J.S., S.K.S. and J.A.A.H.
Edinburgh and New Delhi, 2007

Acknowledgements

Case 4 and Case 5: M Y Rao acknowledges assistance from Robert Rao MBBS, Nuffield Department of Surgery, John Radcliffe Hospital, University of Oxford, UK. Case 8: L Karalliedde acknowledges assistance from Professor S A M Kularatne; photograph by kind permission of Prof Kularatne. Case 13: T Azhar acknowledges assistance from Suhaimi Ayoub MD MMED, International Islamic University of Malaysia, Pahang Darul Makmur, Malaysia. Case 24: Fig 24.1 supplied courtesy of A McMillan and G Scott, 2000, Colour Guide to Sexually Transmitted Infections, Churchill Livingstone, Edinburgh. Case 46: S K Sharma acknowledges assistance from Smriti Hari MD, Department of Radiodiagnosis, AIIMS, New Delhi, India. Cases 47 and 48: T Das acknowledges assistance from Dr Satinath Mukherjee, Department of Endocrinology, IPGMER, Kolkata, India. Case 54: The figure was reproduced with the kind permission of Dr Ian Penman, Department of Gastroenterology, Western General Hospital, Edinburgh. Case 64: Histology section courtesy of Dr Philip P C Ip, Department of Pathology and Clinical Biochemistry, Queen Mary Hospital, Hong Kong. Case 84: The figure was kindly provided by Professor Selim Benbadis, University of South Florida. Case 92: The figure was reproduced from Hunter J H, Savin J A and Dahl M V, *Clinical Dermatology*, 3rd edn, 2002. With permission from Blackwell Publishing.

Contributors

Tofayel Ahmed
MBBS FCPS(Pak) FCPS (Bangladesh)
MRCP FRCP Edin Glas Ire FACP FCCP
Professor of Medicine and Dean,
Postgraduate Faculty of Medicine,
Dhaka University, Bangladesh

Ian D R Arnott
BSc MBChB MD FRCP Edin
Consultant Gastroenterologist
and Honorary Senior Lecturer,
Gastrointestinal Unit, Western
General Hospital, Edinburgh, UK

Tahir Azhar
MBBS FRCP FFRRCS(I)
Dean and Professor of Medicine,
Faculty of Medicine, International
Islamic University Malaysia, Pahang
Darul Makmur, Malaysia

S Banerjee MD
Head of Department of Medicine,
In-charge Diabetes Clinic, NRS
Medical College, Kolkata, India

Peter Bloomfield MD FRCP FACC
Consultant Cardiologist,
Department of Cardiology,
Royal Infirmary of
Edinburgh, UK

Jan D Bos MD PhD FRCP
Professor and Chairman,
Department of Dermatology,
Academic Medical Centre, University
of Amsterdam, The Netherlands

Jane Collier MD FRCP
Consultant Hepatologist,
Department of Gastroenterology and
Hepatology, John Radcliffe Hospital,
Oxford, UK

Jenny I O Craig
MB ChB MD FRCP Edin FRCPath
Consultant Haematologist,
Department of Haematology,
Addenbrooke's Hospital,
Cambridge, UK

Allan Cumming
MBChB MD FRCP
Professor of Medical Education
and Consultant in Renal Medicine,
Department of Renal Medicine,
University of Edinburgh, UK

Mradul Kumar Daga
MD MNAMS
Professor of Medicine and Head
of Medical ITU, Department of
Medicine, Maulana Azad Medical
College, New Delhi, India

D Dalus MD FRCP PhD
Professor of Medicine, Department
of Medicine, Medical College
Hospital, Trivandrum, India

Tapas Das MD
Professor, Department of Medicine,
IPGMER and SSKM Hospital, Kolkata,
India

Richard J Davenport
DM FRCP Edin BMBS BMedSci
Consultant Neurologist and Honorary
Senior Lecturer, Department of
Clinical Neurosciences, Western
General Hospital, Edinburgh, UK

John M Davies
MA MD FRCP FRCPath
Consultant Haematologist and
Honorary Senior Lecturer,
Department of Haematology, Western
General Hospital, Edinburgh, UK

Abul Faiz
MBBS FCPS FRCP PhD
Professor of Medicine and Head,
Department of Medicine,
Dhaka Medical College, Dhaka,
Bangladesh

Michael J Field
MD BS BSc FRACP
Professor of Medicine and Associate
Dean, Northern Clinical School,
Royal North Shore Hospital,
University of Sydney, Australia

Brian M Frier
BSc(Hons) MD FRCP Edin FRCPG
Consultant Diabetologist and
Honorary Professor of Diabetes,
Department of Diabetes, Royal
Infirmary of Edinburgh, UK

Jane Goddard MBChB PhD FRCP Edin
Consultant Nephrologist,
Department of Renal Medicine,
Royal Infirmary of Edinburgh, UK

Neil Grubb MD MRCP
Consultant in Cardiac Electrophysiology,
Cardiovascular Research Unit, Royal
Infirmary of Edinburgh and Honorary
Senior Lecturer,
University of Edinburgh, UK

S B Gunatilake
MBBS MD FRCP Lond FRCP Edin Hon FRACP
Associate Professor and Head of
Medicine, Department of Medicine,
Faculty of Medicine, University of
Kelaniya, Sri Lanka

R Gupta MD DNB FRCP
Associate Professor of Medicine,
Department of Medicine, All India
Institute of Medical Sciences,
New Delhi, India

Adam T Hill MBChB MD FRCP Edin
Consultant in Respiratory Medicine
and Honorary Senior Lecturer,
Department of Respiratory Medicine,
Royal Infirmary of Edinburgh, UK

J A A Hunter OBE BA MD FRCP Edin
Professor Emeritus of Dermatology,
University of Edinburgh, UK

J Alastair Innes
BSc MB ChB PhD FRCP Edin
Consultant Physician and Honorary
Reader in Respiratory Medicine,
Respiratory Unit, Western General
Hospital, Edinburgh, UK

Syed Mohammad Wasim Jafri
MBBS FRCP Lond FRCP Edin FRCP Glas
FACP FACG
Ib-ne-Sina Professor and Chief
of Gastroenterology and Chair,
Department of Medicine,
Aga Khan University, Karachi,
Pakistan

Sanjay Jain
Professor of Internal Medicine,
Postgraduate Institute of Medical
Education and Research,
Chandigarh, India

Alison L Jones
BSc MD FRCP Edin FRCP Fi Biol
Professor of Medicine and Clinical
Toxicology, Faculty of Health,
University of Newcastle, Australia

A L Kakrani MD
Professor and Head, Department
of Medicine, BJ Medical College
and Sassoon General Hospitals,
Pune (Maharashtra), India

Lakshman Karalliedde
MBBS DA FRCA
Visiting Senior Lecturer,
King's College Medical School,
London; Consultant, Chemical
Hazards and Poisons Division, Health
Protection Agency UK, London, UK

Sarah Keir MD FRCP Edin
Consultant, Stroke Medicine, Western
General Hospital, Edinburgh, UK

J A Ker MBChB MMed MD
Deputy Dean, Faculty of Health
Sciences, Department of Internal
Medicine, University of Pretoria,
South Africa

Bhushan Kumar MD MNAMS
Former Professor and Head, Department of Dermatology, Venereology
and Leprology, Postgraduate Institute
of Medical Education and Research,
Chandigarh, India

Ching Lung Lai
MBBS(Hon) MD FRCP FRCP Edin FRCPG
FRACP
Professor of Medicine and Hepatology,
University Department of Medicine,
Queen Mary Hospital, Hong Kong

Christopher A Ludlam
MBChB BSc PhD FRCP FRCPath
Professor of Haematology and
Coagulation Medicine, University
of Edinburgh; Director, Haemophilia
and Thrombosis Centre, Royal
Infirmary of Edinburgh, UK

Christian J Lueck PhD FRCP FRACP
Head, Department of Neurology,
The Canberra Hospital, and
Associate Professor, Australian
National University Medical School,
Canberra, Australia

Govind K Makharia
MD DM DNB MNAMS
Associate Professor, Department
of Gastroenterology and Human
Nutrition, All India Institute of
Medical Sciences, New Delhi, India

Sara E Marshall
MRCP(Eire) FRCPath PhD
Professor of Clinical Immunology,
Department of Immunology,
Ninewells Hospital and Medical
School, University of Dundee, UK

Alexander McMillan MD FRCP FRCP Edin
Former Consultant Physician in
Genitourinary Medicine, Department
of Genitourinary Medicine, Royal
Infirmary of Edinburgh, UK

Euan R McRorie MB ChB FRCP
Consultant Rheumatologist
and Honorary Senior Lecturer,
Rheumatic Diseases Unit, Western
General Hospital, Edinburgh, UK

Alladi Mohan MBBS MD
Chief, Division of Pulmonary
and Critical Care Medicine and
Additional Professor and Head
of Department of Medicine,
Sri Venkateswara Institute
of Medical Sciences, Tirupati,
Andhra Pradesh, India

W F Mollentze MD FCP (SA) MMed FACE
Head of Internal Medicine,
Medical Faculty, University
of the Free State, Bloemfontein,
South Africa

David E Newby
BA BSc PhD BM DM FRCP
Professor of Cardiology, Centre
for Cardiovascular Science,
University of Edinburgh, UK

David Oxenham FRCP FAChPM
Consultant in Palliative Care,
Marie Curie Hospice, Edinburgh, UK

Paul L Padfield MB BCh FRCP
Consultant Physician and
Reader in Medicine, Department
of Endocrinology, Metabolic Unit,
Western General Hospital,
Edinburgh, UK

Prem S Pais MD
Dean and Professor of Medicine,
St John's Medical College,
Bangalore, India

Ian D Penman
BSc MD FRCP Edin
Consultant Gastroenterologist,
Gastrointestinal Unit, Western
General Hospital, Edinburgh, UK

Stuart H Ralston
MB ChB MD FRCP FMedSci FRSE
ARC Professor of Rheumatology,
Rheumatic Diseases Unit,
University of Edinburgh, Western
General Hospital, Edinburgh, UK

Amrany Ramachandran
MD PhD FRCP Dsc MNAMS FICP
Chairman/Managing Director,
Dr A Ramachandran's Diabetes
Hospitals; President, India Diabetes
Research Foundation, Chennai, India

Medha Y Rao
MBBS MD PGDHHM
Professor and Head of Department
of Medicine, M S Ramaiah
Medical College, Bangalore, India

Peter T Reid MD FRCP
Consultant in Respiratory
Medicine and Honorary Senior
Lecturer, Respiratory Medicine Unit,
Western General Hospital,
Edinburgh, UK

Vinay Sakhuja MD DM FAMS
Professor of Nephrology,
Department of Nephrology,
Postgraduate Institute of Medical
Education and Research,
Chandigarh, India

Harsha R Salkar
MD(Internal Med)
Professor and Head of Department
of Medicine, Government Medical
College, Nagpur, India

Rustam Al-Shahi Salman
MA PhD FRCP Edin
MRC Clinician Scientist and
Honorary Consultant Neurologist,
Division of Clinical Neurosciences,
Western General Hospital,
Edinburgh, UK

Olivia M Schofield
MBBS FRCP Edin
Consultant Dermatologist,
Department of Dermatology,
Royal Infirmary of Edinburgh, UK

Gordon R Scott
BSc MBChB FRCP
Consultant Physician, Department
of Genitourinary Medicine, Royal
Infirmary of Edinburgh, UK

K R Sethuraman MD PGDHE
Dean and Senior Professor of
Medicine, Asian Institute of
Medicine, Science and Technology,
Kedah, Malaysia

P S Shankar
MD FRCP FAMS DSc(h c Gul) DSc (h c NTR)
Emeritus Professor of Medicine
and Director, M R Medical College,
Karnataka, India

Surendra Kumar Sharma MD PhD
Chief, Division of Pulmonary, Critical
Care and Sleep Medicine,
Professor and Head, Department
of Medicine, All India Institute of
Medical Sciences, New Delhi, India

Pat Shepherd
MB BCh BAO FRCP FRCPath
Consultant Haematologist, Depart-
ment of Haematology, Western
General Hospital, Edinburgh, UK

Jon Stone
MB ChB FRCP Edin PhD
Consultant Neurologist and Honorary
Senior Lecturer, Department of Clini-
cal Neurosciences, Western General
Hospital, Edinburgh, UK

Mark W J Strachan
BSc MBChB(Hons) MD FRCP Edin
Consultant Physician and Part-time
Senior Lecturer, Metabolic Unit, Western
General Hospital, Edinburgh, UK

Shyam Sundar MD FRCP FNA
Professor of Medicine, Institute
of Medical Sciences, Banaras
Hindu University, Varanasi, India

Michael J Tidman MD FRCP Edin
Consultant Dermatologist,
Department of Dermatology,
Royal Infirmary of Edinburgh, UK

W T Andrew Todd
BSc MB ChB FRCP
Consultant Physician, Lanarkshire
Area Infectious Diseases Unit,
Monklands Hospital, Airdrie, UK

Marc L Turner
MB CLB PLD FRCP FRCPath
Senior Lecturer in Immunohaematol-
ogy and Transfusion Medicine,
Edinburgh and South East Scotland
Blood Transfusion Service, Royal
Infirmary of Edinburgh, UK

A Neil Turner PhD FRCP
Professor of Nephrology,
Medical Renal Unit, Royal Infirmary
of Edinburgh, UK

S Varma MBBS MD
Professor and Head, Department
of Internal Medicine, Postgraduate
Institute of Medical Education and
Research, Chandigarh, India

Simon Walker MB BS MA DM
Senior Lecturer and Honorary
Consultant in Clinical Biochemistry,
University of Edinburgh, UK

Ed Wilkins FRCP FRCPath
Consultant in Infectious Diseases,
Department of Infectious Diseases,
North Manchester General Hospital,
Manchester, UK

Gary A Wittert
MB BCH MD FRACP
Mortlock Professor and Head
of School of Medicine, University
of Adelaide, Australia

M E Yeolekar MD MNAMS FICN FIC
Dean and Professor of Internal
Medicine, Lokmanya Tilak Municipal
Medical College and General
Hospital, Mumbai, India

Abbreviations

AIDS	Acquired immunodeficiency syndrome
ALT	Alanine aminotransferase
ANCA	Antineutrophil cytoplasmic antibodies
ANF	Antinuclear factor
APTT	Activated partial thromboplastin time
AST	Aspartate aminotransferase
CEA	Carcinoembryonic antigen
CRP	C-reactive protein
dsDNA	Double-stranded DNA
ECG	Electrocardiogram
ESR	Erythrocyte sedimentation rate
GGT	Gamma-glutamyl transferase
HBsAg	Hepatitis B surface antigen
HDL	High-density lipoprotein
HIV	Human immunodeficiency virus
LDH	Lactate dehydrogenase
LDL	Low-density lipoprotein
LFTs	Liver function tests
MCV	Mean cell volume
PCV	Packed cell volume
PT	Prothrombin time
RBC	Red blood cells
RF	Rheumatoid factor
SGOT	Serum glutamic oxaloacetic transaminase
SGPT	Serum glutamic pyruvic transaminase
TSH	Thyroid-stimulating hormone
U&Es	Urea and electrolytes
WCC	White cell count

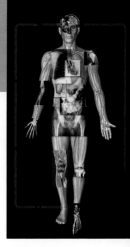

A young woman with intermittent lip swelling and a rash

S.E. MARSHALL

 Presenting problem

A 28-year-old woman is referred for assessment of possible anaphylaxis. Her first episode occurred 2 months previously, when she developed swelling of her lips associated with a generalised itchy rash 20 minutes after eating Chinese-style chicken, vegetables and rice. Her symptoms settled with oral antihistamines and she did not seek medical advice. Six weeks later, she developed sudden onset of flushing, lip swelling, lightheadedness and profound fear while sitting in a café. She collapsed on to the floor and vomited profusely, but did not experience loss of consciousness. Paramedics were called and noted that her blood pressure was 80/50 mmHg. She was taken to the Accident and Emergency department, where she received intramuscular adrenaline (epinephrine) and intravenous chlorphenamine and hydrocortisone. She made a good recovery and was discharged after an overnight stay. On this occasion, her reaction was associated with eating a houmous (chickpea) spread.

She has mild summer hay fever, but no previous history of food allergy, asthma or eczema, and is not on any medication.

What would your differential diagnosis include before examining the patient?

Her history of sudden onset of urticaria, angioedema, breathlessness, and hypotension is very suggestive of an anaphylactic reaction. This is most likely to be associated with a specific food allergy, but other causes of anaphylaxis, including medications, insect stings, latex and exercise, should be considered as possible triggers. Systemic diseases that may present with symptoms similar to anaphylaxis include phaeochromocytoma, carcinoid syndrome and mastocytosis.

 Examination

Physical examination is unremarkable.

Has examination narrowed down your differential diagnosis?

Physical examination is frequently normal in patients with a history of anaphylaxis and so may not narrow down the differential diagnosis.

Investigations

At the time of her acute admission to hospital, blood was taken for serum tryptase. This showed an acute rise in tryptase, concurrent with symptoms and returning to within the normal range over 24 hours (Fig. 1.1). Routine haematology, biochemistry and liver function tests are normal.

Skin prick tests to sesame and chickpeas are performed in the clinic; she develops a positive wheal and flare response to sesame.

Does this narrow down your differential diagnosis?

The sharp rise in serum tryptase at the time of clinical symptoms is pathognomonic of acute mast cell degranulation. However, this does not identify the mechanism (immunoglobulin E (IgE)-mediated or non-IgE-mediated) or the trigger. The finding of a positive skin prick test to sesame in conjunction with a consistent clinical history is very suggestive of specific allergy to sesame.

How will you treat this patient?

Exposure to sesame should be rigorously avoided. Sesame is often used for flavouring and decorative purposes in foods, and thus careful reading of package labelling is required. Sesame is also used in cosmetics, and sesame oil may occasionally be present in pharmaceuticals.

This patient should also be educated in the recognition and management of an allergic reaction in the event of inadvertent exposure. She should be prescribed oral antihistamines to be taken for mild symptoms (e.g. lip swelling). Given her history of anaphylaxis, she should also be prescribed self-injectable adrenaline (e.g. Epipen® or Anapen®1:1000, 0.3 ml × 2 syringes), to be administered intramuscularly if she develops severe symptoms (breathlessness, syncope). Patients and their families should be shown how to use self-injectable adrenaline, and should be provided with written guidelines as to its use. She should also be advised to wear a Medic-Alert bracelet, highlighting her allergy.

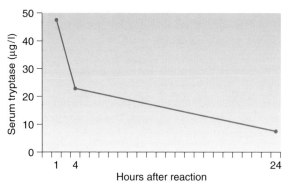

Fig. 1.1 Change in serum tryptase concentrations in the hours following the anaphylactic episode. Normal range 0–14 μg/l.

Global issues

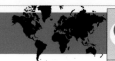

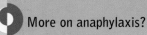 More on anaphylaxis?

See Chapter 4 of
Davidson's Principles and Practice of Medicine
(20th edn)

- Between 1990 and 2005, admissions for anaphylaxis increased by 600% in the UK.

- The prevalence of allergic diseases has reached epidemic proportions in Western countries. In addition, recent studies have shown that the prevalence of allergic disorders in children is rising rapidly in recently industrialised regions, including the Indian subcontinent and Latin America. Urban centres in developing countries may have few resources to implement management programmes for these diseases in the face of multiple other demands.

- The accuracy of food labelling varies in different countries and amongst different manufacturers. In addition, allergen advisory statements, such as 'may contain …' or 'free from …', have no standard definitions. Thus food labelling is often a source of confusion and limits food choices for individuals with allergic diseases.

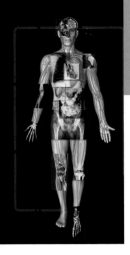

2

Intermittent swelling of the eyelids and mild urticaria in a young man

O. M. SCHOFIELD

Presenting problem

A 35-year-old man presents with a 6-week history of intermittent swelling of the eyelids. The swelling is not itchy or painful, and each episode lasts for about 3 days. It is not associated with any other ocular symptoms. The patient also describes an itchy rash that he describes as being 'like a nettle rash', which has been occurring intermittently over the last 2 months. Oral antihistamines have not been helpful. At no time has he had any swelling of his mouth or tongue. He is otherwise well, except for hypertension for which he takes enalapril. He has no history of any allergies. Direct systems enquiry also reveals that more recently he has developed intermittent abdominal pain associated with the eyelid swelling. He has a sister who has systemic lupus erythematosus and who he thinks has also had problems with eyelid swelling.

What would your differential diagnosis include before examining the patient?

Intermittent eyelid swelling is usually due to angioedema. This can be associated with urticaria and/or dermographism, or can occur in isolation. Angioedema most often occurs as a result of an immunoglobulin E (IgE)-mediated allergic response and in these cases there is usually a history of associated urticaria and a potential trigger for the attacks. The triggers can include allergens such as animals or specific foods, or physical stimuli such as exercise or heat. Certain drugs (e.g. aspirin, non-steroidal anti-inflammatory drugs (NSAIDs), penicillin, angiotensin-converting enzyme (ACE) inhibitors and radiocontrast media) can cause angioedema. When angioedema occurs without urticaria, one has to include the differential diagnosis of hereditary angioedema, in which the attacks start in the second decade, and acquired angioedema (AAE). AAE1 is a rare disorder associated with B cell lymphoproliferative disorders, and AAE2 is an autoimmune condition. Alternative diagnoses to angioedema as a cause of eyelid swelling include lymphoedema and connective tissue disorders such as dermatomyositis. In these situations the eyelid swelling is chronic rather than intermittent.

In this man's case the eyelid swelling is intermittent and associated with some mild urticaria and a family history of both connective tissue disease and possible eyelid swelling. One would therefore consider angioedema to be the most likely diagnosis but the cause needs to be investigated.

Examination

He appears well and has significant swelling of his eyelids, the left more marked than the right (Fig. 2.1). There is no evidence of any urticarial eruption and general examination is unremarkable. His blood pressure is well controlled at 115/70 mmHg.

Further investigations

Blood tests are performed for a full blood count, erythrocyte sedimentation rate (ESR) and C-reactive protein (CRP), urea and electrolytes, liver function tests, creatine kinase (CK) level, thyroid function tests, serum immunoglobulins including IgE, complement levels, antinuclear antibody, anti-double-stranded DNA antibody and C1 esterase inhibitor (C1-INH). The results of these investigations are all within the normal range.

Does this narrow down your differential diagnosis?

The investigations are all within the normal range and therefore have brought us no further forward in terms of establishing the cause of this man's urticaria. The normal CK and C1-INH levels all but rule out diagnoses of dermatomyositis and hereditary angioedema.

How will you treat this patient?

Looking back through his history, it is apparent that temporally his symptoms started soon after commencing enalapril for hypertension. This is an ACE inhibitor and this class of drugs is well known for causing both urticaria and angioedema. In addition a careful history has revealed that he has abdominal pain in association with the attacks of eyelid swelling. Angioedema can affect three predominant sites: subcutaneous tissue (such as around the eyes), abdominal organs (stomach and intestines), and upper airway (which can result in life-threatening laryngeal oedema).

The patient was advised to change his antihypertensive medication from an ACE inhibitor to an alternative class of agent, and within a month his symptoms improved.

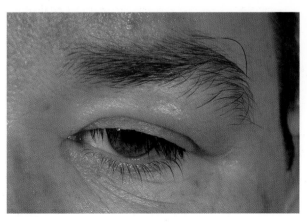

Fig. 2.1 Resolving swelling of the left eyelid. The swelling was intermittent, lasting for just over 24 hours. At its worst the eye was completely closed.

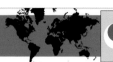
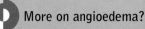

More on angioedema?

See Chapters 4 and 27 of
Davidson's
Principles and
Practice of
Medicine
(20th edn)

- Angioedema is a potentially lethal condition if there is involvement of the tongue or throat due to airways obstruction.

- Oral antihistamines are the mainstay of treatment (both H1 and H2 antagonists).

- Angioedema occurring without any history of urticaria should lead to suspicion of hereditary angioedema.

- Neither hereditary angioedema nor drug-induced angioedema responds well to oral antihistamines.

- Around 1% of individuals on ACE inhibitors develop angioedema. If the drugs are not withdrawn, then attacks become more severe with time.

- The history and examination are the key clues to the diagnosis here. Investigations such as CK, C1-INH and double-stranded DNA antibody are expensive and probably unwarranted in resource-poor settings.

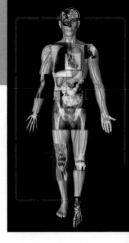

3

A young man with severe malnutrition

G. K. MAKHARIA

Presenting problem

A 20-year-old male presents to the outpatient department with symptoms of generalised weakness, easy fatiguability, tinnitus and anorexia. He has lost about 20 kg weight during the past 6 months. He has bone pain and complains of increasing difficulty in seeing in the dark. He has episodes of burning sensation in his soles and has noticed swelling of both feet. He used to have recurrent intestinal colic with generalised distension of the abdomen, vomiting and intractable constipation. For the last 3 years he has had persistent diarrhoea with occasional bleeding in the stools. He admits to drinking a lot of alcohol.

What would your differential diagnosis include before examining the patient?

This patient is suffering from gross malnutrition. This may be due to many causes, including a poor dietary intake (unavailability of food, poor dentures, dysphagia and neuropsychiatric disorders, including anorexia nervosa), malabsorption syndromes, chronic infections, malignancies and acquired immunodeficiency syndrome (AIDS). The following questions need to be answered: Is there a problem in getting food due to poverty? Is he giving up food in favour of alcohol? Is there an obstruction to the passage of food? Is there any disease of the gastrointestinal tract causing malabsorption? Is there evidence of any systemic inflammatory disease, underlying malignancy, tuberculosis or HIV infection? Does he live alone and neglect himself, or is he depressed or mentally handicapped?

The clue to the cause of this patient's malnutrition comes from his gastrointestinal symptoms. Recurrent intestinal colic with features of abdominal distension, intractable constipation and vomiting suggest the presence of an intestinal stricture. Chronic diarrhoea with bleeding in the stool suggests ulceration in the intestine, most probably in the colon. It also seems likely that his state is being worsened by excessive drinking of alcohol.

Examination

The patient's height, weight and body mass index (BMI) are 157 cm, 31.9 kg (compared with ideal body weight of 57 kg) and 12.9, respectively. He is emaciated, with hollow cheeks and loss of the buccal fat pad. The triceps skin fold thickness is 4.2 mm (normal in males 12.5 mm). The patient is very pale, and has angular cheilitis and stomatitis. His tongue has a magenta colour. His skin is dry, scaly and lustreless and has a rough texture, while his body hairs are lustreless and sparse. Examination of the eyes reveals the presence of Bitot's spots. His nails are white and opaque, and there is koilonychia and vertical ribbing. There is a widening of the wrist joints and he has knock knees. His face is swollen and he has bilateral pitting oedema of his lower legs. The costochondral angle is wide and there is fixed indrawing of the lower ribs, causing symmetrical horizontal grooves — Harrison's sulci. The liver is enlarged 3 cm below the costal margin but abdominal examination is otherwise unrevealing. Examination of the nervous system reveals evidence of a peripheral neuropathy in that he has reduced sensation in a 'glove and stocking' distribution.

Has examination narrowed down your clinical diagnosis?

A careful physical examination helps to characterise the extent of malnutrition and specific nutrient deficiencies (Box 3.1). In this case, the physical examination suggests that the young man has a severe degree of malnutrition. He has lost much of his body fat, has a very low muscle mass (suggesting a deficiency of somatic proteins) and has anasarca (suggesting loss of visceral protein). He has features of multiple vitamin deficiencies, including vitamin A (night blindness, dry skin and Bitot's spots), riboflavin (angular cheilitis, magenta-coloured tongue), vitamin B_6 (peripheral neuropathy), iron and folic acid (anaemia), and vitamin D (knock knees and widening of the wrist joints). The presence of

---

BOX 3.1

Clinical characteristics of nutritional deficiencies

Body part/organ	Characteristic	Deficient nutrient
General	Wasting	Calories
Skin	Pallor	Iron, folic acid, vitamin B_{12}
	Hyperpigmentation	Niacin, protein
	Thickening and dryness	Essential fatty acid
	Bruising	Vitamins C, K
Hair	Sparse and thin	Protein
Eyes	Pallor	Iron, folic acid, vitamin B_{12}
	Bitot's spot	Vitamin A
	Corneal vascularisation	Riboflavin
Nails	Koilonychia	Iron
	White nails	Protein
	Transverse lines	Protein
Oral cavity	Glossitis	Riboflavin, niacin, vitamin B_{12}
	Angular cheilitis	Riboflavin
	Bleeding gums	Vitamins C, K
Bones and joints	Knock knees	Vitamin D
	Widening of wrists	Vitamin D

Harrison's sulci and widening of the costochondral angle suggests that vitamin D deficiency has been present since childhood.

Further investigations

The results of blood tests are shown in Box 3.2. Bone mineral densitometry reveals osteoporosis in the spine and hip bones (T-scores −3.8 and −3.4 respectively). Colonoscopic examination reveals deep longitudinal ulcerations in the sigmoid colon and caecum (Fig. 3.1). Histology of a colonic lesion shows the presence of non-caseating granulomas, cryptitis and crypt abscesses. A barium contrast study shows multiple intestinal strictures with thickening of the intestinal wall; other organs are normal.

BOX 3.2	
Further investigations	
Haemoglobin	65 g/l (6.5 g/dl)
MCV	64 fl
WCC	3.4×10^9/l (10^3/mm^3) with lymphopenia
Platelets	345×10^9/l (10^3/mm^3)
Sodium	145 mmol/l (meq/l)
Potassium	3 mmol/l (meq/l)
Urea	4.2 mmol/l (25.2 mg/dl)
Creatinine	23 µmol/l (0.26 mg/dl)
Total protein	60 g/l (6.0 g/dl)
Albumin	25 g/l (2.5 g/dl)
Calcium	1.59 mmol/l (6.38 mg/dl)
Phosphate	0.8 mmol/l (2.48 mg/dl)
Iron	5 µmol/l (27.9 µg/dl)
Transferrin saturation	17%
Folate	1.6 µg/l (ng/ml)
Serum B$_{12}$	110 pg/l
Coeliac serology	Negative
HIV serology	Negative

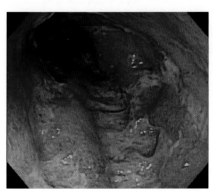

Fig. 3.1 Colonoscopic examination showing multiple deep longitudinal ulcers in the sigmoid colon. These are characteristic features of Crohn's disease.

Does this narrow down your differential diagnosis?

Laboratory investigations confirm severe malnutrition secondary to Crohn's disease.

How will you treat this patient?

There are two goals of treatment in a patient with malnutrition: (1) restoration of the body composition to normal by supplying macronutrients (carbohydrates, protein and fat) and micronutrients (minerals and vitamins); (2) treatment of the primary disease that has led to malnutrition.

Treatment of severe malnutrition is divided into two stages. The objective of the first phase includes correction of fluid and electrolytes and acid–base imbalances and treatment of hypocalcaemia, hypophosphataemia and hypoglycaemia. The objective of the second phase is to supply nutrients to restore normal body composition; their administration should be initiated at a slow pace and then gradually accelerated.

To start with, calories derived from carbohydrate, fat and protein are supplied at a rate of 30 kcal/kg/day and protein at the rate of 0.8 g/kg/day. Once this food is tolerated, the calories may be increased to 35–50 kcal/kg/day and protein to 1–1.5 g/kg/day. In addition, this man should be provided with supplements of calcium, iron, folic acid, vitamins (both fat- and water-soluble) and other micronutrients. His daily dietary intake should be recorded. He should be assessed regularly to gauge improvement in his nutritional status. Dietary supplements should be guided by a dietitian.

The malnutrition in this patient has been caused by Crohn's disease. He requires treatment for this, including immunosuppressive drugs and mesalamines. He should be counselled to stop drinking alcohol.

Global issues

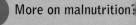 More on malnutrition?

- Alcohol (with self-neglect), anorexia nervosa and organic disease of the bowel are the main causes of malnutrition in the developed world.

- Malnutrition not only may be caused by chronic infections such as parasitic infestations, tuberculosis and HIV, but also predisposes an individual to chronic infections.

See Chapters 5 and 23 of
Davidson's Principles and Practice of Medicine (20th edn)

- Malnutrition associated with chronic illness leads to frequent hospitalisation and produces a huge socioeconomic burden in resource-poor countries.

- Malnutrition increases in-hospital morbidity and mortality.

- Almost half of elderly hospitalised patients in industrialised countries have some degree of malnutrition; the proportion is higher still in developing countries.

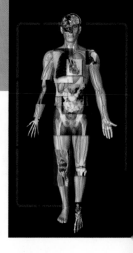

4

An elderly woman with repeated falls

MEDHA Y. RAO

Presenting problem

A 75-year-old lady is referred from home complaining of inability to stand or walk and pain in the left hip, following a fall while getting out of a taxi. On questioning, she says that she has tripped a few times in the recent past without major consequences. She also gives a past history of a stroke, at the age of 69, from which she recovered completely. There is no history of dizziness or visual disturbance. She is not known to have diabetes, but she has always been frail and was a heavy smoker prior to the stroke. She currently takes aspirin, bendroflumethiazide, ramipril and simvastatin. At 72, she was diagnosed with thyrotoxicosis secondary to a multinodular goitre, when she presented with atrial fibrillation. This was successfully treated with radio-iodine therapy and she reverted spontaneously to sinus rhythm. The results of laboratory investigations performed by her GP are detailed in Box 4.1.

BOX 4.1	
Initial investigations	
Haemoglobin	136 g/l (13.6 g/dl)
WCC	14.2×10^9/l (10^3/mm^3)
Differential count	
Neutrophils	82%
Lymphocytes	10%
Eosinophils	6%
Monocytes	2%
PCV	0.42
ESR	50 mm/1st hr
Blood glucose (fasting)	4.44 mmol/l (80 mg/dl)
Urea	3.927 mmol/l (11 mg/dl)
Serum creatinine	45.756 μmol/l (0.6 mg/dl)
Sodium	140 mmol/l (140 meq/l)
Potassium	3.7 mmol/l (3.7 meq/l)
TSH	0.3 mU/l

What would your differential diagnosis include before examining the patient?

Given the predominance of pain, a soft-tissue or bony injury must be excluded — most notably a fractured neck of femur. Why did this woman fall, though? It might have been a simple trip, but there is a history of this having happened on more than one occasion. Nothing is known about her vision, so it will be important to check that there is no problem here. With a previous history of stroke, reduced mobility of the affected leg and impaired proprioception would clearly increase her risk of falling.

In older people who have fallen, one of the first questions to ask is, 'What drugs does this person take?' The potential for polypharmacy and multiple drug interactions/side-effects in this age group is enormous. This lady is on two antihypertensive agents. Could she have postural hypotension? It is also important to exclude intercurrent illness. Could she have developed a urinary tract infection or a chest infection that has impaired her walking? There is no history of vertigo. The possibilities are almost endless, but careful examination and simple investigations should help.

Examination

Examination reveals a frail elderly lady, clinically non-icteric and mildly pale. Her left lower limb appears externally rotated and shortened, with tenderness over the greater trochanter. She does not have peripheral oedema or clinically significant lymphadenopathy. Her blood pressure is 130/80 mmHg, with no postural drop, and her pulse is regular at 90 beats/min. She has no murmurs and chest auscultation is clear. Examination of her higher mental functions is unremarkable. She does not have a visual field defect, but corrected vision is 6/18 in the right eye and 6/24 in the left; fundal examination reveals bilateral cataracts. There is slight reduction in power in the right arm and leg (4+/5), and careful sensory examination reveals impairment of proprioception in the right foot. There are no distal peripheral vascular deficits in either limb nor any clinical evidence of thyroid overactivity.

Have examination and initial investigations narrowed down your differential diagnosis?

Clinical examination points to a left fractured neck of femur. There is subtle evidence of a residual deficit from the previous cerebrovascular accident, of which the patient was unaware. This might have contributed to the fall, but it seems unlikely that, on its own, this would have been sufficient to cause it. There is no postural drop in blood pressure, so on this occasion her medication cannot be blamed. Despite her initial assertion, her vision is not good. She has cataracts and, of course, there may also be an element of age-related macular degeneration. She is clinically and biochemically euthyroid, but her white cell count and erythrocyte sedimentation rate are elevated. Could there be some intercurrent infection?

Further investigations

X-ray of the left hip confirms an intertrochanteric fracture of the left femur (Fig. 4.1). A dual-energy X-ray absorptiometry (DEXA) scan confirms the diagnosis of osteoporosis, with a T-score at the hip of −3.1 and −2.9 in the lumbar vertebrae. A 12-lead electrocardiogram (ECG) and chest X-ray are unremarkable. Urinalysis reveals blood++; protein ++; leucocytes +++ and nitrate +++, and subsequent urine culture grows numerous *Escherichia coli* organisms.

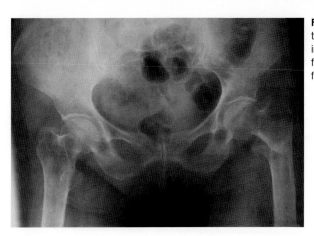

Fig. 4.1 X-ray of the hip showing an intertrochanteric fracture of the left femur.

Has the diagnosis been clinched?

Yes; she has a fracture of the left femoral neck. The trauma was relatively trivial and this is in keeping with it being an insufficiency (osteoporotic) fracture. She has several risk factors for osteoporosis — most notably her post-menopausal status, her previous history of thyrotoxicosis and her heavy smoking history.

As is often the case in elderly people, the fall was almost certainly multifactorial in nature. The circumstances were crucial; getting out of a car is never easy for older people, who often have back pain or arthritic joints. On top of that she has a residual subtle neurological deficit from her stroke that will have impaired her joint position sense. Her eyesight is poor and she had an intercurrent urinary tract infection. Occam's Razor ('there is usually a unifying diagnosis to explain a person's symptoms') is therefore disproved!

How will you treat this patient?

The fractured neck of femur should be treated surgically by closed reduction with internal fixation under spinal block (preferable) or general anaesthesia. If the latter is chosen, the patient will need a good anaesthetist. Bisphosphonate therapy and supplemental calcium and vitamin D should be prescribed to reduce the risk of further osteoporotic fractures.

A fractured neck of femur is often a major turning point in an individual's life. It can mark the end of functional independence and may be the start of a general decline in physical (and mental) status. Post-operatively, this lady will need a lot of input from physiotherapists and occupational therapists. A careful assessment of her care needs will be required prior to discharge. Will she be able to return home? If so, will she need aids for bathing and toileting there? With regard to her mobility, she will probably need to walk with a stick or walking frame. If her mobility and functional status are poor, she will need support from relatives or 'home helps' as far as shopping and cleaning are concerned; alternatively, she may require placement in sheltered housing or a care home. The implications for this woman are potentially enormous.

With regard to the falls, the urinary tract infection should be treated with appropriate antibiotic therapy. The patient might just need a good pair of glasses to improve her eyesight, but she should be reviewed by an ophthalmologist for consideration of cataract surgery, if her condition following hip replacement makes this appropriate.

Global issues

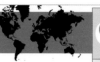

- Falls are common in older people and are usually multifactorial in aetiology.

- Polypharmacy, particularly in Western countries, is an increasing problem and is often responsible for falls.

- Osteoporosis prophylaxis should be considered in elderly people, particularly those at high risk: for example, those with previous insufficiency fractures, premature menopause or a strong family history of osteoporotic fractures.

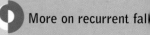

More on recurrent fall

See Chapter 7 of
Davidson's Principles and Practice of Medicine
(20th edn)

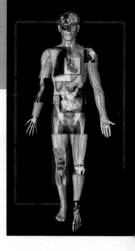

5

An elderly man with acute confusion

MEDHA Y. RAO

Presenting problem

A 74-year-old man is brought to the Accident and Emergency department, as he is found to be confused, disoriented and delirious. He lives independently and has previously been socially active. As he had not telephoned his family in the preceding 2 days, his son entered his apartment and found him lying on the floor, covered in urine and faeces. The patient is conversant, but confused and drowsy. He was a healthy man with no previous medical problems. He does not take any regular medications and has not sought any medical care for many years. He is a chronic cigarette smoker (1 pack per day) and occasionally drinks alcohol.

What would your differential diagnosis include before examining the patient?

When an elderly person suddenly becomes confused, the diagnostic possibilities include infectious, metabolic/endocrine, neurological, toxic and other causes. A collateral history from a relative, friend or carer is often extremely useful in determining the sequence of events in the days leading up to admission and can give valuable information about the underlying diagnosis.

Infections in the elderly can present without fever. The chest and the urinary tract are the most common sites of infection in this setting, but acute meningitis, encephalitis and intra-abdominal infection must also be considered. As the patient is a chronic smoker, lung cancer, presenting as a post-obstructive pneumonia or with cancer-induced hypercalcaemia, should also be considered in the differential diagnosis.

Metabolic/endocrine possibilities include hypoglycaemia, hyponatraemia, hyperosmolar coma and uraemia. Acute alcohol withdrawal should also be considered, particularly if there is a history of chronic excess consumption. There may not be such a history, though, as elderly people can be extremely clever at hiding significant alcohol intake from friends and family. Neurological causes include ischaemic or haemorrhagic stroke, subdural haematoma and cerebral contusion. There is no history of any medication or recreational drug use, but iatrogenic causes of confusion, e.g. a recent prescription of opiate medication for back pain, should always be sought. It should also be remembered that elderly patients with acute myocardial infarction can sometimes present with an acute confusional state.

Examination

On general physical examination, the patient appears moribund and dishevelled. He gives his name correctly and remembers where he lives, but does not know the name of the hospital where he is presently nor the date, day of the week or the year. He is able to recall the name of only one of three objects mentioned. He is malnourished with a body mass index (BMI) of 15.4 kg/m^2. He is afebrile, but has mild central cyanosis and his tongue is dry. His heart rate is 110 beats/min, respiratory rate is 24 breaths/min and blood pressure is 130/70 mmHg. The optic fundi appear normal and there is no papilloedema.

The trachea is central but the left side of the chest moves less with respiration. The inframammary, infra-axillary and infrascapular areas on the left side are dull on percussion. High-pitched tubular bronchial breath sounds are heard in these areas. There is increased resistance to passive flexion of the neck. The cranial nerves and motor and sensory system examinations are normal, deep tendon reflexes are symmetric in the upper and lower extremities and the plantar reflexes are flexor on both sides. His abdomen is soft without tenderness, rigidity or hepatosplenomegaly, and the bowel sounds are present. Cardiovascular examination is unremarkable but for the tachycardia.

His son says that over the past week the patient has had a chesty cough and 4 days ago he tripped over in the house and sustained a relatively minor bang to the head; there was no loss of consciousness.

Has examination narrowed down your differential diagnosis?

It seems highly likely that this patient's acute confusional state is due to left lower lobe pneumonic consolidation. Dehydration, hyponatraemia, hypoglycaemia and hypoxaemia may also be contributing to his delirium; all need to be investigated. The meningeal irritation needs to be looked into and, since there is a history of fall, a subdural haematoma should be ruled out.

Investigations

The results of the investigations carried out in the Accident and Emergency department are shown in Box 5.1. A 12-lead electrocardiogram (ECG) does not suggest an acute coronary event. A chest X-ray shows homogeneous opacity in the left mid- and lower zones (Fig. 5.1). An arterial blood gas (ABG) analysis while breathing room air yields the following results: PaO$_2$ 7.3 kPa (54 mmHg); PaCO$_2$ 4.6 kPa (34.6 mmHg); bicarbonate 21.9 mmol/l (21.9 meq/l); hydrogen ion 37.2 nmol/l (pH 7.41); oxygen saturation is 89%. A computed tomogram (CT) of the head without contrast reveals age-related cerebral atrophy. Lumbar puncture reveals normal cerebrospinal fluid (CSF). Serological tests for *Mycoplasma*, *Chlamydia*, *Legionella*, common viral infections and syphilis are negative. Pneumococcal antigen is not detected in the serum. A sputum culture is sterile, but blood culture grows *Haemophilus influenzae* sensitive to co-amoxiclav.

Does this narrow down your differential diagnosis?

A neutrophilic leucocytosis supports the diagnosis of an acute bacterial infection. Biochemical investigations confirm hyponatraemia, but rule out hypoglycaemia and uraemia. Hyponatraemia may be dilutional or depletional — easy to write, but often difficult to determine in practice. In this case, though, the patient does appear clinically dry and this is supported biochemically by the elevated

BOX 5.1	
Initial investigations	
Haemoglobin	100 g/l (10 g/dl)
WCC	16×10^9/l (10^3/mm^3)
Differential count	
Neutrophils	85%
Lymphocytes	10%
Eosinophils	3%
Monocytes	2%
PCV	0.32
Blood glucose	5.55 mmol/l (100 mg/dl)
Blood urea	10.71 mmol/l (30 mg/dl)
Serum creatinine	88.4 µmol/l (1.0 mg/dl)
Sodium	128 mmol/l (128 meq/l)
Potassium	4.3 mmol/l (4.3 meq/l)

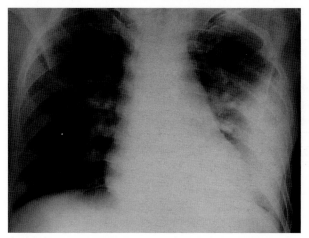

Fig. 5.1 Chest X-ray showing left mid- and lower zone consolidation.

urea:creatinine ratio. A normal CSF analysis and a normal CT of the head exclude neurological causes. There seems little doubt that the patient has left-sided pneumonic consolidation, caused by *H. influenzae*, with an acute confusional state due to the infection, dehydration, hyponatraemia and type I respiratory failure.

How will you treat this patient?

This man should be admitted to a high-dependency unit. As there is no evidence of carbon dioxide retention, high-flow humidified oxygen therapy may be administered through a ventimask, maintaining the arterial oxygen saturation (SaO_2) above 90%. Intravenous co-amoxiclav (1.2 g i.v. 8-hourly) and clarithromycin (500 mg i.v. 12-hourly) should be commenced and intravenous fluids administered. The patient's serum sodium level should be monitored closely to ensure that it returns to normal as he is rehydrated. Once his clinical state has improved, he will need input from members of the multidisciplinary team, to assess his ongoing care needs on discharge. Given his smoking history, it will be important to confirm radiological resolution of the consolidation with a follow-up chest X-ray after 6–8 weeks. If radiological signs persist, the possibility of an underlying bronchogenic neoplasm should be actively considered.

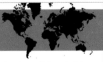

Global issues

 More on pneumonia?

- Respiratory infections are the most important and treatable cause of acute confusion in the elderly. These infections are often missed in the absence of a high index of suspicion. Clinical presentation of pneumonia in the elderly may be atypical and fever is frequently absent. Therefore, if no other obvious cause is evident, it may be appropriate to initiate empirical antibiotic treatment once cultures have been taken.

See Chapter 19 of **Davidson's Principles and Practice of Medicine** (20th edn)

- In areas where tuberculosis (TB) is highly endemic, miliary TB (especially cryptic miliary TB) and TB meningitis should also be considered in the differential diagnosis, especially if the individual is HIV-positive.

- Alcohol intoxication and withdrawal are important causes of acute confusion in the elderly in countries where alcoholism is common.

- An acute confusional state may not only be due to the effects of alcohol ingestion, but may also be a consequence of alcoholism. For example, an elderly person intoxicated with alcohol can sustain a fall and consequently develop an acute confusional state due to a subdural haemorrhage.

6

An elderly woman with sudden onset of dizziness

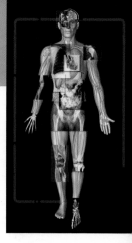

D. DALUS

Presenting problem

A 70-year-old female is admitted, complaining of swaying, unsteadiness and lightheadedness. She is a known hypertensive but is on irregular treatment. For the past few years she has experienced neck pain aggravated by movement. On the advice of her GP, some initial investigations have been carried out; the results are detailed in Box 6.1.

What would your differential diagnosis include before examining the patient?

Repeated episodes of dizziness affect at least 30% of people aged over 65 years. Older people often find it difficult to describe the sensation they feel; therefore assessment can be very frustrating. Acute dizziness in the elderly can result from several causes. This patient is known to be hypertensive but is irregular in taking antihypertensive drugs. Inadequately controlled blood pressure itself can produce dizziness. Postural hypotension (a sustained drop in systolic (≥ 20 mmHg) or diastolic (≥ 10 mmHg) blood pressure within 3 minutes of standing from the supine position) can result from the use of antihypertensive drugs. Other drugs producing postural hypotension include diuretics, antidepressants, phenothiazines, narcotics, barbiturates and calcium channel blockers. The history may reveal an underlying cause for the dizziness, such as diabetes mellitus,

BOX 6.1	
Initial investigations	
Urea	6 mmol/l (36 mg/dl)
Creatinine	100 µmol/l (1.12 mg/dl)
Sodium	136 mmol/l (136 meq/l)
Potassium	4.2 mmol/l (4.2 meq/l)
Cholesterol (total)	7.3 mmol/l (280 mg/dl)
Blood glucose (fasting)	5.2 mmol/l (94 mg/dl)
TSH	3.5 mU/l
ECG	No evidence of left ventricular hypertrophy, arrhythmia or myocardial infarction

Parkinson's disease or cardiac failure. Hypoglycaemia can also produce dizziness. Acute dizziness can also result from hypotension due to an arrhythmia, acute myocardial infarction, gastrointestinal bleeding or pulmonary thromboembolism. Absence of chest pain and no past history of coronary artery disease rule out significant cardiac disease. Absence of chest pain and dyspnoea does not support the diagnosis of thromboembolism. Furthermore, the normal ECG rules out a persistent arrhythmia and myocardial infarction.

An acute posterior fossa stroke can produce dizziness. Vestibular neuronitis is another cause and this symptom is frequently accompanied by nausea (sometimes with vomiting) and jerky nystagmus; the dizziness frequently increases with rapid head movements and patients try to hold their head still. This patient has a history of painful neck movements; this might point to a diagnosis of cervical spondylosis with vertebrobasilar insufficiency.

Examination
The patient looks apprehensive. She is obese and has a supine blood pressure of 160/100 mmHg with no significant postural hypotension. Neurological examination reveals impaired tandem walking and an absent right biceps jerk.

Has examination narrowed down your differential diagnosis?
As mentioned above, the cause of dizziness is often multifactorial. Nevertheless, the most effective way of establishing the cause is to determine which one of the following is the dominant symptom, even if more than one is present. Lightheadedness suggests presyncope and the presence of vertigo suggests labyrinthine or brain-stem disease, while unsteadiness or poor balance suggests joint or neurological disease. The history of neck pain with an absent biceps jerk favours the possibility of cervical spondylotic radiculopathy. The presence of gait ataxia, as suggested by impaired tandem walking, suggests the clinical diagnosis of posterior fossa stroke. So the present episode may be due to an acute posterior fossa stroke.

Further investigations
Holter monitoring (ambulatory ECG for 24 hours) reveals no significant abnormality. A CT of the brain and cervical spine shows a localised area of decreased density in the right cerebellar hemisphere (Fig. 6.1). The spine shows degenerative changes involving the C5–C6 and C6–C7 vertebrae.

Has the diagnosis been clinched?
Investigation has confirmed the clinical diagnosis of acute posterior fossa stroke with cervical spondylotic radiculopathy.

How will you treat this patient?
Management of acute stroke is aimed at minimising the volume of brain that is irreversibly damaged, preventing complications, reducing the patient's disability and handicap through rehabilitation, and minimising the risk of recurrent episodes. If this woman had presented within 3 hours of onset of symptoms, she might have been a candidate for intravenous thrombolysis with recombinant tissue plasminogen activator (rt-PA). An antiplatelet drug, such as aspirin (300 mg daily), should be started immediately after an ischaemic stroke unless rt-PA has been given, in which case it should be withheld for at least 24 hours.

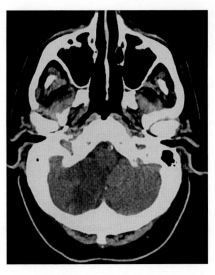

Fig. 6.1 CT of the brain showing an area of low density in the right cerebellar hemisphere, consistent with an acute stroke.

To reduce the risk of further strokes, a statin (if total cholesterol is over 3.5 mmol/l) and an antihypertensive drug (if blood pressure is over 130/70 mmHg 1–2 weeks after onset) should be given. Lifestyle modification should be strongly recommended. Regarding cervical spondylotic radiculopathy, conservative treatment with analgesics and physiotherapy results in the reduction of symptoms in the great majority of patients, but a few need surgery in the form of foraminotomy/disc excision.

Global issues

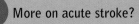 More on acute stroke?

- Dizziness affects 30% of those aged over 65 years.

- After persistent stroke, aspirin started within 48 hours of insult improves long-term outcome. Treating 1000 patients for 2 weeks prevents 13 dying or becoming dependent by 6 months.

- Lowering blood pressure even to the 'normal range' reduces the risk of a recurrent stroke, myocardial infarction and vascular deaths. Treating 1000 patients for 1 year prevents about 22 strokes.

See Chapter 26 of

Davidson's Principles and Practice of Medicine (20th edn)

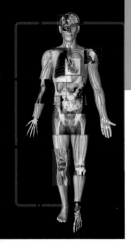

7

Unexplained weight loss in an elderly woman

A. MOHAN

Presenting problem

A 74-year-old lady presents with anorexia and weight loss of 15 kg over the preceding 3 months. There is no history of fever or diarrhoea. She is an otherwise healthy lady who has never visited a hospital till the present episode of ill-health. She does not smoke or drink alcohol and is not taking any medication.

What would your differential diagnosis include before examining the patient?

When an elderly lady presents with gradual onset of anorexia and weight loss without accompanying fever, the differential diagnosis (Box 7.1) would include organic causes such as underlying malignant disease, chronic infections,

---

BOX 7.1

Causes of weight loss in an elderly patient

Physiological causes
- Anorexia of ageing

Organic causes
- Underlying malignant disease (primary or metastatic)
- Endocrine disorders (hyperthyroidism, diabetes mellitus, Addison's disease)
- Renal failure
- Chronic infections such as tuberculosis, HIV/AIDS, brucellosis and parasitic infestations
- Gastrointestinal problems (e.g. malabsorption syndrome, inflammatory bowel disease, pernicious anaemia, cirrhosis)
- Chronic obstructive pulmonary disease
- Chronic congestive cardiac failure
- Parkinsonism

Other causes
- Alcohol and drugs (metformin, levodopa and angiotensin-converting enzyme (ACE) inhibitors)
- Psychiatric problems (e.g. depression, dementia)
- Unknown

---

gastrointestinal disorders, chronic obstructive pulmonary disease, diabetes mellitus, hyperthyroidism, chronic renal failure, depression and dementia. Though not applicable to this case, alcoholism and drug-induced weight loss would also have to be considered as causes in the appropriate setting.

Examination

Physical examination reveals a frail, pale-looking, emaciated elderly lady whose body mass index (BMI) is 13. She is well oriented in time, place and person, and her mini-mental status examination (MMSE) score is 26. She can clearly understand her problem and is worried as to why she is losing weight. There is no evidence of peripheral lymphadenopathy or hepatosplenomegaly. Pelvic examination is normal. The rest of the physical examination is also unremarkable.

Has examination narrowed down your differential diagnosis?

Other than evidence of wasting and pallor, there are no clues to help in the localisation of this lady's weight loss. This is often the case. Given that she is well oriented and has clear thinking, depression, dementia and other psychological problems and physiological anorexia of ageing seem unlikely. Even though fever is absent, infection cannot be excluded, as fever sometimes may not be evident in elderly individuals with chronic low-grade infections.

Investigations

The following blood results are obtained: haemoglobin 72 g/l (7.2 g/dl), a total leucocyte count of 2.8×10^9/l (10^3/mm³) and a platelet count of 90 $\times 10^9$/l (10^3/mm³). Peripheral smear examination shows a normocytic normochromic picture and pancytopenia. The erythrocyte sedimentation rate (ESR) is elevated (80 mm at the end of the first hour, Westergren method). Serum biochemistry, including electrolytes and urine examination, is normal. Urine culture is sterile. An oral glucose tolerance test rules out diabetes mellitus. Stool examination for parasites and occult blood is negative on three occasions. A tuberculin skin test (TST) with 5 TU (tuberculin units) of purified protein derivative (PPD) is negative. She is human immunodeficiency virus (HIV)-seronegative. The thyroid profile is within normal limits. The chest X-ray on admission (Fig. 7.1) is reported to be normal. Abdominal ultrasonography reveals kidneys with normal size and echo texture and no intra-abdominal lymphadenopathy or focal lesions in liver, spleen or other viscera. The patient

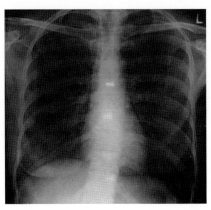

Fig. 7.1 A normal X-ray (postero-anterior view) on the patient's admission.

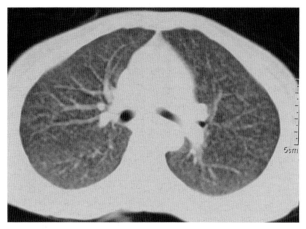

Fig. 7.2 High-resolution CT of the chest of the same patient, showing a classical miliary pattern.

undergoes upper gastrointestinal endoscopy and colonoscopy, and these tests are also unremarkable.

In view of the pancytopenia, trephine biopsy of the bone marrow is performed. It reveals granulomas with caseous necrosis and acid-fast bacilli (AFB). Subsequently, a fundus examination performed following mydriatic administration reveals choroidal tubercles. A high-resolution computed tomogram (HRCT) of the chest (Fig. 7.2) reveals a classical miliary pattern. Lumbar puncture is also performed and the cerebrospinal fluid analysis is documented as normal.

Does this narrow down your differential diagnosis?

The patient has 'cryptic miliary tuberculosis'. Unlike in classical miliary tuberculosis, fever may sometimes be absent, especially among the elderly, and patients may present with progressive wasting, mimicking a metastatic carcinoma. In these patients, the chest X-ray may be normal and the TST is often negative. Blood dyscrasias such as pancytopenia may sometimes be evident. This constitutes a valuable diagnostic clue and would call for bone marrow examination, which may confirm the diagnosis as in this case. In earlier days, cryptic miliary tuberculosis was often diagnosed at autopsy. However, with the availability of HRCT, many of these cases are now diagnosed during life.

How will you treat this patient?

Miliary tuberculosis is fatal if untreated and antituberculosis treatment remains the essential treatment strategy. In the absence of associated meningeal involvement, 6 months of treatment (a 2-month intensive phase with isoniazid, rifampicin, pyrazinamide and ethambutol, followed by a 4-month continuation phase with isoniazid and rifampicin) appears to be adequate. In the presence of associated tuberculosis meningitis, treatment needs to be given for at least 12 months. In view of the high frequency of associated tuberculosis meningitis in miliary tuberculosis, all patients with miliary tuberculosis should undergo a lumbar puncture so that they receive treatment of the optimum duration. The World Health Organization endorses the use of directly observed treatment, short-course (DOTS) therapy for all patients with tuberculosis.

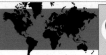

Global issues

 More on weight loss?

- Clinical presentation of miliary tuberculosis in the elderly can be misleading. Absence of fever and the presence of anorexia and weight loss mimicking metastatic carcinoma all delay the diagnosis of miliary tuberculosis.

- Miliary tuberculosis is increasingly being encountered in elderly patients. The HIV/AIDS pandemic, widespread use of immunosuppressive drugs, the modulating effect of BCG (bacille Calmette–Guérin) vaccination, increasing use of CT, and wider application of invasive diagnostic methods may all be relevant in explaining some of this demographic shift.

- Choroidal tubercles, if present, are pathognomonic of miliary tuberculosis and offer a valuable clue to the diagnosis. Therefore, systematic ophthalmo-scopic examination after mydriatic administration must be performed in every patient in whom the diagnosis is suspected.

- Disseminated histoplasmosis, especially in HIV/AIDS patients, can also produce a similar appearance on HRCT of the chest.

- Several other diseases can also produce a miliary pattern on HRCT of the chest. These include miliary metastasis from thyroid malignancy and pneumoconiosis.

See Chapter 22 of
Davidson's Principles and Practice of Medicine
(20th edn)

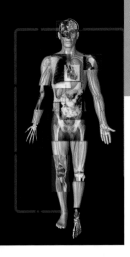

8

A man who has been bitten by a snake

L. KARALLIEDDE

Presenting problem

A 55-year-old Sri Lankan farmer is rushed to his local hospital late one evening after collapsing whilst working in the fields. A co-worker reports that, before he collapsed, he screamed in apparent pain and shouted out that a snake had bitten him on the leg.

What would your differential diagnosis include before examining the patient?

If the man says he has been bitten by a snake, then it is reasonable to assume that is indeed what has happened! The key to his clinical course and to your subsequent management is to identify the species of snake that attacked him. Some people will be able to describe or identify the snake to rescuers or medical staff. However, if the bite occurred, for example, while walking through long grass, the snake may not have been seen. There may be a clue in the timing of the bite — cobra (*Naja naja*) bites generally occur during the daytime, while Russell's viper (*Daboia russelli russelli*) bites and krait (*Bungarus caeruleus, Bungarus ceylonicus*) bites typically occur at night. Examination may also provide crucial information. Significant local tissue swelling is seen following cobra and Russell's viper bites, but is not typically observed following bites by kraits. Neurotoxicity is a feature of envenoming by elapid (krait, cobra) snakes and the Russell's vipers of Sri Lanka and India. In contrast to Elapidae, viper bites are nearly always associated with a coagulopathy.

Examination and initial investigations

The patient is drowsy, but responds to commands. The most striking finding is that he has a bilateral complete ptosis (Fig. 8.1). His pupils are of normal size, with normal direct and consensual reactions to light. He has weakness of the external ocular muscles (external ophthalmoplegia) and there is partial weakness of the facial and pharyngeal muscles. The patient finds it extremely difficult to raise his head from the pillows because of weakness of the flexor muscles of the neck. His respiratory rate is 18 breaths/min, with a tidal volume of 350 ml. There is swelling of the right foot up to the mid-leg, with oozing of blood from a puncture wound on the lateral side of the right ankle.

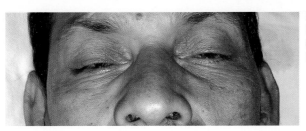

Fig. 8.1 Complete bilateral ptosis following a bite from a Sri Lankan Russell's viper.

Urea and electrolytes and a full blood count are normal. No abnormality is seen on chest X-ray.

Have examination and initial investigations narrowed down your differential diagnosis?

The finding of an oozing lesion in the leg strongly supports a diagnosis of envenoming. There are clear signs of significant neurotoxicity, which could be due to a bite from either an elapid or a viper. The timing of the bite and the significant soft tissue reaction would both favour the latter. The main difference between Elapidae and Viperidae envenoming is that the latter is most often associated with a coagulopathy. Further investigation is necessary.

Further investigations

A coagulation screen is performed. The international normalised ratio (INR) is 4 and the bleeding time is 3 minutes (normal range: up to 5 minutes). The whole blood clotting test 20 (WBCT20) is more than 20 minutes. The D-dimer test is positive. The following were also found: urine microscopy – red cells ++, haemoglobin +, myoglobin +.

Does this narrow down your differential diagnosis?

The finding of a coagulopathy, in conjunction with the obvious neurotoxicity, is strong evidence that the bite was caused by a Russell's viper. Its venom contains a mixture of components, about 90% of which are proteins. The main protein is phospholipase A_2, of which there are at least seven isoenzymes; this exhibits a wide range of clinical effects, including haemolysis, rhabdomyolysis, neurotoxicity, platelet damage, vasodilatation and release of autacoids. Russell's viper venom activates different coagulation factors, and this leads to a consumptive coagulopathy, i.e. consumption or depletion of coagulation factors. This takes place as soon as the venom enters the circulation, but bleeding occurs with a latency that is largely unpredictable, as it depends on the dose of the venom and also on the state of health of the victim.

An increased bleeding time indicates a defect in the vessel wall or in the quantity or quality of the platelets (not the case here). The clotting time indicates the activity of the clotting factors, an increase pointing to a depletion or deficiency of the clotting factors. The 20-minute clotting test, which was developed as a bedside test for developing countries by David Warrell, indicates a clotting defect in a non-specific manner and serves as an aid to diagnosis; it also guides treatment in environments where laboratory facilities for coagulation studies are not available.

How will you treat this patient?

Russell's viper bites caused a substantial number of deaths before the advent of antivenin. Polyspecific and monospecific antivenins are being used in the region, but these products of animal origin are associated with considerable risk of allergy and anaphylaxis. Adrenaline (epinephrine) should therefore be near at hand during antivenin testing and treatment. After a negative intradermal test dose, Russell's viper antivenin (10 vials diluted in 500 ml of normal saline) should be administered intravenously, with close observation for anaphylactic reactions. The bedside clotting test is repeated in 6 hours, and if the test is positive, a repeat infusion of the antivenin is administered. The antivenin only inactivates the venom and prevents the venom from using up the clotting factors. The coagulopathy may be reversed with appropriate clotting factors, but ultimately the return of the clotting factors to normal following envenoming will be dependent on the synthetic potential of the victim's liver.

For this man, the immediate need is to monitor his respiratory function (oxygen saturation, tidal volume and blood gases) and to prepare for intubation and ventilation if respiratory failure sets in. The patient should be aggressively rehydrated with intravenous fluids to ensure an adequate urine output. The wound must be cleaned with an antiseptic and a dressing applied to reduce the risk of secondary infection.

Global issues

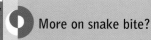

More on snake bite?

- Viper bites are nearly always associated with a coagulopathy, except those from the European adder.

- Russell's viper is distributed in 10 Asian countries, including Sri Lanka, India, Myanmar, Thailand, Pakistan and Bangladesh.

- There are marked geographical variations in the manifestations following a Russell's viper bite. The subspecies *Vipera russelli siamensis*, found in Myanmar, causes severe coagulopathy, increased generalised capillary permeability, hypotension and shock, but does not cause neurotoxicity. The same subspecies found in Thailand does not cause hypotension and shock.

See Chapter 9 of
Davidson's Principles and Practice of Medicine
(20th edn)

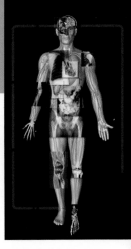

9

A young woman who has been stung by a scorpion

L. KARALLIEDDE

Presenting problem

A woman aged 25 years who lives in a small village in the south of India is rushed to the Accident and Emergency department of her local hospital. She was gathering firewood in the forest behind her cottage when she was stung on her right index finger by a scorpion hiding in the dead wood. She has been in good health until this incident and is not on any medication.

What would your differential diagnosis include before examining the patient?

Scorpions are nocturnal animals; their natural habitat is under stones or dead wood. In areas where scorpions are found, though, it is necessary to watch out for dark hiding places indoors: for example, in cupboards, under the duvet and bed, in baseball gloves, in caps and in shoes. Scorpions do not attack human beings spontaneously, but sting when they feel trapped or are stepped on or disturbed. This lady comes from a part of the world where scorpions live, and if she says that she has been stung by a scorpion, then there should be no cause to doubt this.

Examination

On examination the patient is restless and agitated — she is visibly in pain. Her right hand is very tender to the touch, and on tapping the affected finger, there is excruciating pain. Her pupils are dilated, and she is sweating profusely and is vomiting. Her pulse is 130 beats/min and blood pressure is 179/112 mmHg. In the short time that she has been in the Accident and Emergency department her condition has deteriorated rapidly. She becomes increasingly tachypnoeic, her oxygen saturation (on high-flow oxygen) falls to 89%, and widespread crepitations are heard in the chest.

Has examination narrowed down your differential diagnosis?

There are 46 known species of scorpion in India, and unless the patient (or relatives) brings the offending scorpion into hospital with them, it is usually impossible to know which particular species was responsible. Stings from some of these species simply cause minor skin irritation, akin to a sting from a bee or wasp.

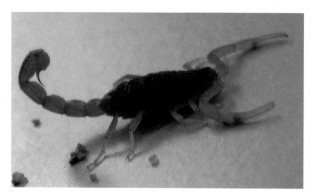

Fig. 9.1 The Indian red scorpion.

As with stings from insects, scorpion stings can cause anaphylactic reactions in susceptible individuals.

Some species of scorpions, however, have a highly toxic venom that can be fatal. *Mesobuthus tamulus* (Indian red scorpion) is the most lethal species in the Buthidae family of scorpions (Fig. 9.1). Indian red scorpion venom contains neurotoxins that block sodium channels and thus cause spontaneous depolarisation of parasympathetic and sympathetic nerves. This results in an 'autonomic storm', characterised by transient cholinergic symptoms (vomiting, sweating, salivation, priapism (persistent and painful erection of the penis) in males, bradycardia and ventricular ectopics) and then sustained sympathetic stimulation (hypertension, tachycardia, pulmonary oedema, hyperglycaemia and shock), which is usually fatal. This lady is clearly extremely unwell and is deteriorating fast. This does not look like an anaphylactic reaction — there is no urticarial rash or wheeze. Unfortunately, it seems as though she is having a major toxic reaction to the scorpion sting.

Investigations

A 12-lead ECG shows sinus tachycardia and a chest X-ray reveals changes consistent with pulmonary oedema. Blood gas results are shown in Box 9.1. Routine biochemistry is normal and there is no coagulopathy. Blood glucose is 14.4 mmol/l (259 mg/dl).

Does this clinch the diagnosis?

This lady has all the hallmarks of an 'autonomic storm' response to the scorpion sting — most probably from an Indian red scorpion. Her prognosis is not good. She has a metabolic acidosis, which will almost certainly be a lactic acidosis — a direct consequence of tissue hypoxia. The pulmonary oedema is most likely due to acute left ventricular failure from myocardial toxicity and profound vasoconstriction and hypertension.

How will you treat this patient?

This lady is in extremis and requires urgent action to save her life. If the necessary facilities and expertise are available, she should be transferred to an intensive care unit where facilities for monitoring and assisted ventilation are available. Antivenin for a red scorpion sting is available in some parts of India. This is a solution of enzyme-digested, refined antibodies prepared from equine blood; 1 ml of the reconstituted serum neutralises 1 mg of dried red scorpion venom. However, there are problems with scorpion anti-venin that limit its clinical use. Antivenins themselves can cause serious anaphylactic reactions; moreover, they are species-specific and, as has already been noted, in most instances the precise species of scorpion causing the sting is not known. An alternative to administering anti-venin is to give the α-blocker, prazosin (0.5 mg 8-hourly orally or through a nasogastric tube, until all symptoms subside); indeed, randomised controlled studies have not proved that antivenin is more efficacious than prazosin in the management of Indian red scorpion stings.

Prazosin is a vasodilator and this should help the pulmonary oedema. Short-acting intravenous β-blockers (e.g. esmolol or metoprolol) may be used cautious-ly to control the tachycardia. Loop diuretic treatment will also be required and there is the option of additional vasodilator therapy such as nitrates or sodium nitroprusside. The next 24 hours will be critical; the patient's relatives will need support and counselling, and will need to know that the outlook is grave, even with the best possible supportive therapy.

BOX 9.1

Blood gas results on 60% oxygen

PO_2	6.9 kPa (52 mmHg)
PCO_2	3.1 kPa (23 mmHg)
H^+	64 nmol/l (pH 7.19)
HCO_3	19 mmol/l (meq/l)

Global issues

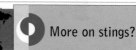

- Scorpions are found in South, West and North Africa; North, Central and South America; India; the Middle East; and the Caribbean.

- They can also be transported from their natural habitats to foreign countries with foodstuffs and other cargo.

- Fatal stings may be caused by scorpions of the gen-era *Androctonus*, *Buthus* and *Leiurus* (found in North Africa and the Middle East), *Parabuthus* (found in South Africa), *Mesobuthus* (found in India) and *Centruroides* and *Tityus* (found in North, Central and South America and the Caribbean).

- Caribbean scorpions cause severe abdominal pain, vomiting and even haematemesis following envenoming.

- Scorpions from the Middle East (particularly the *Hemiscorpius* genera found in Iraq and Iran) can cause severe local reactions, including necrosis.

More on stings?

See Chapter 9 of
**Davidson's
Principles and
Practice of
Medicine**
(20th edn)

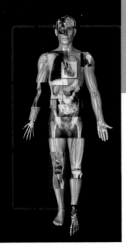

10

A young man who is semiconscious in the Accident and Emergency department

A. FAIZ

Presenting problem

A 30-year-old man is admitted to hospital in a state of reduced consciousness (Glasgow Coma Scale 9) with froth coming out of his mouth and laboured respiration. According to his family members, he was found collapsed in his room 1 hour ago. He is an otherwise healthy man taking no regular medication. The accompanying person also brought an unlabelled empty container, found in the same room, which is reported to store pesticides. The man's clothing is soaked with vomitus. A strong pungent garlic-like odour is apparent and is found to come from the patient's body; the container also has a similar smell. Further questioning reveals a family dispute the previous night. The patient has no past history of psychiatric illness.

What would your differential diagnosis include before examining the patient?

With the background of a family quarrel, self-poisoning is top of the list in an otherwise healthy young man. The history and presenting features of acute illness are suggestive of a deliberate suicidal attempt, most likely with some kind of organophosphorus (OP) compound. Other agents like organochlorines are not available nowadays. Pyrethroid insecticides rarely cause severe poisoning. Aluminium phosphide ingestion should be considered in areas where it is common (e.g. Northern India). It has a characteristic odour of rotten fish.

Examination

The patient is found to be cyanosed and dyspnoeic, with small pinpoint pupils. There are muscle fasciculations and reduced tendon jerks. His pulse is 102/min and blood pressure is 80/60 mmHg. He has bilateral crepitations.

Has examination narrowed down your differential diagnosis?

The findings of typical garlic odour, miosis and muscle fasciculations are so pathognomonic that there should be no doubt about OP poisoning. Altered consciousness, muscle fasciculations and cyanosis stratify the case as severe. The accompanying persons should be interrogated about the amount and the brand ingested. Lung crepitations can be attributed to bronchorrhoea and aspiration of secretions from salivation due to the muscarinic effects of an acute cholinergic syndrome. Bradycardia is typical but tachycardia may occur in 20% of cases.

Further investigations

Laboratory confirmation of OP poisoning is neither necessary nor always possible before starting treatment. In doubtful cases a test dose of atropine (1 mg i.v.) may be helpful. (A marked increase in heart rate and skin flushing eliminate the possibility of OP poisoning.) Pulse oximetry and cardiac status should be monitored. Urea and electrolytes are unremarkable. Arterial blood gases on high-flow oxygen are shown in Box 10.1. Blood should also be sent for cholinesterase estimation.

BOX 10.1

Arterial blood gas results on high-flow oxygen	
PaO_2	7.4 kPa (55 mmHg)
$PaCO_2$	3.1 kPa (23 mmHg)
H^+	34 nmol/l (pH 7.47)
HCO_3^-	24 mmol/l (meq/l)

How will you treat this patient?

The patient is hypoxic despite high-flow oxygen and should be managed in an intensive care unit. Establishment of an airway is the priority. Suction and endotracheal intubation, followed by assisted ventilation with a high concentration of oxygen, will be necessary. Atropine should be started immediately at a dose of 3 mg i.v. bolus and doubled every 5 minutes, until atropinisation (clear lungs, dry tongue, normal heart rate and blood pressure) has occurred. Following atropinisation, an atropine infusion is given every hour at 20–30% of the dose required for atropinisation (~5 mg/hr). The patient should be observed frequently and the atropine dose titrated. Pralidoxime (which reactivates acetylcholinesterase) should be given as a 1 g i.v. bolus in 30 min, followed by an infusion of 0.5 g/hour. Convulsions should be controlled with intravenous diazepam. Meticulous nursing care is mandatory. After the initial resuscitation, decontamination should be undertaken by changing the clothing and washing the skin with soap and water. The eyes should be irrigated; gastric lavage with charcoal may be tried at this stage. The patient should be observed regularly and carefully for early detection of the intermediate syndrome (IMS; Fig. 10.1); this is rapidly progressive weakness from the ocular muscles to the neck, proximal limbs and respiratory muscles, occurring within 48–72 hours, and develops in 20% of the patients. Early recognition and intervention with endotracheal intubation are required. Recovery from IMS is complete. Organophosphate-induced delayed polyneuropathy (OPIDN), characterised by cramping, numbness and paraesthesia in distal limbs, with weakness, gait apraxia and foot or wrist drop, is a recognised late complication. It usually occurs about 1–3 weeks after acute exposure due to degeneration of long myelinated nerve fibres. Recovery from OPIDN is incomplete. Before discharge this patient should have psychiatric evaluation to identify any underlying psychiatric illness.

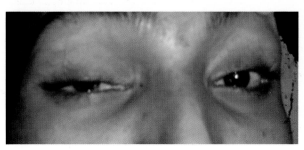

Fig. 10.1 A young woman with intermediate syndrome following organophosphorus poisoning. She is unable to keep her eyes open due to muscular weakness.

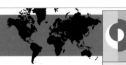

More on organo-phosphorus poisoning?

See Chapter 9 of
Davidson's Principles and Practice of Medicine
(20th edn)

- Pesticides or insecticides used by victims differ in various parts of the world according to local use and availability.

- OP pesticide intoxications are estimated at 3 million per year worldwide, with approximately 300 000 deaths.

- Case fatality varies and is higher in developing countries. In Asia it ranges from 20% to 70%, depending on the season and availability of health services.

11

A young woman who has taken an overdose of paracetamol (acetaminophen)

A. L. JONES

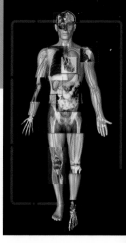

Presenting problem

A 23-year-old lady, who is 34 weeks pregnant with her first child, is seen in the Accident and Emergency department after taking 28 paracetamol (500 mg) tablets 2 hours ago. She is 62 kg in weight. She did not co-ingest any other drug or alcohol. She complains of nausea and intermittent vomiting, but this has been consistent throughout her pregnancy.

What would your differential diagnosis include before examining the patient?

There is no real diagnostic difficulty in this case. The issue of greatest concern is that she has probably ingested 225 mg/kg of paracetamol, i.e. more than 150 mg paracetamol per kg of body weight. Hence she is at risk of developing hepatotoxicity and/or (more rarely) nephrotoxicity. The additional risk is that paracetamol can cross the placenta and this places the baby at risk. The onset of vomiting in this case is too early to be due to paracetamol-induced liver damage if, as she states, the timing of ingestion was only 2 hours ago. Paracetamol overdose per se, as well as pregnancy itself, can cause early-onset vomiting.

Examination

All her clinical observations (heart rate, blood pressure etc.) are within normal limits. She has no renal angle tenderness and no right upper quadrant tenderness. (Such signs might occur if she had taken the overdose at an earlier interval than stated, or in a staggered way, and was beginning to develop signs of renal or hepatic injury, respectively.) Her uterus is of a size that is in keeping with her stated gestation. She has a very low mood and odd affect.

Has examination narrowed down your differential diagnosis?

Examination of the patient reveals no evidence of current hepatotoxicity or nephrotoxicity, in keeping with the patient's history of *recent* ingestion of paracetamol. However, if left untreated, she would be expected to develop liver damage from paracetamol within the next 24–36 hours. Her low mood indicates the need to apply the Beck's depression scale (or to undertake some other form of immediate mood assessment), in order to determine her risk on the ward and the appropriate degree of nursing/psychiatric support. In view of the fact that she is pregnant, she may also have obstetric needs.

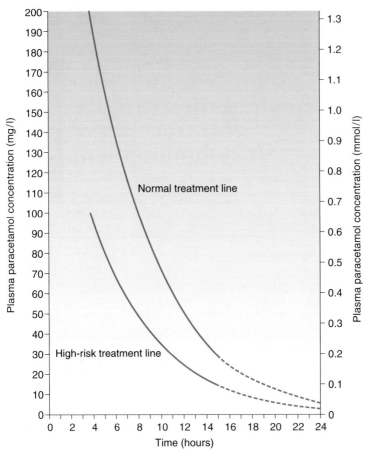

Fig. 11.1 Paracetamol treatment graph. Patients whose plasma paracetamol concentration is above the normal treatment line should receive antidote. The high-risk treatment line is used in individuals who may develop paracetamol toxicity at lower levels (see text). After 15 hours (dotted lines) the prognostic accuracy is uncertain. (Source: University of Wales College of Medicine Therapeutics and Toxicology Centre).

Initial investigations

Paracetamol levels are checked 4 hours after ingestion and the concentration plotted on a paracetamol treatment normogram (Fig. 11.1). Prothrombin ratio, liver function tests and venous bicarbonate concentrations are normal (Box 11.1).

Serum paracetamol concentrations should be measured in any patient who admits to taking excess paracetamol, anyone who has ingested white tablets and any patient with unexplained coma. Paracetamol concentrations within 4 hours of ingestion are not interpretable. Prothrombin ratio (PTR) is the most sensitive marker of ensuing liver dysfunction in paracetamol poisoning; it becomes elevated at 18–24 hours after significant ingestion, with ensuing hepatotoxicity. Prothrombin time is checked in this case, because of the need to be certain that ingestion has not taken place earlier than the patient states, i.e. to establish that there is no evidence of liver damage from paracetamol at presentation. Plasma venous bicarbonate is a useful early screening test for metabolic acidosis and can warn of impending liver damage from paracetamol.

How will you treat this patient?

This patient requires a full course (20¼ hours) of the antidote for paracetamol poisoning, because her paracetamol level at 4 hours is above the normal treatment line (Fig. 11.1). She is not glutathione-deplete (e.g. due to alcoholism, anorexia or known human immunodeficiency (HIV) disease) or on enzyme-inducing agents (e.g. carbamazepine, phenobarbital, phenytoin or rifampicin) and so the lower, 'high-risk' treatment line is not used.

The antidote, intravenous N-acetylcysteine, will protect her liver and kidneys from paracetamol-induced hepatotoxicity. The dose is 150 mg/kg over 15 minutes, then 50 mg/kg over 4 hours and then 100 mg/kg over 16 hours. During infusion of the first two bags of N-acetylcysteine, up to 5% of patients develop an anaphylactoid reaction (flushing and wheezing). Watch out for this, and if it occurs, stop the infusion for at least 30 minutes and give an antihistamine drug. At the end of the infusion the patient needs to be clinically examined for upper quadrant tenderness or renal angle pain; if she is clinically well, however, she does *not* require further blood tests because N-acetylcysteine given within 10 hours of paracetamol ingestion offers virtually 100% protection from liver/renal injury.

There are, of course, two patients here: mother and fetus. Both paracetamol and N-acetylcysteine cross the placenta, and fortunately the fetus is fully protected by treating the mother with the antidote. Neither N-acetylcysteine nor paracetamol is known to be teratogenic (harmful) to the fetus. The mother will require a treatment for nausea that will not harm the baby — such as cyclizine. She also needs psychiatric evaluation to assess her ongoing suicidal risk. If you are in doubt about the care of a poisoned or potentially poisoned patient, doctors at a poisons information centre are there to help guide you on such issues. Keep a note of the poisons centre number with you.

BOX 11.1	
Initial investigations	
Paracetamol level at 4 hours after ingestion	350 mg/l
U&Es	Normal
LFTs	Normal
Prothrombin time	Normal
Plasma venous bicarbonate	Normal

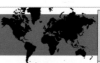

Global issues

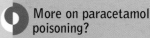
More on paracetamol poisoning?

- Paracetamol poisoning is extremely common in the UK but also occurs in other parts of the world; paracetamol is called acetaminophen in the USA.

- Availability of the antidote N-acetylcysteine is not global. Up to 10 hours after an overdose, oral methionine (12 g orally 4-hourly, to a total of four doses) is a suitable alternative antidote for paracetamol poisoning if intravenous N-acetylcysteine is neither available nor affordable.

- The incidence of acute liver failure developing from paracetamol does not appear to be the same in every country. In Australia acute liver failure from paracetamol is rare but in the UK it is much more common; many factors dictate this risk.

- Do not forget the potential of drowsy patients having ingested a paracetamol/opioid combination. Check the paracetamol level in such patients!

See Chapter 9 of
Davidson's Principles and Practice of Medicine
(20th edn)

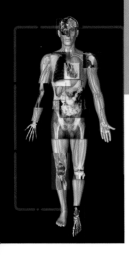

12

A young woman with chest pain

K. R. SETHURAMAN

Presenting problem

A 30-year-old school teacher, looking for relief from troublesome pain in her chest, seeks a third medical opinion. The pain is 'severe and stabs through her heart' several times a day, lasting for minutes to hours. She points to her left mammary region as the site of maximum pain. The pain does not radiate to any other part of the body. At times, deep slow breathing tends to ease her pain. Episodes of chest pain are triggered by household chores on occasions and at other times by emotional upset. She has been to a hill temple for worship recently (on foot) and did not have any pain then.

The pain first started when she was 15 years old. She recalls it as 'a tough day at school followed by a tiff with my mother who scolded me for coming home late'. The pain recurred in school and later in college when she was 'forced to do outdoor exercises'. She negotiated with the administrators and got permission to abstain from outdoor physical activities.

When she was newly married, she had episodes of abdominal aches with a bloating sensation, for which no cause could be found. She got married at the age of 21 years and divorced 4 years later by mutual consent. She is not willing to talk about it, other than to say, 'With our separation, my stomach aches disappeared, only to reappear in my chest.'

Her mother is alive and active. When the woman was 10 years old, her father died at the age of 40 of some heart problem. She has a younger brother, who is 27 years old and quite healthy.

The patient attained menarche when she was 13. She has severe pain during the first 2 days of her periods. She has not conceived, and has remained single and celibate after her divorce.

There are no problems with her sleep and appetite. The young woman has worked as a school teacher from the age of 22 years. She is satisfied with her career, though at times 'The work load gets too much for comfort.' She has never smoked or consumed alcohol.

The patient has spoken to her friends and looked on the Internet, and feels that she may be 'suffering from a floppy mitral valve'. She has already consulted two other physicians. One reassured her and refused her request for a scan. The other doctor carried out an echocardiogram and told her, 'It is all in your mind, madam.' She has chosen to consult you now because you have treated her friends to their satisfaction. She wants a complete work-up to diagnose her chest pain.

What would your differential diagnosis include before examining the patient?

In view of the woman's age, the atypical nature of the chest pain and her gender, angina pectoris is unlikely. Moreover, she has recently been to a hill temple without any physical discomfort. Depression with somatisation is unlikely because her sleep, appetite and energy levels seem to be unaffected.

Two possibilities could be considered: atypical chest pain of mitral valve prolapse (MVP) syndrome and somatoform pain. MVP syndrome needs to be carefully looked for during the physical examination.

The only 'red flag' in the historical detail is the death of her father at the age of 40. If this was due to premature coronary artery disease, you need to look for coronary risk factors that are genetically transmitted, such as familial hypercholesterolaemia.

 Examination

The physical examination is normal. There are no xanthomas or xanthelasmas. Blood pressure is 116/72 mmHg. There are no auscultatory findings to suggest MVP syndrome. On isometric handgrip exercise and on squatting down, cardiac auscultation is negative for the click–murmur of MVP.

Has examination narrowed down your differential diagnosis?

Physical examination has ruled out MVP syndrome. Somatoform pain is the clinical diagnosis that would explain the patient's symptoms in the absence of any abnormal physical findings.

She could be started on treatment for somatoform pain. However, in order to convince her that she does not have MVP, you might consider using echocardiography to document normal mitral valve motion during isometric handgrip.

In view of her father's premature death, it is prudent to investigate her for any coronary risk factor and advise appropriate primary prevention.

Investigations

The patient's results are shown in Box 12.1.

Does this narrow down your differential diagnosis?

Yes. MVP syndrome has been ruled out by echocardiography during isometric handgrip. A final diagnosis of somatoform chest pain can be made in this case.

This young woman's biochemical tests have ruled out two risk factors for coronary artery disease: namely, diabetes mellitus and hypercholesterolaemia. In view of her low coronary risk score, she should be advised not to have a treadmill test done, as it will have a low positive predictive value in her case.

How will you treat this patient?

Management of medically unexplained complaints is quite a challenge. Demonstrate by words and non-verbal clues that you believe that your patient's pain is genuine, even if there is no medical label that can be attached to it. Try to establish a collaborative therapeutic partnership to manage the chest pain. Educate the lady on the mind–body connection and how stress can provoke somatic pain without any organic disease. Being a school teacher and familiar with the Internet, she can be guided to appropriate Web links to learn more about somatoform disorders. Encourage her to be fully functional in the knowledge that

BOX 12.1

Initial investigations

Haemoglobin	125 g/l (12.5 g/dl)
Blood glucose	
Fasting	5.0 mmol/l (90 mg/dl)
2 hrs post-prandial	6.1 mmol/l (120 mg/dl)
Cholesterol	
Total	4.7 mmol/l (181 mg/dl)
HDL	1.2 mmol/l (48 mg/dl)
ECG	Normal tracing
Echocardiography at rest and during isometric hand grip	Normal study of mitral valve and left ventricle

her coronary risk is negligible at present and that floppy mitral valve has been excluded in her case.

If chest pain interferes with her functioning, you may offer medications to try to control it. If she accepts it, you might try a tricyclic antidepressant in small doses or an anticonvulsant such as carbamazepine or gabapentin.

Subject to its availability, she may be referred to undergo cognitive behaviour therapy (CBT).

Global issues

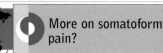

More on somatoform pain?

- Somatoform disorders are a global problem and form a large portion of the illness burden.

- About 40% of presenting problems in primary care practice are likely to be medically unexplainable. Therefore, a primary healthcare provider has to acquire the competence and skills to manage these cases.

- Patients with somatoform pain may be referred for CBT. However, be cautious in traditional communities where referral to a psychiatric service has stigma attached to it.

See Chapter 10 of **Davidson's Principles and Practice of Medicine** (20th edn)

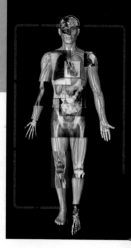

13

A middle-aged woman with facial rash, joint swelling and hepatomegaly

T. AZHAR

Presenting problem

A 47-year-old lady presents with a history of progressive lethargy associated with an erythematous rash involving the face and hands. The rash developed about 8 months ago and was associated with painless swelling of the finger joints. She has since become progressively lethargic, with generalised muscle weakness over the last few months. There is no history of photosensitivity or oral ulcers. There is a history of diffuse thinning of hair with loss of appetite and weight.

What would your differential diagnosis include before examining the patient?

Some form of connective tissue disorder seems very likely, particularly systemic lupus erythematosus (SLE). The facial rash, joint swelling and hair thinning are common features of SLE. The age of onset is a little older than usual, since SLE commonly presents in the second or third decade.

Examination and initial investigations

On examination, the patient is found to be pale, cachectic and afebrile. There is no jaundice or clubbing. Cervical and axillary lymph nodes are not palpable. In the inguinal region some shotty nodes are palpable. Macular erythematous lesions are noted over the malar region with sparing of the upper eyelid and the nasolabial folds, and there is just a hint of infraorbital oedema. There are streaks of erythema overlying the extensor tendons on the backs of the hands and dusky erythema of the proximal nail folds. Tortuous capillaries in the proximal nail folds and flat-topped papules on the digits are especially striking (Fig. 13.1, from another patient). The scalp shows diffuse non-scarring alopecia. There are no oral ulcers. Neck examination reveals a 1 cm non-tender, solitary right thyroid nodule. There are no palpable breast lumps. There is hepatomegaly of 5 cm below the right subcostal margin, which is firm in consistency with a nodular surface. The spleen is not palpable and there are no other masses palpable in the abdomen. Respiratory and cardiovascular examination is unremarkable. Blood pressure is 130/80 mmHg and pulse is 80/min. Results of initial investigations are provided in Box 13.1.

Have examination and initial investigations narrowed down your differential diagnosis?

Considering the muscle weakness and skin signs, dermatomyositis with an underlying malignancy is top of the list. The enlarged firm nodular liver is compatible with a multicentric primary hepatocellular carcinoma or secondaries

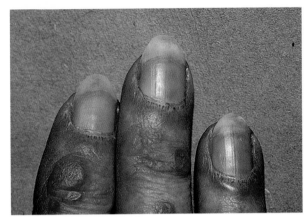

Fig. 13.1 The erythema, dilated and tortuous nail capillaries in the proximal nail folds, and the flat-topped (Gottron's) papules on the digits are important diagnostic features of dermatomyositis.

BOX 13.1

Initial investigations

Haemoglobin	93 g/l (9.3 g/dl)
WCC	7.3×10^9/l (10^3/mm^3)
Platelets	340×10^9/l (10^3/mm^3)
ESR	52 mm/1st hour
Blood smear	Normochromic, normocytic anaemia with aniso-poikilocytosis; no target cells, sickling, nucleated red blood cells or Howell–Jolly bodies
Blood urea, sodium, potassium, serum creatinine	All normal
Bilirubin	4.3 µmol/l (0.26 mg/dl)
Albumin	32 g/l (3.2 g/dl)
ALT	26 U/l
AST	96 U/l
Alkaline phosphatase	181 U/l
CRP	6.7 mg/l (normal < 6)
Creatine kinase	96 U/l (normal 24–195)
Rheumatoid factor, antinuclear antibody, HBsAg, Anti-HCV antibody, HIV antibody	All negative

---

from elsewhere. SLE can cause hepatomegaly but not nodularity. The right thyroid nodule needs to be investigated. Small differentiated thyroid malignancies (follicular and papillary) do not normally metastasise early and tend to constitute a locoregional disease in the early stages. This may not be true of tumours with an anaplastic histology where haematogenous dissemination can occur early. The patient is a little young to develop an anaplastic carcinoma of the thyroid.

Initial investigations show a mild normocytic normochromic anaemia, associated with a moderately elevated erythrocyte sedimentation rate (ESR), but these are non-specific findings. The creatine kinase level is not raised; this is unusual in dermatomyositis but can occasionally happen when the brunt of the reaction involves skin rather than muscles. Underlying malignancy is now high on the differential diagnosis list and the obviously enlarged nodular liver needs to be investigated.

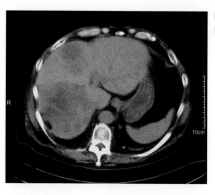

Fig. 13.2 CT showing multiple lesions in the liver compatible with metastatic deposits.

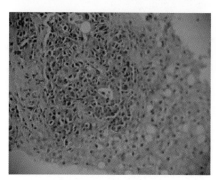

Fig. 13.3 Histopathological examination of one of the masses in the liver shows malignant cells arranged in a glandular formation.

Further investigations

Computed tomography (CT) of the abdomen reveals multiple heterogeneous lesions scattered in both lobes of the liver and ranging from 1 to 5 cm in diameter. The main portal vein is intact. There is partial compression of the inferior vena cava. The spleen, pancreas, kidneys and uterus are normal. There is no para-aortic lymphadenopathy. The bowels are normal and no ascites is detectable.

An ultrasound-guided liver biopsy is carried out. Histopathological examination of the biopsy specimen reveals malignant cells arranged in sheets with some glandular formation (Figs 13.2 and 13.3). The stain for mucin is positive.

Imaging studies of potential primary sites are undertaken. An ultrasound scan of the thyroid shows that the nodular lesion is primarily cystic; an ultrasound-guided fine needle aspiration reveals no cytological features of malignancy. An ultrasound of the breast is normal. Transvaginal ultrasound shows normal uterus and ovaries and no adnexal masses. Upper gastrointestinal endoscopy shows mild pan-gastritis, with no ulcers or masses. A colonoscopy and a barium enema are entirely normal. A CT of the neck and thorax is entirely normal, except for the previously documented right thyroid nodule. Results of serum tumour markers are provided in Box 13.2.

BOX 13.2
Serum tumour markers
Alpha-fetoprotein	9.15 µg/l (ng/ml) (normal < 15)
CA-125	13 kU/l (U/ml) (normal < 35)
CEA	5176 µg/l ng/ml) (normal < 5)

Does this narrow down your differential diagnosis?

Yes. The presenting symptoms of a facial/hand rash and joint swelling associated with muscle weakness can be attributed to a paraneoplastic dermatomyositis syndrome.

Dermatomyositis appearing after the age of 40 should always make a physician suspicious of underlying malignancy. Different series report different risks but the increased risk in this patient is not less than threefold. The biopsy findings are suggestive of an underlying mucin-secreting adenocarcinoma. Primary liver tumours (hepatocellular carcinoma) are not mucin-secreting. These must be metastatic deposits from another primary site such as the lung, the breast or the gut. Further imaging and endoscopic investigations did not reveal any obvious primary site. The very high levels of carcinoembryonic antigen (CEA) are compatible with a tumour arising from the gut, although breast and lung tumours can also lead to high CEA levels.

How will you treat this patient?

A two-pronged approach should be taken. First of all, systemic corticosteroid treatment should help the woman's myositis and make her feel generally much better and less lethargic. Occasionally, if progress is slow, prednisolone needs to be supplemented with an immunosuppressive agent.

Second, consideration needs to be given to the treatment of the metastatic adenocarcinoma of unknown origin. This is a difficult situation and the evidence base for management is poor. Clearly, there is a distinction between patients with an unknown primary who have been insufficiently investigated and those in whom exhaustive investigation has been unhelpful. In most instances, this represents the end stage of the natural history of the malignancy. If an individual has a good performance status, then chemotherapy can be considered. The choice of regimen may be determined by the pattern of disease. Thus, for example, isolated peritoneal disease in a woman should generally be managed as ovarian cancer; isolated axillary lymph nodes in a woman should be managed as breast cancer; and isolated malignant pleural effusion should be managed as primary lung cancer (but mesothelioma needs to be excluded).

In this case, the elevated CEA is consistent with, but by no means diagnostic of, a gastrointestinal primary. The main aim of management is palliation, along with the provision of both physical and emotional support for the lady and her family. This being so, a few cycles of 5-fluorouracil (5-FU) could be recommended, and with this a significant clinical response may be seen. The treatment itself is generally well tolerated. Some oncologists favour a more aggressive regimen of either oxaliplatin and 5-FU or cisplatin and gemcitabine, but this is clearly associated with a higher side-effect profile.

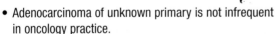

Global issues

More on malignant disease?

- Adenocarcinoma of unknown primary is not infrequent in oncology practice.

- Common presenting sites are the head and neck region, and the regional nodes; rarely, the skin may be involved.

- In the majority of cases the primary is never established, even at postmortem.

See Chapter 11 of **Davidson's Principles and Practice of Medicine** (20th edn)

- Careful pathological analysis is a vital part of the investigation of these patients. Immunocytochemical profiling (including CK7, CK20, TTF1 and CEA) is available in many centres and may help to indicate a likely site of origin.

- No fewer than 30% of adults with dermatomyositis have an underlying malignancy. Hunt for this in the middle-aged and elderly, but not in juvenile cases.

14

A 40-year-old man with urinary retention

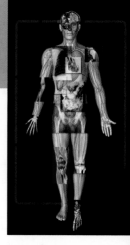

D. OXENHAM

Presenting problem

A 40-year-old man presents to hospital, having not passed urine for the previous 24 hours. He is acutely uncomfortable and has a large suprapubic mass. A urinary catheter is inserted and drains 1200 ml of clear urine. He was diagnosed 1 year ago with non-small cell lung cancer, which was initially treated with radical radiotherapy. At diagnosis there was no evidence of metastases and initial treatment appeared successful. Over the last 4 months he has developed increasingly severe lower back pain, which has been partially controlled with codeine, paracetamol and diclofenac.

What would your differential diagnosis include before examining the patient?

Any patient presenting with back pain and known or suspected metastatic cancer should be presumed to have spinal cord compression until proved otherwise. The presence of sphincter disturbance makes cord compression the most important diagnosis to exclude. Non-oncological causes of spinal cord compression (rheumatoid arthritis, osteoporosis, Paget's disease of bone) should also be considered, although they are unlikely in this patient.

The other possible explanation for urinary retention in this situation would be constipation or a side-effect of medications (e.g. amitriptyline or opioids). It would be foolish to assume these diagnoses; if you fail to investigate this patient adequately, he may develop an avoidable paralysis.

Examination and initial investigations

On examination, the man has some tenderness over his first lumbar vertebra. Neurological examination is entirely normal with no areas of sensory deficit or signs of motor weakness. There is no loss of perineal sensation or reduction in anal tone.

The lumbar spine X-ray is normal. A full blood count reveals a mild anaemia of chronic disease (104 g/l, or 10.4 g/dl) and biochemistry is normal, except for a low albumin (31 g/l, or 3.1 g/dl).

Have examination and initial investigations narrowed down your differential diagnosis?

In this situation, a normal neurological examination should not reduce your suspicion of cord compression. If you wait until the cord compression has progressed to produce a classic clinical picture of flaccid lower limb paralysis and loss of sensation below the level of compression (a 'sensory level'), you will have failed your patient miserably. Treatment is likely to preserve function but unlikely to reverse significant neurological deficit. A normal plain X-ray of the lumbar spine does not exclude either bone metastases or cord compression. On the other hand, an abnormal X-ray would make the diagnosis almost certain.

Further investigations

The investigation of choice is magnetic resonance imaging (MRI) of spine; this will demonstrate any significant cord compression. In this gentleman there is a metastasis protruding into the spine at the level of L1 (Fig. 14.1).

How will you treat this patient?

Spinal cord compression is a medical emergency and treatment should be started quickly to avoid unnecessary neurological damage. All treatment should balance potential benefit and harm, but in most situations where metastatic spinal cord compression is suspected, the correct initial therapy would be 16 mg intravenous dexamethasone. This will reduce any surrounding oedema and reduce the risk of further damage.

Further management would depend on local services, but options would be either urgent radiotherapy or surgical decompression. This should be discussed urgently with local specialists and managed according to their advice.

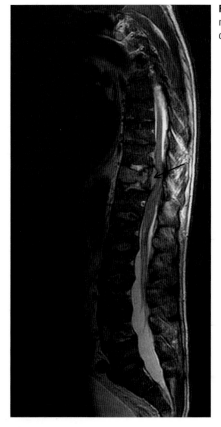

Fig. 14.1 MRI of the spine demonstrating a metastasis at the level of L1 (arrow), which is causing compression of the spinal cord.

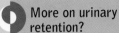

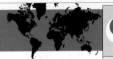

Global issues

More on urinary retention?

- Tuberculosis is a significant cause of cord compression in developing nations. Lower thoracic and lumbar vertebrae are commonly involved. Early diagnosis and treatment are rewarding, but often the diagnosis is made at a stage when the patient has developed paralysis.

See Chapter 11 of
Davidson's Principles and Practice of Medicine (20th edn)

- Spinal epidural abscess commonly occurs in the thoracic or lumbar spine. Patients usually have comorbid conditions such as diabetes mellitus or HIV infection. Early diagnosis and treatment with antibiotics and surgical drainage can prevent neurological sequelae.

- CT and MRI are important diagnostic tools for an early diagnosis; however, access to these investigations may be limited in developing nations.

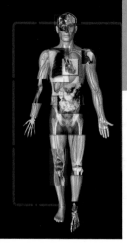

15

A young man from Bangladesh with a pyrexia of unknown origin

T. AHMED

Presenting problem

A 32-year-old man is readmitted to a tertiary care hospital because of persistent fever. The story is complicated. He was admitted to the same hospital 3 months ago with an evening rise of temperature of 2 months' duration. His temperature had risen to a maximum of 38.9°C and was associated with night sweats. He had lost 5 kg body weight during the previous 2 months, but had no other symptoms except mild anorexia. He denied extramarital sexual encounters. He said that there were no cats and dogs in the family. There were no other positive findings on physical examination. Extensive investigations were carried out and these are summarised in Box 15.1.

The patient was treated empirically with a four-drug regimen of anti-tuberculosis chemotherapy. Not only did the fever persist, but he also developed clinical jaundice after 6 weeks of anti-TB chemotherapy. The jaundice disappeared after stopping the drugs. A detailed history taken on this admission does not reveal any additional information.

BOX 15.1	
Initial investigations	
Haemoglobin	100 g/l (10 g/dl)
WCC	20×10^9/l (10^3/mm³), 77% neutrophils
Blood film	No malarial parasites identified; no abnormal cells
ESR	110 mm/1st hr
U&Es, LFTs	Normal
Serum protein electrophoresis	Polyclonal gammopathy
Urinalysis	Normal
Blood and urine culture	No growth
Chest X-ray, upper and lower GI endoscopies, echocardiography, abdominal ultrasound, isotope bone scintigraphy and bone marrow examination	Normal
Tuberculin skin test (TST) with 5 tuberculin units (TU)	Negative

What would your differential diagnosis include before examining the patient?

The patient was extensively investigated on his initial admission. No cause for his fever was found and he was prescribed anti-TB chemotherapy on an empirical basis, as TB is the most common infectious cause of a pyrexia of unknown origin (PUO) in this part of the world. The fever did not respond to the prescribed treatment and, moreover, the young man probably developed a drug-induced hepatitis, which resolved spontaneously after stopping the drugs. The risk of hepatotoxicity during anti-TB drug therapy is variable, ranging from 5% to 33%, and is influenced by several factors such as advancing age, a low serum albumin concentration and the extent of the pulmonary TB.

The causes of PUO vary with age, geography and subpopulations and the list is a very long one, although infections always top the list (Box 15.2). Amongst the infective causes, other than TB, an occult abscess (which may not have been detected initially on abdominal ultrasound) is a strong possibility. Culture-negative bacterial endocarditis (due to previous use of antibiotics), fungal infections and sarcoidosis should also be considered. Amongst the malignant causes, lymphoma and renal carcinoma are possibilities. This patient's presentation and the available investigations make a connective tissue disorder most unlikely.

Examination

Physical examination reveals that the patient is pale but not icteric. His axillary temperature is 38.1°C and he is sweating profusely; he appears chronically ill and thin. The liver edge is palpable 1 cm below the right costal border and is mildly tender; the spleen is also palpable 1.5 cm below the left costal margin. There are no peripheral lymph nodes. A grade 2/6 ejection systolic murmur is heard best at the lower left sternal border. The remainder of the examination is normal.

Has examination narrowed down your differential diagnosis?

Physical examination reveals hepatosplenomegaly as a new sign. The murmur may be either organic or functional. There are no other localising clues. Lymphoma and bacterial endocarditis top the list of possibilities, but other infective conditions such as hepatosplenic abscesses, mycobacterial and fungal diseases, malaria and kala-azar should still be considered. Enteric fever usually does not persist for such a long period. For further narrowing down of the differential diagnosis the focus of investigations should be the liver and spleen.

BOX 15.2

Aetiology of pyrexia of unknown origin (PUO)

- Infections 30%
- Malignancies 20%
- Connective tissue disorders 15%
- Miscellaneous 20%
- No diagnosis or spontaneous resolution 15%

Further investigations

The results of blood tests are listed in Box 15.3. Chest radiography and trans-oesophageal echocardiography are normal. Abdominal ultrasonography reveals mild splenomegaly with a small rounded hypo-echoic lesion (19 mm) within the spleen. The liver is also enlarged with multiple rounded hypo-echoic lesions of varying sizes involving both lobes. There are also multiple para-aortic, pre-aortic, precaval, retrocaval, mesenteric and peri-pancreatic lymph nodes (Fig. 15.1). A rounded hypo-echoic space-occupying lesion near the uncinate process of the head of the pancreas raises the possibility of a primary malignant tumour in the pancreas. A small amount of fluid is also seen in the pelvis. A contrast-enhanced computed tomogram

Further investigations on readmission	
Haemoglobin	84 g/l (8.4 g/dl)
Total WCC	50.2 × 10⁹/l (10³/mm³), 95% mature neutrophils
ESR	115 mm/1st hr
Blood film	No malarial parasites identified
Serological tests for *Salmonella typhi*, *Brucella*, *Leptospira* and *Leishmania*, HIV types 1 and 2, HBsAg, anti-HCV antibody	Negative
Blood and urine cultures	Negative
U&Es and calcium	Normal
LFTs (including LDH)	Normal, except for ALT 64 U/l

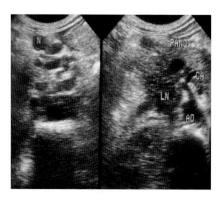

Fig. 15.1 Multiple para-aortic, pre-aortic, precaval, retrocaval, mesenteric and peri-pancreatic lymph nodes on abdominal ultrasonography. (N and LN = lymph nodes; CA = coeliac artery; AO = aorta; PANC = pancreas)

(CT) of the abdomen and pelvis confirms the ultrasound findings, with peripheral enhancement of the lesions in the liver and spleen. A CT of the chest is normal.

Has the diagnosis been clinched?

Abdominal imaging with ultrasonography as well as CT in this young man with PUO reveals multiple hypo-echoic lesions involving the liver and spleen, along with multiple enlarged para-aortic, mesenteric and peri-pancreatic lymph nodes. Ultrasonography may not be sufficient in the evaluation of structural lesions of various organs and the use of CT provides additional information, such as the presence of necrosis and calcification in TB and fungal infections. The differential diagnosis at this stage should include TB, fungal infections, sarcoidosis, lymphoma and metastatic carcinoma, as all these conditions can produce hypo-echoic lesions in the liver and spleen and have associated lymphadenopathy. This patient has been treated with anti-TB drugs without a significant response, thus TB is unlikely; drug-resistant TB (DR-TB), however, cannot be excluded (especially in extrapulmonary paucibacillary disease). A chest X-ray reveals classical bihilar lymphadenopathy and right paratracheal lymphadenopathy in most patients with sarcoidosis. A normal chest X-ray in this patient makes the diagnosis of sarcoidosis unlikely. TB, fungal infections and lymphoma can also produce mediastinal lymphadenopathy on the chest X-ray. A tissue specimen from the liver or spleen or any of the lymph nodes, under image guidance, should reveal the definitive diagnosis. Ideally, this would be a core biopsy, but fine needle aspiration cytology (FNAC) is an alternative if the necessary expertise to perform the former is not available.

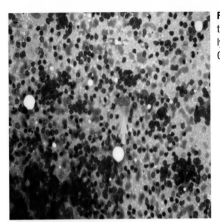

Fig. 15.2 Ultrasound-guided fine needle aspiration cytology (FNAC) from the retroperitoneal lymph nodes showing a Reed–Sternberg cell on Giemsa stain.

Definitive diagnosis

An ultrasound-guided FNAC from a retroperitoneal lymph node reveals predominantly small lymphocytes admixed with binucleate Reed–Sternberg cells, which have enlarged vesicular nuclei and prominent nucleoli (Fig. 15.2). Therefore, the cytomorphological features in this patient are those of Hodgkin's lymphoma and imaging investigations indicate stage IV B disease.

How will you treat this patient?

This patient requires combination chemotherapy with 6–8 cycles of either ChlVPP (chlorambucil, vinblastine, procarbazine and prednisolone) or ABVD (adriamycin, bleomycin, vinblastine and daunorubicin). The latter regimen is more potent, but is also more expensive. The patient should be informed about the side-effects of this chemotherapy. The stage of the disease, along with the presence or absence of systemic symptoms, influences the response to treatment. In the UK, a young man such as this, with extensive disease at presentation and treated with an ABVD regimen, would have a greater than 80% 5-year survival. The treatment response should be evaluated by clinical criteria, as well as by repeat CT examination. Positron emission tomography (PET), if available, is the most sensitive means of documenting remission.

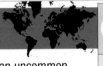

Global issues

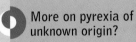
More on pyrexia of unknown origin?

- PUO is more likely to be caused by an uncommon presentation of a common problem than by a rare disorder.

- Causes of PUO vary in different geographical areas and also depend on the extent of the initial investigations.

See Chapter 13 of
Davidson's Principles and Practice of Medicine
(20th edn)

- TB is the most common cause of PUO worldwide, particularly in the developing world and immigrants from those countries.

- The first step in the evaluation of a patient with PUO for the physician, who has not seen the case previously, is to elicit the history carefully and to repeat the physical examination.

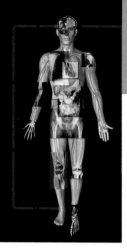

16

A young man with fever, jaundice and a purpuric rash

A. FAIZ

Presenting problem

A 35-year-old farmer from a rural area is admitted to the medical unit with a history of fever for 5 days and yellowish discoloration of the eyes. He has noticed darkening of the urine for 2 days, and over the last 24 hours has developed red spots over his body. The fever is high-grade and continuous; the patient is mentally alert. He does not take any regular medication. Prior to referral, a private practitioner carried out some routine blood tests. The results of these tests are detailed in Box 16.1

What would your differential diagnosis include before examining the patient?

This combination of the presenting problems — fever, jaundice and rash — warrants the consideration of a wide range of diseases in the differential diagnosis, depending on place, period and prevalence. This is a particularly common problem in the tropics, though it may occur anywhere in world. The possibilities are *falciparum* malaria, leptospirosis, dengue, viral hepatitis and septicaemia. Severe *falciparum* malaria and leptospirosis should always be borne in mind in endemic areas. Jaundice and renal involvement are recognised complications in both conditions but a rash is unusual in malaria. However, patients with *falciparum* malaria can develop purpuric spots due to thrombocytopenia. A patient with viral hepatitis leading to hepatic failure or dengue may present with this type of picture. In viral hepatitis, fever usually precedes jaundice and bleeding, but this is not an absolute rule. Similarly, in dengue haemorrhagic fever (DHF), bleeding usually occurs once the febrile episode is over, but hepatic involvement may complicate the initial febrile phase. Septicaemia culminating in disseminated intravascular coagulation is also a strong possibility. Rickettsial diseases should also be considered in areas where such infections are prevalent. Patients may have a tell-tale eschar and brain involvement. Yellow fever should also be considered in areas where the disease is common; the disease does not occur in Asia. Bradycardia and leucopenia are observed.

The initial investigations in this patient show leucocytosis and mild renal impairment. These two features favour the diagnosis of leptospirosis, but may also occur in septicaemia and severe malaria. A leucocytosis is unlikely in dengue and viral hepatitis.

BOX 16.1	
Initial investigations	
WCC	$16 \times 10^9/l$ ($10^3/mm^3$)
Bilirubin	105 µmol/l (5 mg/dl)
AST	120 U/l
Urea	13.5 mmol/l (81 mg/dl)
Creatinine	159 µmol/l (1.8 mg/dl)
Urine examination	
Albumin	+
RBC	+
Cast	+

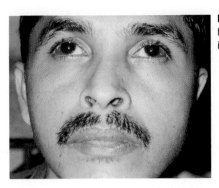

Fig. 16.1 Bilateral conjunctival haemorrhages and scleral jaundice in a patient with leptospirosis.

Examination

The patient is slightly pale and icteric. He has a widespread purpuric rash with conjunctival hyperaemia (Fig. 16.1). His pulse and blood pressure are normal. The liver is enlarged but there is no splenomegaly. The lungs are clear.

Has examination narrowed down your differential diagnosis?

Anaemia, jaundice, renal dysfunction and hepatomegaly are common in leptospirosis and severe malaria. Purpuric rashes and conjunctival congestion are features of leptospirosis and DHF. Dengue infections are a major cause of morbidity and mortality in the tropical and subtropical regions of the world. Although sporadic cases of dengue can occur, disease outbreaks or epidemics are much more common. The patient can have back pain and severe myalgia ('break-bone fever'). The illness may be mild and self-limiting, but severe forms of disease such as DHF or dengue shock syndrome (DSS) can occur. The severe form is characterised by hypovolaemia, raised haematocrit and low platelet counts. Endothelial permeability and subsequent plasma leakage are important pathological features of DHF. Patients can develop unilateral or bilateral pleural effusions, ascites or a perihepatic collection of fluid. Typically, gallbladder wall thickening occurs. These findings can be detected on ultrasonography of the abdomen and chest. The exact cause for the drop in the platelet count is not known. Mechanisms include transient suppression of haematopoiesis and immune-mediated platelet clearance. Bleeding can occur from several sites, such as the gastrointestinal tract, lungs and nose. Intracranial haemorrhage can be fatal. Hypotension or shock occurs in severe cases.

Leptospirosis requires serious consideration in this patient because he has a leucocytosis and hepatic and renal dysfunction, in addition to a purpuric rash. Leptospirosis is common in the tropics. Recent large outbreaks have been described in Asia, Central and South America, and the USA. The disease appears to be ubiquitous in wildlife and in many domestic animals. The most frequent host is a rodent, especially the common rat. The organisms persist indefinitely in the convoluted tubules of the kidney without causing apparent disease, and are shed into the urine periodically. Leptospires can enter their human hosts through intact skin or mucous membranes, but entry is facilitated by cuts or abrasions. This spirochaete can survive in water for months. Our patient is a farmer; certain occupational groups are at high risk and these include agricultural workers, sewage workers, veterinarians, workers in abattoirs and those in the fishing industry. People engaged in recreational water activities are also likely to acquire the infection. After a brief period of bacteraemia, leptospires are distributed throughout the body. The main organs affected in humans are the kidneys, liver, meninges and brain. Leptospires damage the wall of small vessels, leading to vasculitis, which is ultimately responsible for several manifestations of the disease, including haemorrhages and hypovolaemia. This patient has a purpuric rash and hepatic and renal dysfunction. Leptospirosis does not usually cause severe hepatocellular necrosis. However, it can produce severe disease, known as Weil's syndrome, characterised by hepatic and renal dysfunction with bleeding manifestations. Centrilobular necrosis with Kupffer cell hyperplasia is seen in the liver histopathology.

Hepatic involvement in leptospirosis requires differentiation from viral hepatitis. In leptospirosis, fever and jaundice occur concomitantly, whereas in acute viral hepatitis fever is frequently low-grade and is followed by the onset of jaundice. In contrast to acute viral hepatitis, leptospirosis produces large increases in serum bilirubin and alkaline phosphatase, and a modest increase in hepatic enzymes (up to 200 U/l), whereas viral hepatitis causes a several-fold increase in the hepatic enzymes (often > 1000 IU/l) and a modest increase in serum bilirubin. In addition, creatine phosphokinase may be elevated during the first week in nearly half of cases of leptospirosis. In severe cases, rhabdomyolysis occurs and contributes to renal dysfunction. Rarely, a fatal pulmonary syndrome may occur in severe leptospirosis due to haemorrhage in the lungs. This syndrome may produce acute respiratory failure. Narrowing down of the differential diagnosis requires further investigations.

 Further investigations

The results of further investigation are provided in Box 16.2.

Does this narrow down your differential diagnosis?

The negative results of thick and thin films, as well as the 'dipstick' test for malaria, make it most unlikely that the patient is suffering from severe malaria. Dengue and rickettsial fever have also been excluded. Leptospirosis remains a strong possibility in this case, but definitive diagnostic tests are required for its confirmation.

The definitive diagnosis of leptospirosis depends upon the isolation of the organism, serological tests or detection of specific DNA. Blood cultures may be

BOX 16.2

Further investigations

Thick and thin peripheral blood film for malarial parasites	Negative
Immunochromatographic 'dipstick' test for *falciparum* malaria	Negative
Bilirubin	105 μmol/l (5 mg/dl)
ALT	170 U/l
AST	240 U/l
Prothrombin time	12 secs (control 12 secs)
Haemoglobin	90 g/l (9 g/dl)
Platelets	150×10^9/l (10^3/mm^3)
Blood culture	Negative
Blood tests for dengue antigen and antibody	Negative
Rickettsia group-specific microscopic agglutination test	Negative

positive if taken before the 10th day of the illness and leptospires appear in the urine during the second week of illness. The serological investigation of choice is the microscopic agglutination test (MAT). Enzyme-linked immunosorbent assay (ELISA) and immunofluorescent assays are also available. Polymerase chain reaction (PCR) shows great promise in detecting leptospiral DNA in blood in early symptomatic disease; it is positive in the urine from the eighth day onward and remains positive for many months afterwards.

Definitive investigations

Leptospires are isolated from a urine specimen and so the final diagnosis is leptospirosis.

How will you treat this patient?

Intravenous benzylpenicillin is administered as 1.5 mega-units 6-hourly for 1 week or doxycycline in oral doses of 100 mg 12-hourly for 1 week. Parenteral ceftriaxone 1 g daily is equally effective as penicillin. The patient's renal failure should be monitored closely; if deterioration occurs, peritoneal or haemodialysis may be life-saving. The general care of the patient is critically important. Blood should be taken early for grouping and cross-matching. Episodes of bleeding should be treated by prompt blood transfusion.

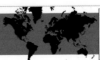

Global issues

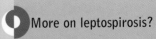

More on leptospirosis?

- Dengue is endemic in South-east Asia and India, and is also seen in Africa.

- Malaria occurs throughout the tropics and subtropics at altitudes below 1500 metres.

- Leptospirosis has emerged as an important public health problem during the last few years.

- Leptospirosis is one of the most common zoonotic diseases, favoured by a tropical climate and flooding during monsoons.

See Chapter 13 of
Davidson's
Principles and
Practice of
Medicine
(20th edn)

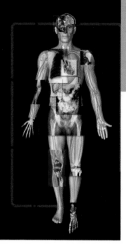

17

An Indian farmer with a high fever

S. SUNDAR

Presenting problem

A 30-year-old farmer is brought to an Accident and Emergency department in Delhi on a hot July afternoon with a high-grade fever and altered conscious level. He was found in a disoriented state by co-workers in the field. His wife reports that he is normally very fit and well, but that he has had a very high temperature for the past 8 days and was febrile when he went out to work this morning. She gives no history of severe headache, loss of consciousness or seizures.

What would your differential diagnosis include before examining the patient?

This patient presented with a very high temperature and reduced conscious level, with a history of manual labour under the hot tropical sun. Heat stroke is very high up the list of potential differential diagnoses and must be treated immediately. However, the preceding history of fever should arouse suspicion of other potential causes.

The differential diagnosis of short-duration, high-grade fever in the tropics is extensive. Malaria is one of the most common infections, and so cerebral malaria, which is a medical emergency, has to be considered. Enteric fever usually presents with altered consciousness by the end of the second week. Encephalitis and meningitis (tuberculous, other bacterial and viral) are other possibilities, although extreme elevation of temperature is uncommon in meningitis. Japanese B encephalitis is endemic in India, South-east Asia, Japan and China. It has a case fatality of 25–50%, and survivors are left with disabling neurological sequelae. Other common causes of fever in the tropics, like dengue and leptospirosis, should also be considered while examining this patient, though the level of consciousness is seldom affected in these conditions.

Examination

The patient's rectal temperature is recorded to be 40°C and his skin is hot and dry. His Glasgow Coma Scale (GCS) is 7, but there is no meningism and no focal neurological signs. Pulse rate is 120/min and blood pressure is 94/52 mmHg. The spleen is palpable 2 cm below the costal margin. The rest of the examination is normal.

BOX 17.1

Initial investigations

Haemoglobin	70 g/l (7 g/dl)
WCC	$16.4 \times 10^9/l$ ($10^3/mm^3$)
Platelets	$167 \times 10^9/l$ ($10^3/mm^3$)
Urea	36 mmol/l (100 mg/dl)
Creatinine	120 µmol/l (1.36 mg/dl)
Glucose	4.5 mmol/l (81 mg/dl)
Bilirubin	34.2 µmol/l (2 mg/dl)
AST (SGOT)	75 U/l
ALT (SGPT)	92 U/l
Alkaline phosphatase	200 U/l

The patient's clothes are removed, his entire body is sprayed with water in front of a fan and ice packs are applied. After a venous blood sample is taken, intravenous fluids are started. With this treatment, the patient's temperature normalises in 45 minutes, but there is only mild improvement in his conscious level (GCS 10).

Has examination narrowed down your differential diagnosis?

The failure of the farmer's conscious level to improve significantly following cooling makes heat stroke unlikely. The absence of conjunctival hemorrhage, icterus and signs of meningeal irritation makes leptospirosis or meningitis less probable. Dengue usually presents with a transient morbilliform rash, severe aches ('breakbone fever') and circulatory failure, or with haemorrhagic signs like petechiae, ecchymosis or gastrointestinal bleeding in its infrequent haemorrhagic form. The absence of any of these features practically rules out dengue. The presence of splenomegaly makes malaria and enteric fever more likely possibilities. The sequelae of viral encephalitis are so serious that it must be formally excluded.

Investigations

Initial blood test results are shown in Box 17.1. Blood cultures and a Widal test are negative. Magnetic resonance imagining (MRI) of the brain and cerebrospinal fluid (CSF) examination are normal. CSF testing for Japanese B encephalitis virus is negative. Thick and thin peripheral blood smears show high levels (> 5% infected red blood cells) of ring forms of *Plasmodium falciparum* (Fig. 17.1).

Does this narrow down your differential diagnosis?

MRI findings of bilateral thalamic lesions are quite characteristic of Japanese B encephalitis. The absence of these features and the negative antigen tests exclude this important diagnosis. The presence of ring forms of *Plasmodium falciparum* in the peripheral smear of a patient with impaired consciousness, where other encephalopathies have been ruled out, clinches the diagnosis of cerebral malaria.

How will you treat this patient?

As cerebral malaria is associated with significant mortality and persistent neurocognitive impairments in survivors (especially children), it is a medical emergency and requires careful and urgent management with parenteral

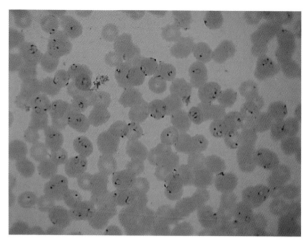

Fig. 17.1 Peripheral blood smear of the patient showing numerous erythrocytes infected with ring forms of *Plasmodium falciparum*. The size of the erythrocytes is normal, with several of them infected with multiple parasites; this is characteristic of *falciparum* infection.

antimalarial therapy. The airway should be maintained, dehydration should be corrected with intravenous fluids and the patient should be nursed on his side. Intravenous quinine should be commenced: a loading dose of 20 mg/kg in 5% glucose over 4 hrs, followed by 10 mg/kg 8-hourly, until the patient can take drugs orally. Hypoglycaemia is an important and serious complication of cerebral malaria and occurs as a result of malaria itself or its treatment with quinine. This complication is more common in children and pregnant women. Intravenous or intramuscular artesunate is a relatively safe alternative to quinine. Once the patient is able to take oral medication, doxycycline 100 mg daily should be administered for 7 days. Clindamycin should be substituted for doxycycline during pregnancy. Fresh blood should be transfused if the patient has a severe anaemia.

Blood pressure, urine output, blood glucose, parasite count and haematocrit should all be monitored regularly so that other complications of severe *falciparum* malaria (hypoglycaemia, severe anaemia, acute renal failure, acute respiratory distress syndrome, peripheral circulatory failure and shock) can be detected and managed early.

Global issues

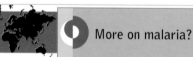

More on malaria?

- Infection with *Plasmodium falciparum* can lead to life-threatening complicated malaria with multi-organ involvement.

- In residents of the tropics or travellers returning from endemic countries, fever with an altered conscious level should arouse suspicion of complicated malaria.

See Chapter 13 of
Davidson's Principles and Practice of Medicine
(20th edn)

- Malarial retinopathy, characterised by whitening of the macula (sparing of the central fovea), peripheral retina, retinal vessels, papilloedema and haemorrhages occurs more commonly in children with cerebral malaria (> 60%) and indicates a poor prognosis.

- A high incidence of both transient and permanent neurological deficits in children with cerebral malaria produces a huge socioeconomic burden in countries with limited resources. Therefore, early diagnosis and treatment are crucial.

- As chloroquine resistance is quite common in malaria-endemic regions of the world, treatment of complicated malaria should only be initiated with either quinine or artemisinin derivatives and it is usually prudent to add a second antimalarial drug. Steroids should not be administered, as they are harmful.

- Prevention of malaria should be a priority and diligent efforts must continue to develop efficient insecticides and vaccines.

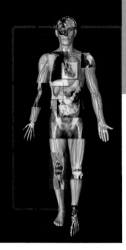

18

An elderly woman with sudden diarrhoea

W. T. A. TODD

Presenting problem

A 63-year-old caucasian woman is admitted to hospital 2 weeks after she returned home from a visit to Spain. Whilst there, she had symptoms of a urinary tract infection and at a local clinic was given a 7-day course of co-amoxiclav, which she completed before departure. For 1 week she has had intermittent fevers and shivers and has had profuse diarrhoea, such that her bowels have been opening 8–10 times daily. The diarrhoea is watery and, over the last 72 hours, she has noticed some fresh blood in the stool. She also complains of colicky lower abdominal pain relieved by defaecation. Her general practitioner sent a stool sample for bacterial culture and the patient was given a 3-day course of ciprofloxacin, but she remains symptomatic despite having completed this. She is normally well, smokes 10 cigarettes per day, drinks only social alcohol and her only regular medication is omeprazole for reflux oesophagitis. Her partner had loose stools for 3–4 days on return from holiday, but is now better.

What would your differential diagnosis include before examining the patient?

There are numerous potential causes of blood-stained diarrhoea, but the history of fever and rigors, the recent holiday abroad and similar symptomatology in a family contact all suggest an infective cause. The most likely culprits would be: *Campylobacter*, non-typhoidal salmonellae, verocytotoxigenic *Escherichia coli* (VTEC), e.g. *E. coli* O157, *Shigella* (rare) and *Clostridium difficile*. The possibility of non-infectious diarrhoea must also be considered, and in this regard, diverticular disease, inflammatory bowel disease and new-presentation of bowel malignancy would all be possible.

Examination and initial investigations

On examination, the lady is pyrexial, with a temperature of 38.1°C, and is clinically dehydrated. Pulse is 89/min, respiratory rate 16 breaths/min and blood pressure 114/67 mmHg. Her abdomen is not distended, but she is tender in the infra-umbilical region and there are active bowel sounds. A rectal examination reveals loose brown liquid stools with admixed fresh blood. Initial blood test results are shown in Box 18.1. Chest and abdominal X-rays are normal. The stool culture from the sample sent from the GP surgery grows a *Salmonella* species.

BOX 18.1

Initial investigations

Haemoglobin	142 g/l (14.2 g/dl)
WCC	9.5×10^9/l (10^3/mm^3)
Platelets	410×10^9/l (10^3/mm^3)
Sodium	138 mmol/l (meq/l)
Potassium	3.4 mmol/l (meq/l)
Chloride	103 mmol/l (meq/l)
Bicarbonate	28 mmol/l (meq/l)
Urea	9.7 mmol/l (27.17 mg/dl)
Creatinine	100 µmol/l (1.13 mg/dl)
AST	29 U/l
ALT	43 U/l
LDH	396 U/l
Alkaline phosphatase	104 U/l
GGT	71 U/l
Bilirubin	13 µmol/l (0.78 mg/dl)

Have examination and initial investigations narrowed down your differential diagnosis?

Clinical examination is notoriously unhelpful in differentiating infective from other causes of acute diarrhoea. The lack of definitive surgical features on abdominal examination is reassuring. The stool culture, however, has confirmed *Salmonella* gastroenteritis. In view of the patient's age and ongoing fever, plus her medication with a proton pump inhibitor, the possibility of *Salmonella* bacteraemia must be considered.

She may still have background diverticular disease, although this is less likely to be implicated in her presentation on this occasion. Infective gastroenteritis from any cause can produce symptoms and signs of colonic inflammation, but usually salmonellae tend to produce small bowel disease.

Further investigations

Blood cultures reveal *Salmonella* species in the aerobic bottles. A trans-thoracic echocardiogram is normal and, in particular, the aortic root dimension is normal. An ultrasound examination of the abdomen is unremarkable. Plain X-rays of the cervical, thoracic and lumbar spines are normal. Erythrocyte sedimentation rate (ESR) is 49 mm/hour and C-reactive protein (CRP) is 65 mg/l.

Does this narrow down your differential diagnosis?

This lady has *Salmonella* bacteraemia; at her age this can have serious consequences, with possible endovascular and distant bone infection. Blood cultures are positive in approximately 5% of the population and the elderly and immuno-compromised are at greater risk of both bacteraemia and metastatic infection.

Endovascular infection occurs in 10–25% of persons over 50, and usually involves the aorta.

Any cause of hypochlorhydria, including proton pump inhibitor therapy, removes the body's primary defence against food poisoning bacteria, including salmonellae.

How will you treat this patient?

Initially, she needs adequate fluid to replace both her established losses and, additionally, to cover for ongoing fluid loss from persistent diarrhoea. If she can take oral fluid, then she should have 1–2 litres of oral rehydration solution (ORS), followed by 200 ml per each loose stool; this is in addition to her normal maintenance fluid requirements. If she cannot take oral fluid, then intravenous fluid replacement should be given to replace established losses rapidly (1–2 litres in the first 4 hours), then fluid maintenance should continue, with additional allowance for any ongoing diarrhoeal losses.

High-dose ciprofloxacin remains the treatment of choice. Oral therapy should be sufficient, unless she has persistent vomiting or evidence of sepsis or endovascular/bony infection. A prolonged (2–3-week) course should be prescribed to minimise the possibility of seeding of infection. Endovascular or bone infection requires prolonged therapy, guided by microbiological and clinical expertise.

The microbiology laboratory must be asked to confirm antimicrobial susceptibility of this isolate since, notoriously, *Salmonella* originating from the Mediterranean has increased levels of ciprofloxacin resistance.

Global issues

More on diarrhoea?

- Non-typhoidal (or food poisoning) *Salmonella* remains, worldwide, a very common cause of food-borne disease.
- Many different foods are implicated, ranging from faecal contaminated vegetables and crops to dairy products. Meat products, particularly those containing chicken or uncooked eggs, are the most important and the serotypes most often involved are *S. typhimurium*, dt.104 and *S. enteritidis*, phage type 4.

See Chapter 13 of **Davidson's Principles and Practice of Medicine** (20th edn)

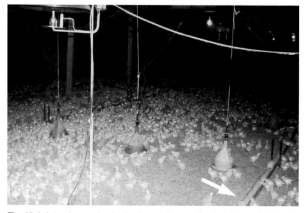

Fig. 18.1 Intensive rearing in sheds with thousands of birds together promotes the spread of salmonellae. The continuous feed belt (arrow) is open to faecal contamination.

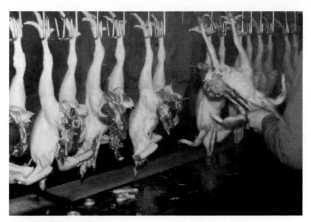

Fig. 18.2 Mass slaughter operations clearly add to the potential for cross-contamination of carcasses.

- The spread of these serotypes has been facilitated by both intensive rearing conditions (Fig. 18.1) and mass production of broiler chickens (Fig. 18.2) prevalent in parts of the developed world. Free-range birds found throughout the world in smallholdings pose a much-reduced risk in this respect.

- An embargo on uncooked egg dishes, coupled with an aggressive culling and vaccination policy in the UK and Scandinavia, has significantly reduced the incidence of *Salmonella* food poisoning over the last decade. This is not so in parts of the world where no such action has been undertaken.

- Quinolone resistance is widespread in some developing nations where these drugs are freely available as over-the-counter preparations (without prescription) and consequently used with indiscretion.

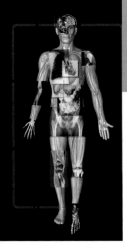

19

A young Indian with eosinophilia, nocturnal dry cough and progressive breathlessness

S. VARMA

Presenting problem

A 32-year-old male of Indian origin is referred to the chest clinic with a 6-month history of progressive breathlessness and dry cough that is worse at night. There is no history of fever, chest pain, haemoptysis or wheezing. The patient complains of anorexia and weight loss, but was apparently normal 6 months ago. He is not on any medication. He denies any associated joint pain or swelling, focal sensory or motor symptoms, rashes or the passage of worms in his stools. There is no family history of atopy or asthma. A chest X-ray, performed on the advice of his general practitioner, was normal. Sputum smears for acid-fast bacilli have been negative on three occasions. A complete blood count is subsequently carried out and an increased eosinophil count is identified (Box 19.1).

What is your differential diagnosis before examining the patient?

The patient has eosinophilia (peripheral blood eosinophil count $> 5.0 \times 10^9/l$ $(10^3/mm^3)$; this is common in many settings such as parasitic infections, drugs (sulphonamides, penicillins, cephalosporins etc.), allergies (hay fever, asthma, allergic bronchopulmonary aspergillosis etc.) and malignancies (chronic myeloid leukaemia, Hodgkin's disease etc.). Peripheral blood eosinophilia can be classified into secondary (cytokine-driven reactive phenomenon), clonal (presence of a bone marrow histological, cytogenetic or molecular marker of a myeloid malignancy) and idiopathic (neither secondary nor clonal) categories (Box 19.2). However, a moderate $(1.5–5.0 \times 10^9/l \; (10^3/mm^3))$ to marked $(> 5.0 \times 10^9/l \; (10^3/ mm^3))$ increase in the eosinophil count is often associated with Loeffler's syndrome, idiopathic hyper-eosinophilic syndrome, tropical pulmonary eosinophilia, eosinophilic pneumonia, allergic bronchopulmonary aspergillosis (ABPA) and clonal eosinophilic disorders, such as eosinophilic leukaemia.

Loeffler's syndrome is a benign disorder characterised by transient migratory pulmonary infiltrates and peripheral blood eosinophilia, generally lasting for 3 weeks and associated with the passage of larvae during the life cycles of *Ascaris lumbricoides*, hookworms (*Necator americanus* and *Ancylostoma duodenale*) and *Strongyloides stercoralis* through the lungs. Marked eosinophilia with pulmonary symptoms is also known to occur in association with visceral or cutaneous larva migrans, infection with lung flukes and haematogenous spread of *Trichinella spiralis* or schistosomal infections.

ABPA is characterised by bronchial hyper-reactivity, pulmonary infiltrates and central bronchiectasis in a patient with long-standing asthma or cystic fibrosis and hypersensitivity to the conidial colonisation of *Aspergillus fumigatus*. The Churg–Strauss syndrome is a systemic antineutrophil cytoplasmic antibody (ANCA)-associated vasculitis that involves small- and medium-vessel arteries and is characteristically accompanied by asthma and peripheral blood eosinophilia. Eosinophilic pneumonias (acute and chronic) are a rare group of steroid-responsive pulmonary eosinophilic disorders.

The idiopathic hyper-eosinophilic syndrome represents a heterogeneous group of disorders with the common feature of prolonged eosinophilia of unknown cause and multi-organ dysfunction, including the heart, central nervous system, kidneys, lungs, gastrointestinal tract and skin. Tropical pulmonary eosinophilia is a symptom complex of dyspnoea, fever, intense eosinophilia,

---

BOX 19.1

Initial investigations

Haemoglobin	110 g/l (11 g/dl)
WCC	28.8×10^9/l (10^3/mm^3)
Differential count	
Polymorphs	36%
Lymphocytes	12%
Monocytes	1%
Eosinophils	51%
Absolute eosinophil count	14.7×10^9/l (10^3/mm^3)
Peripheral blood film	No atypical cells

BOX 19.2

Causes of peripheral blood eosinophilia

Secondary

- Parasitic infections (mostly helminthic — hookworm, roundworm etc.)
- Drugs (anticonvulsants, sulphonamide group of drugs, allopurinol etc.)
- Pulmonary infiltrates with eosinophilia (idiopathic eosinophilic pneumonias, Loeffler's syndrome, Churg–Strauss syndrome, tropical pulmonary eosinophilia etc.)
- Malignancy (metastatic cancer, Hodgkin's disease)
- Endocrinopathies (Addison's disease, growth factor deficiency etc.)
- Others (HIV, human T-cell lymphotropic virus 1 (HTLV1), systemic sclerosis, polyarteritis nodosa, sarcoidosis, inflammatory bowel disease, chronic pancreatitis, eosinophilia–myalgia syndrome, eosinophilic fasciitis)

Clonal disorders

- Acute leukaemia, chronic myeloproliferative, myelodysplastic syndrome etc.

Idiopathic

- Hyper-eosinophilic syndrome

pulmonary infiltrates, with or without wheezing, and weight loss. Characteristics of tropical eosinophilia include an extreme degree of peripheral blood eosinophilia (generally $\geq 30 \times 10^9/l$), high titres of antifilarial antibody and extreme elevation of serum immunoglobulin (Ig) E, typically more than 1000 IU/ml. Classically, there is an absence of circulating microfilariae in the presence of high antifilarial antibody titres. Eosinophilic leukaemia is now considered a chronic myeloproliferative disorder and is grouped with chronic myeloid leukaemia. It may occur as part of an established chronic myeloproliferative disorder such as chronic myeloid leukaemia; at times it accompanies acute leukaemia or it may be unclassified.

Examination

Physical examination does not reveal any skin lesions, lymphadenopathy or hepatosplenomegaly. Examination of the chest and cardiovascular and other systems is unremarkable.

Has examination narrowed down your differential diagnosis?

No, not at all! In some haematological abnormalities such as eosinophilia, there are no characteristic physical signs or so-called 'easy spot' diagnoses (e.g. a patient with acromegaly or Cushing's syndrome). Further diagnosis, as in this case, will often depend on investigations directed towards common conditions such as parasitic infestations, ABPA and so on. Also, unlike with many other disorders, there are no initial key discriminatory tests and a battery of investigations has to be performed before the diagnosis can actually be 'hit'.

Further investigations

A stool examination is normal and an immediate hypersensitivity skin test against *Aspergillus fumigatus* is negative. Echocardiography is normal and so is an ultrasound examination of the abdomen. Spirometry is suggestive of mild airflow obstruction without any significant bronchodilator reversibility. High-resolution computed tomography (HRCT; Fig. 19.1) shows randomly scattered 'miliary' nodular opacities distributed throughout the lung fields with

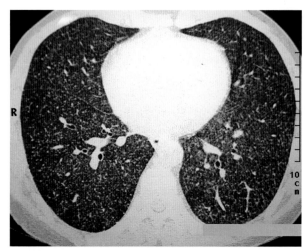

Fig. 19.1 High-resolution computed tomography shows bilateral, randomly scattered, miliary nodular opacities and patchy ground-glass opacities.

areas of patchy ground-glass opacities. The patient undergoes a fibreoptic bronchoscopy. A differential cell count in the bronchoalveolar lavage fluid reveals an eosinophil count of 35%; bronchoscopic lung biopsy reveals a bronchocentric eosinophilic infiltrate. The total serum IgE level is significantly elevated at 4500 IU/ml (normal 0–300 IU/ml). An enzyme-linked immuno-sorbent assay (ELISA) for antifilarial antibody (antibodies against *Wuchereria bancrofti*) is positive.

Does this narrow down your differential diagnosis?

A diagnosis of tropical pulmonary eosinophilia is made.

How will you treat this patient?

This young man is started on diethylcarbamazine at a dosage of 6 mg/kg/day for 3 weeks. With this he shows complete resolution of symptoms. HRCT of the chest is repeated after 4 weeks and shows almost complete clearance of the lesions. Repeat spirometry, performed 6 weeks after treatment, is reported to be normal. The response to treatment confirms the final diagnosis of tropical pulmonary eosinophilia.

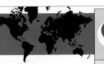

Global issues

 More on eosinophilia?

- Parasitic infections, especially by tissue-dwelling helminths, are the most common cause of marked eosinophilia in endemic areas. Elsewhere, allergic phenomena and drug hypersensitivity are frequent causes. Other causes include connective tissue diseases, neoplasia, idiopathic hyper-eosinophilic syndrome and primary bone marrow disorders like chronic myeloproliferative disorder or leukaemia.

See Chapter 13 of
Davidson's Principles and Practice of Medicine (20th edn)

- A travel history, as well as epidemiological information about parasitic infection, is important in all patients with eosinophilia. In persons with a history of travel to tropical countries, parasitic diseases should be actively pursued.

- Eosinophilia is more marked in patients with tissue-dwelling helminths. Stool examination is generally non-informative in such cases. Serological or molecular tests are needed to confirm the diagnosis.

- Relapses after successful treatment may occur in tropical pulmonary eosinophilia. Retreatment with diethylcarbamazine is usually successful in such cases.

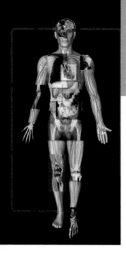

20

Fever in a man with human immunodeficiency virus (HIV)

E. Wilkins

Presenting problem

A 35-year-old white British homosexual man is admitted with a 3-week history of fevers, sweats, and pain on swallowing. He was diagnosed with HIV infection 1 month previously, following presentation with weight loss and chronic frequent watery diarrhoea. At that time, his CD4 count was found to be 24 cells/mm^3 and viral load > 1 million copies/ml. Antiretroviral (ARV) combination therapy with lopinavir/ritonavir, tenofovir and emtricitabine was started and he is tolerating this well. Co-trimoxazole prophylaxis for *Pneumocystis* pneumonia was also commenced, but had to be discontinued because of a hypersensitivity rash. He denies any other symptoms of note. His admission investigations are detailed in Box 20.1.

What would your differential diagnosis include before examining the patient?

The two most common causes of fever in later-stage HIV infection are mycobacterial infection (either disseminated *Mycobacterium avium intracellulare* (MAI) or tuberculosis (TB)) and lymphoma. The presence of frequent diarrhoea and weight loss in addition to this patient's fever may indicate a single aetiology (e.g. MAI, cytomegalovirus (CMV) or *Salmonella* infection) or reflect two or more coexisting causes (e.g. TB causing fever, and *Cryptosporidium* or lopinavir/ritonavir causing diarrhoea). Similarly, his anaemia may indicate a disseminated process such as mycobacterial infection or lymphoma, but could also reflect Kaposi's sarcoma (KS) involvement of his gastrointestinal tract. Although not discriminatory features, they do identify potential investigations where the diagnosis may be confirmed (stool culture, endoscopy and bone marrow). Disseminated CMV infection is an infrequent but recognised cause of prolonged fever and needs to be considered. Fever without breathlessness makes *Pneumocystis* pneumonia unlikely, and without headache, cryptococcal infection is unlikely. Secondary syphilis is improbable but should be excluded. Finally, the recent commencement of ARV therapy raises the possibility of immune reconstitution syndrome (IRS), which occurs in approximately 15% of patients with mycobacterial co-infection.

BOX 20.1

Initial investigations	
Haemoglobin	70 g/l (7.0 g/dl)
Film	Hypochromic, microcytic
WCC	2.7×10^9/l (10^3/mm^3)
Differential count	
Lymphocytes	0.38×10^9/l (10^3/mm^3)
Neutrophils	1.91×10^9/l (10^3/mm3)
Platelets	207×10^9/l (10^3/mm^3)
ALT	42 U/l
GGT	114 U/l
Albumin	17 g/l (1.7 g/dl)
Prothrombin ratio	1.0

Examination

The patient is febrile, but comfortable at rest. He is wasted, with lesions that resemble cutaneous and oral KS; he also has perianal herpes simplex and severe oropharyngeal candidiasis. He has two-finger breadth hepatosplenomegaly but no abdominal tenderness; rectal examination reveals an empty rectum. There is no lymphadenopathy and no localising signs for his infection. Dilated funduscopy demonstrates no evidence of retinitis.

Has examination narrowed down your differential diagnosis?

Detailed examination in patients with HIV, particularly of the skin, mouth, genitals and perianal area, is often rewarding. The presence of lesions consistent with KS may explain the anaemia but not the leucopenia, and the likelihood is that its cause is multifactorial. The presence of oropharyngeal candidiasis makes oesophageal candidiasis a probable cause of his pain on swallowing. The hepatosplenomegaly is consistent with mycobacterial infection, visceral KS and lymphoma, and is therefore not discriminatory in determining the aetiology of his fever, but it is a significant finding.

Further investigations

Blood and stool cultures at 48 hours are negative. The patient's CD4 count is 32 cells/mm^3 and viral load is 1200 copies/ml. Cryptococcal antigen and treponemal antibody blood tests are negative, as is immunoglobulin (Ig) M antibody for CMV. Induced sputa are negative on direct examination for *Pneumocystis jirovecii* and acid-fast bacilli, and there is no growth on standard culture. A chest X-ray is normal, but a computed tomogram (CT) of the chest reveals numerous enlarged lymph nodes 2–5 cm in diameter in the mediastinum. An upper gastrointestinal endoscopy demonstrates oesophageal candidiasis and gastric KS (Figs 20.1 and 20.2).

Does this narrow down your differential diagnosis?

These results are consistent with the two most likely diagnoses, mycobacterial infection and lymphoma. CMV, cryptococcal infection and syphilis are now extremely unlikely. In patients from the developing world, the differential

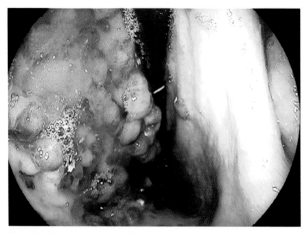

Fig. 20.1 Kaposi's sarcoma of the stomach.

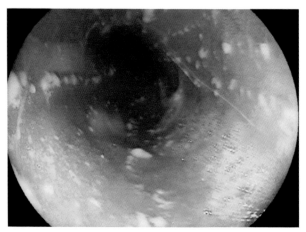

Fig. 20.2 Oesophageal candidiasis.

diagnosis at this stage would still include fungal infections, e.g. histoplasmosis, and visceral leishmaniasis.

Definitive investigations

A bone marrow aspiration is performed and numerous acid-fast bacilli are identified on a Ziehl–Nelsen stain. Three weeks later, blood cultures grow mycobacterial organisms.

Does this further narrow down your differential diagnosis?

With the identification of mycobacteria in blood and bone marrow, the differential lies between TB and MAI. The normal chest X-ray points more towards this being MAI, although extrapulmonary and disseminated presentations of TB are far more common in HIV, especially in late-stage disease. Rapid distinction between the two mycobacterial species and detection of rifampicin resistance if *Mycobacterium tuberculosis* is confirmed will depend upon molecular techniques (e.g. polymerase chain reaction (PCR)). Subsequent rapid sensitivity testing will allow rationalisation of therapy.

How will you treat this patient?

While awaiting identification of the species, it is important to consider choosing a combination of drugs that provides treatment for both mycobacterial species. It is also necessary to examine potential drug interactions with his antiretroviral agents. Ritonavir is a potent inhibitor of the cytochrome P450 complex and rifampicin a potent inducer. Because of this, protease inhibitors should not ordinarily be prescribed with rifampicin, although rifabutin, which has equal potency to rifampicin against *M. tuberculosis* but is also active against MAI, is the preferred rifamycin. Pyrazinamide and isoniazid, although first-line anti-TB drugs, have no significant activity in clinical disease associated with MAI, whereas ethambutol and certain quinolones (e.g. ciprofloxacin) have proven activity against both mycobacteria. Lastly, both azithromycin and clarithromycin have activity against MAI and one should be included. Hence, although several combinations are possible, a suitable one would include rifabutin, azithromycin, ethambutol, ciprofloxacin and pyrazinamide. Treatment can then be modified when identification is established (dropping pyrazinamide if MAI is confirmed and switching to standard four-drug therapy if it is *M. tuberculosis*). His culture PCR confirms MAI, which is successfully treated, as is his KS, which is treated with cyclical liposomal doxorubicin. The oesophageal candidiasis is successfully treated with a 14-day course of fluconazole.

Global issues

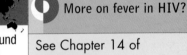

More on fever in HIV?

- The causes of fever in late-stage HIV can vary around the world, depending upon the local prevalence of certain infections. Fever in late-stage HIV is highly likely to indicate TB in a person living in, or coming from, a TB-endemic area.

See Chapter 14 of
Davidson's Principles and Practice of Medicine (20th edn)

- The incidence of MAI infection has fallen by 90% since the advent of highly active antiretroviral (HAART) combination therapy. *M. tuberculosis* is the most common opportunistic infection in HIV/AIDS in the developing world.

- Kaposi's sarcoma is uncommon in certain parts of the world (and extremely rare in India).

- The national AIDS control programmes of some countries do not include protease inhibitors in antiretroviral therapy regimens because of high cost. Instead, non-nucleoside reverse transcriptase inhibitors (either efavirenz or nevirapine) are used, along with two nucleoside reverse transcriptase inhibitors.

- Drug interactions are common when combining antimycobacterial and anti-HIV drugs. Regimens containing efavirenz are safe in patients receiving anti-TB drugs; however, nevirapine should be used in place of efavirenz during pregnancy.

- When nevirapine is co-administered with rifampicin, therapeutic drug monitoring (TDM) of nevirapine levels is indicated. However, access to TDM is seldom available in resource-limited settings where both HIV and TB are common.

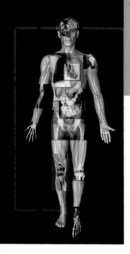

21

A young woman with vulval pain and dysuria

A. McMILLAN

Presenting problem

A 25-year-old white woman is referred to a genitourinary medicine clinic with a 2-day history of vulval pain and pain on passing urine. She has also noticed tender lumps in both groins. A few days before the onset of these symptoms, she had felt generally unwell with malaise and mild fever. She has no other symptoms and, other than using the combined contraceptive pill, she does not take any medication or use recreational drugs. The lady has not used any deodorants or similar chemical agents on the affected areas. Her last menstrual period was 8 days prior to the development of her symptoms and was normal. Using a mirror, she has noticed sores on her genitals. She has been married for 18 months to a businessman who travels frequently to Uganda. They had sexual intercourse 1 week previously, on the night he had returned from Africa. Intercourse was not traumatic. Her husband is in good health and has no genital symptoms or signs.

What would your differential diagnosis include before examining the patient?

The clinical features are suggestive of primary genital herpes, caused by herpes simplex virus (HSV). Candidiasis can cause superficial genital ulceration, but itch rather than pain is the principal symptom and lymph node enlargement is not a feature. Trauma secondary to intercourse seems unlikely, as is ulceration caused by drugs or chemicals. The patient's husband has travelled frequently to Africa, where ulcerative conditions such as syphilis, lymphogranuloma venereum (LGV) and chancroid are more prevalent than in the UK. If he has had sexual contact with a local person there, these conditions need to be considered.

Examination

The patient walks with some difficulty because of pain. Her temperature is 37.4°C. The inguinal lymph nodes are enlarged and tender bilaterally. On the mucosal surface of the vulva, there are multiple white plaques, and vesicles and shallow tender ulcers are noted on the labia, perineum and inner aspects of the upper thighs (Fig. 21.1). The ulcers are not indurated and do not bleed when touched. It is impossible to pass a vaginal speculum because of pain. Neither a rash nor oral ulceration is evident.

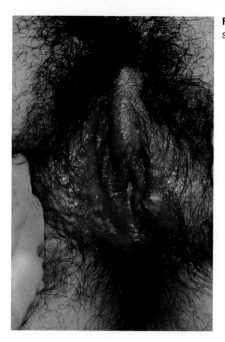

Fig. 21.1 Primary herpes simplex of the vulva.

Has examination narrowed down your differential diagnosis?

The clinical appearance is consistent with genital herpes. Primary syphilis usu-ally presents with a solitary, painless, indurated genital ulcer and, although atypical presentations are not uncommon, this seems an improbable diagnosis. Secondary syphilis is often associated with mucosal ulceration, but this is usu-ally painless and in most cases a maculopapular or papular rash is also found. Lymphogranuloma venereum, caused by *Chlamydia trachomatis* genovar *lym-phogranuloma venereum*, is unlikely. This condition is uncommon in women and is associated with transient painless genital ulceration followed several weeks later by unilateral lymph node enlargement. Chancroid, caused by *Haemophilus ducreyii* and common in Africa, is associated with multiple genital ulcers that bleed easily, and with inguinal lymphadenopathy. In the absence of other fea-tures, systemic conditions such as erythema multiforme and Behçet's syndrome are unlikely.

Has the diagnosis been clinched?

The clinical picture is almost diagnostic, but the diagnosis should always be confirmed so that the most appropriate management can be provided.

Further investigations

Herpes simplex virus type 1 DNA is detected in material obtained from one of the vesicles. Serological tests for syphilis, including an anti-treponemal IgM enzyme immunoassay to detect early infection, are negative. As culture for *H. ducreyii* and nucleic acid amplification methods for the detection of specific DNA sequences are only available in a limited number of centres, these tests are not undertaken in this case.

How will you treat this patient?

When the diagnosis is reasonably certain, antiviral therapy should be initiated before receiving the laboratory results. Aciclovir, given in an oral dosage of 200 mg five times per day for 5 days, is the most widely used and cheapest drug. It is well tolerated with few adverse effects, although a rash may occasionally complicate therapy. The use of aciclovir decreases healing time, new lesion formation and viral shedding; all symptoms are shorter than if the individual is untreated. Treatment, however, does not decrease the likelihood of subsequent recurrence. There is no place for topical aciclovir in the treatment of primary genital herpes. In addition to specific antiviral treatment, mild analgesics should be prescribed for pain, and the individual should frequently bathe the affected area with physiological 0.9% saline.

Oral valaciclovir and famciclovir are alternative antiviral agents that are as effective as aciclovir.

Counselling and support are essential in the management of the newly diagnosed individual with first-episode genital herpes. It is also helpful to give written information. Patients should be given the opportunity to return within a few days to discuss their anxieties and fears, and it is sometimes helpful to have a joint counselling session. In this case, the infection is likely to have been acquired from oral–genital contact with her husband, who is a symptomless excretor of the virus. There is no indication that he has been unfaithful.

Global issues

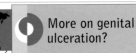

- In many countries an increasing proportion of cases of genital herpes are caused by herpes simplex virus type 1.

- An increasing proportion of genital ulcer disease in developing countries is caused by herpes simplex virus.

- Genital herpes is recognised as an important factor facilitating the transmission of the human immunodeficiency virus (HIV).

More on genital ulceration?

See Chapter 15 of
Davidson's Principles and Practice of Medicine
(20th edn)

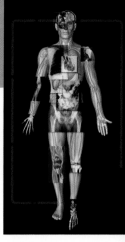

22

A man with a urethral discharge

G. R. SCOTT

Presenting problem

A 34-year-old man presents in your GP surgery in the UK complaining of a urethral discharge that started the day before. He describes this as pus coming from the end of his penis, associated with severe pain when passing urine. You know he is married and that he works in the hotel trade.

What would your differential diagnosis include before examining the patient?

Chlamydia trachomatis is by far the most common sexually transmitted infection (STI) seen in men presenting with urethritis in the UK. However, the severity of this man's symptoms, also reflected in his rapid attendance for treatment, makes gonorrhoea a significant possibility. *Trichomonas* is a rare cause of urethral discharge in the UK and, although herpes simplex virus infection may present with urethritis, external genital ulceration is much more common. Non-specific urethritis, perhaps due to *Mycoplasma* or *Ureaplasma*, is also a possibility.

Further history and examination

You advise this man to attend the local genitourinary medicine (GUM) clinic but he asks you to manage him yourself. What essential questions must be asked? You must take a sexual history, perhaps prefacing this by saying, 'I understand you are married. When did you last have sex with your wife?' The next question should be, 'When did you last have sex with anyone else?' Let's say he answers somewhat gloomily, 'Last week.' The questioning should continue along the following lines: 'Is this a regular partner or was it more of a 'one-off'?'; 'Was this local, within the UK or abroad?', 'Did you use a condom?' and 'Was this partner female or male?'

The last question is essential and should be asked in a neutral tone that does not infer one answer or the other. The fact that the patient is married does not exclude the possibility that he has had sex with a man. It transpires that he has had unprotected, insertive and receptive anal sex with another man 8 days ago.

General examination is unremarkable. Examination of the genitalia confirms the presence of a purulent urethral discharge (Fig. 22.1). Rectal examination is normal.

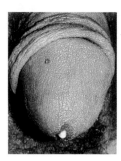

Fig. 22.1 Urethral discharge.

Has examination narrowed down your differential diagnosis?

Gonorrhoea is relatively more common among men who have sex with men (MSM) than it is among heterosexual men in the UK, although chlamydia remains a distinct possibility. The findings on examination are consistent with either.

Many cities in the UK have seen increased numbers of cases of syphilis among MSM over the last 5 years. Hepatitis B is more common among MSM, and of course human immunodeficiency virus (HIV) infection is a major concern. It is important to remember that multiple concurrent STIs may be diagnosed.

Investigations

A urethral swab for culture of *Neisseria gonorrhoeae* is sent in the appropriate transport medium to the local laboratory. This must reach the laboratory on the day it is taken; otherwise any gonococci will die in transit. If there is any doubt about transport delay, a slide of the urethral discharge may be sent for microscopy, ensuring careful packaging. A first-voided urine specimen is also sent for chlamydia examination.

Swabs from the rectum are sent for gonorrhoea and chlamydia testing because this man has had receptive anal sex; a pharyngeal swab is also sent for gonorrhoea testing.

Blood is taken for serological tests for syphilis and hepatitis B, with a view to vaccination against the latter if there is no evidence of current or past infection.

Blood is also taken for an HIV test, after an explanation of the procedure to be followed should the test be positive (pretest counselling), and arrangements are made to give the result in person.

How will you treat this patient?

Treatment should be given prior to confirmation of the microbiological diagnosis. There is no single agent that cures both gonorrhoea and chlamydia with sufficient certainty to be recommended. In GUM clinics in the UK, a currently recommended regime would be cefixime 400 mg stat, to cover gonococcal infection, and azithromycin 1 g for possible co-infection with chlamydia.

The urethral swabs grow gonococci. All other swabs are negative. He should be advised to abstain from sexual contact until cure has been confirmed, and sexual partners should be advised to attend for investigation. If he has had sex with his wife since acquiring gonorrhoea, she will need to be tested as well. Advice on safer sex would be particularly important in this case, and again referral to your local GUM service would be appropriate.

All serological tests are negative. These will need to be repeated in due course, as his most recent sexual contact was within the window period for these infections. His risk of HIV infection will depend on local prevalence of HIV, the number of (male) partners that he has had sex with, and the type of sex. Anal sex carries the greatest risk of transmission, especially for the receptive partner. The presence of others STIs, such as gonorrhoea, increases risk of transmission. A single episode of insertive anal sex in a UK city with an HIV prevalence of ~5% would carry a relatively low risk, but a test for HIV should be recommended nevertheless.

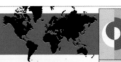

Global issues

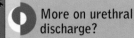
More on urethral discharge?

- There is a wide range of human sexual expression in all parts of the world. Some married men will have sex with other men. This may range from low-risk sexual activity such as mutual masturbation, through oral sex to unprotected anal sex.

- A thorough risk assessment is essential in order to diagnose and treat infections for which a man is at risk, and to give advice and support in adhering to safer sexual practice in the future.

See Chapter 15 of
Davidson's Principles and Practice of Medicine
(20th edn)

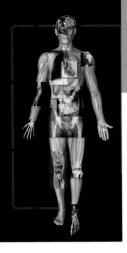

23

A man with constipation, pain on defaecation and rectal bleeding

A. McMILLAN

Presenting problem

A 43-year-old white man presents to a genitourinary medicine clinic with a 10-day history of constipation, painful defaecation, streaking of the stools with slime, a feeling of incomplete emptying of his bowels, and the passage of blood anally to a degree that it splashes in the toilet pan. His health is otherwise good and he has not had previous bowel problems. At the age of 35 years he had acute hepatitis B, and 3 years before the current illness he was treated for urethral gonorrhoea and giardiasis. Otherwise he has had no significant illnesses in the past. He has never been tested for human immunodeficiency virus (HIV) infection. His most recent sexual contact was 3 weeks previously at a party in Amsterdam, when he had unprotected receptive anal intercourse with an unknown male.

What would your differential diagnosis include before examining the patient?

The clinical features are strongly suggestive of proctitis. As the onset was acute in an individual with no previous history of intestinal disease and, as there appears to be a temporal relationship between the onset of symptoms and the episode of unprotected anal intercourse, a sexually transmitted infection (STI) seems to be the most likely cause. Box 23.1 shows the STIs that can cause proctitis. As the symptoms are severe, infection with *Chlamydia trachomatis* genovar *trachoma* is unlikely. An outbreak of cases of severe proctitis caused by *C. trachomatis* genovar *lymphogranuloma venereum* (LGV), however, has been described recently amongst men who have sex with men (MSM) in Western Europe, including the Netherlands. Primary syphilis usually has a pre-patent period of about 6 weeks, making this infection a less likely cause of this patient's symptoms. Primary herpetic proctitis is usually associated with perianal ulceration, but there is no history of this. Perirectal cellulitis following traumatic anal intercourse usually presents sooner, and there are often systemic features that are absent in this case.

BOX 23.1

Sexually transmitted organisms causing proctitis

- *Neisseria gonorrhoeae*
- *Chlamydia trachomatis*
  Genovar *trachomatis*
  Genovar *lymphogranuloma venereum*
- *Treponema pallidum*
- Herpes simplex virus

Examination

The patient looks well and is apyrexial. There is no abdominal tenderness or guarding, and no masses are felt; neither liver nor spleen is palpable. The perianal region appears normal with no ulceration. At sigmoidoscopy, the rectal mucosa is markedly oedematous and friable, with mucopus in the lumen. These inflammatory changes extend to about 12 cm from the dentate line, the more proximal mucosa appearing normal. Two ulcers, each about 1.5 cm in diameter, are noted within the inflamed mucosa.

Has examination narrowed down your differential diagnosis?

The diagnosis of distal proctitis is confirmed — the inflammatory changes do not extend beyond the rectosigmoid junction, unlike the appearance in proctocolitis. Although rectal gonorrhoea can produce acute proctitis, prominent ulceration is unusual. In most, but by no means all, cases of primary herpetic proctitis there is perianal ulceration and the patient is usually pyrexial. Infection with *C. trachomatis* genovar *trachomatis* usually causes minimal symptoms and signs, and is an unlikely cause of the proctitis in this case. The LGV genovar of *C. trachomatis*, however, is commonly associated with severe disease, and this must be high on the list of differential diagnoses. Primary syphilis also needs to be considered. The lack of abdominal tenderness and fever argues against a diagnosis of perirectal cellulitis.

Further investigations

A nucleic acid amplification test for *C. trachomatis* is positive, and genotyping shows infection with the LGV genovar, clinching the diagnosis of LGV proctitis. Negative culture for *Neisseria gonorrhoeae* and a negative polymerase chain reaction (PCR) assay for herpes simplex virus (HSV) DNA exclude concurrent infection with these organisms. Syphilis serology, including an anti-treponemal IgM test to detect early infection, is negative. To exclude incubating syphilis, however, it would be necessary to repeat serological tests 1 and 3 months later.

Rectal biopsy is not likely to be helpful, as the histological changes associated with these infections are non-specific. The granulomatous changes found in LGV proctitis (Fig. 23.1) closely resemble those of Crohn's disease.

Serological tests show that this patient is infected with HIV. He is only moderately immunocompromised, with a CD4+ T-cell count of 387 per mm^3 (normal range 500–1500 per mm^3). An antibody test for hepatitis C virus is negative, but to exclude infection acquired at the same time as LGV, serology should be repeated in 3 and 6 months' time.

How will you treat this patient?

As the proctitis is severe, treatment should not be withheld until laboratory test results are available. The most likely diagnosis from the history and examination is LGV proctitis, and doxycycline in an oral dosage of 100 mg 12-hourly for 3 weeks should be prescribed. Aciclovir, given orally in a dose of 200 mg five times per day for 5 days, should also be prescribed to treat possible HSV infection (while awaiting the serology results). As multiple rectal infections, including gonorrhoea, are common in MSM, it also seems prudent to treat this man with a single oral dose of cefixime (400 mg) or with a single intramuscular injection of ceftriaxone (250 mg). He will require counselling regarding the new diagnosis of HIV and will clearly need long-term follow-up. No antiretroviral therapy is indicated at this stage.

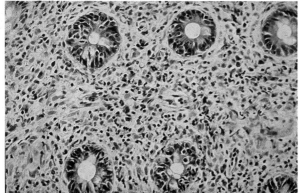

Fig. 23.1 Granulomatous proctitis in lympho-granuloma venereum. There is infiltration of the lamina propria of the rectum with lymphocytes, histiocytes and plasma cells. Early granuloma formation is also shown.

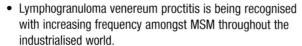

Global issues

- Lymphogranuloma venereum proctitis is being recognised with increasing frequency amongst MSM throughout the industrialised world.

- Lymphogranuloma venereum proctitis has been recognised for many years amongst women in developing countries, and has been associated with considerable morbidity.

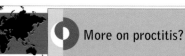

More on proctitis?

See Chapter 15 of **Davidson's Principles and Practice of Medicine** (20th edn)

24

A young woman with a vaginal discharge

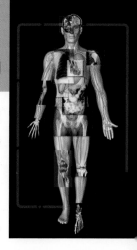

G. R. SCOTT

Presenting problem

You are visiting a sub-Saharan African country to assist in the training of local staff in the delivery of antiretroviral therapy for human immunodeficiency virus (HIV). In a community-based clinic, a 23-year-old woman presents to you with a complaint of vaginal discharge and vulval itch. She is not known to have any ongoing health problems and does not take any regular medication.

What would your differential diagnosis include before examining the patient?

In the UK the most likely diagnoses would be candidiasis or bacterial vaginosis, with the presence of itch making the former more likely. However, it is essential to assess the risk of a sexually transmitted infection (STI) by taking a sexual history. You quickly establish that this lady has had a regular male partner for several months. They are not using condoms, or indeed any form of contraception. In many parts of the world, condom use is not widespread among men. The patient should, therefore, be considered to be at risk of having an STI.

Trichomonas vaginalis (TV) is the most common treatable STI in the world with an estimated 170 million cases each year. The main symptom of TV is a vaginal discharge, often accompanied by vulval itch and/or irritation. Gonorrhoea and chlamydia are also common, with 62 and 90 million cases respectively world-wide per annum, but vaginal discharge is a less common symptom with both.

Examination

General physical examination reveals no abnormal findings. Vaginal examination reveals a yellow discharge at the entrance to the vagina. You have a speculum but no light source; so ascertaining whether the discharge is vaginal or cervical is impossible.

Has examination narrowed down your differential diagnosis?

Not really! A discharge emanating from the cervix would make gonorrhoea or chlamydia more likely. A vaginal discharge would be more in keeping with TV, bacterial vaginosis and candidiasis. The only way to determine the underlying diagnosis is to examine a specimen of the discharge.

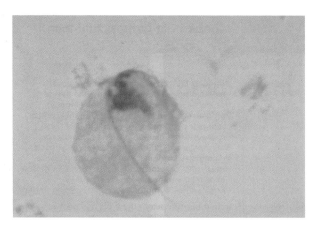

Fig. 24.1 Wet mount of vaginal discharge demonstrating *Trichomonas vaginalis* organisms.

Investigations

Fortunately, there is a microscope to hand, along with facilities for carrying out simple Gram staining. Motile, flagellated organisms are identified in a wet-mount preparation (Fig. 24.1). Gram staining of the discharge reveals mixed organisms consistent with anaerobic infection.

Does this narrow down your differential diagnosis?

The organisms identified on the wet mount are typical of TV. Examination of *cervical* discharge for Gram-negative diplococci has a sensitivity of about 50% in the diagnosis of gonorrhoea, so the positive yield from a blind vaginal swab is going to be even lower. Culture of the discharge and automated nucleic acid amplification tests (NAATs) would increase the likelihood of detecting gonococci, but these facilities are not available. Both candida and bacterial vaginosis can be diagnosed accurately by microscopy of vaginal discharge.

How will you treat this patient?

Clearly, appropriate treatment should be given for any infection diagnosed by microscopy, in this case TV. However, multiple diagnoses are not uncommon. If local prevalence of gonorrhoea and chlamydia is known to be high, then effective antimicrobials for these infections should be given, even if the organisms are not identified. This woman should be prescribed metronidazole 2 g for TV, cefixime 400 mg or ciprofloxacin 500 mg for gonorrhoea, and either azithromycin 1 g stat or doxycycline 100 mg twice daily for 7 days for chlamydia; she should also be offered treatment for candida. Treatment would also be recommended for her partner, but persuading him to attend may be difficult.

A discussion about having an HIV test would also be routine practice in the UK for anybody diagnosed with an STI. Unhindered access to antiretroviral therapy (ART) makes a proactive approach easy to justify. Unfortunately, some parts of the developing world have limited programmes for delivering ART. As you are actively working with local staff to create treatment access, this lady should be offered an HIV test. Her partner should also be encouraged to attend the clinic for HIV testing.

Finally, the patient is not using any form of contraception. If she does not wish to become pregnant, long-acting injectable methods of contraception are more effective in preventing pregnancy than short-acting methods such as the oral contraceptive pill.

Global issues

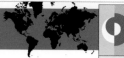

More on vaginal discharge?

See Chapter 15 of
**Davidson's
Principles and
Practice of
Medicine**
(20th edn)

- Accurate diagnosis is the bedrock of managing STI, allowing precise treatment and informed tracing of sexual contacts.

- Laboratory support is taken for granted in the developed world, but routine culture or automated NAATs are rarely available in most countries.

- Affordable, accurate, rapid point-of-care tests, such as those now available for the diagnosis of HIV infection, would significantly improve management of STI.

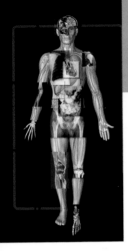

25

Hyponatraemia discovered in an elderly man in a neurosurgical ward

M. J. FIELD

Presenting problem

A consultation is requested on the neurosurgery ward for a 71-year-old man who has become confused and aggressive on the ward. He was admitted 14 days previously following a motor vehicle accident in which he received numerous injuries to the head and trunk. An intracerebral haematoma in the left parietal lobe was identified on computed tomography (CT) (Fig. 25.1) and evacuated 8 days following his admission. In the immediate post-operative period he was ventilated in the intensive care unit and, following discharge from there, he developed a right lower lobe pneumonia which was treated with intravenous antibiotics. His behaviour has been deteriorating for several days by the time of consultation, and routine biochemistry has shown that the plasma sodium has fallen from 136 mmol/l (meq/l) on the day of admission to 117 mmol/l (meq/l).

What would your differential diagnosis include before examining the patient?

Hyponatraemia generally indicates a relative excess of water in relation to sodium in the extracellular fluid. It can develop in a context where the total body sodium content is low, normal or high. In the present clinical situation, it is possible

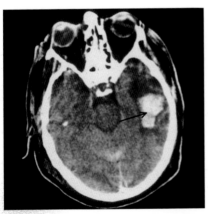

Fig. 25.1 Cerebral CT scan of the patient, showing an intracerebral haematoma (arrow) in the left parietal lobe.

that a disturbance of total body sodium (and hence extracellular fluid volume) has occurred during his period of hospital treatment, but it is even more likely that he has developed water retention without a major underlying disturbance of sodium balance. It is important to check that he has not been given an excess of sodium-free intravenous fluids, such as 5% glucose, which would aggravate any tendency to water retention. Both cerebral injury and lung pathology have the potential to stimulate the release of antidiuretic hormone (vasopressin) from the hypothalamus–posterior pituitary axis. Therefore, the syndrome of inappropriate secretion of antidiuretic hormone (SIADH) seems the most likely working diagnosis.

Examination

On examination, the patient is disoriented and somewhat aggressive to those around him. There is a dressing over his craniotomy wound. On examination of the cardiovascular system the blood pressure is normal and there is no evidence of dehydration, or of peripheral oedema suggestive of sodium retention. Examination of the lung fields reveals some reduction of air entry and crepitations at the right base, consistent with resolving pneumonia. There are no focal neurological signs, although complete examination is difficult because of his confused state. The intravenous fluid charts show that no sodium-free fluids have been administered since his admission to hospital.

Has examination narrowed down your differential diagnosis?

The hyponatraemia appears to have developed here in the context of normovolaemia; in the absence of a large administered load of free water, the most likely diagnosis remains SIADH. If the hyponatraemia had developed more insidiously and over a longer time period, hypothyroidism and impaired adrenocortical function would need to be considered. A number of drugs can cause SIADH (e.g. carbamazepine, phenothiazines and clofibrate), but none has been used in this patient.

Further investigations

Repeat plasma biochemistry analysis is shown in Box 25.1. A single urine specimen is taken at the same time as the above blood specimen and shows: urine sodium 53 mmol/l (meq/l), urine osmolality 603 mmol/kg. Plasma ADH concentration is 3.2 pmol/l (3.5 pg/ml).

Does this narrow down your differential diagnosis?

The low plasma osmolality confirms that the measured hyponatraemia is real, rather than being an artefact, and it suggests that the patient's disturbed mental function is likely to reflect a degree of cerebral oedema. (The head injury itself and the chest infection may also be contributing to his confusion.) The finding of a high urine osmolality, associated with a high urine sodium concentration, is consistent with SIADH rather than a hypovolaemic cause of water retention or an oedema-forming hypervolaemic state, both of which are typically associated with low urine sodium concentrations. The ADH concentration is elevated above the near-zero levels that would be expected in the face of the low plasma osmolality. In the present context this is consistent with SIADH, as there is no hypovolaemic stimulus to its release.

BOX 25.1	
Further investigations	
Sodium	116 mmol/l (meq/l)
Chloride	84 mmol/l (meq/l)
Potassium	4.1 mmol/l (meq/l)
Urea	4.9 mmol/l (13.7 mg/dl)
Creatinine	115 µmol/l (1.3 mg/dl)
Uric acid	0.21 mmol/l (3.53 mg/dl)
Plasma osmolality	243 mmol/kg (normal range 285–294)

How will you treat this patient?

The mainstay of treatment for SIADH is fluid restriction. Carefully supervised restriction of fluid intake to 600 ml per day is the appropriate first step in management of this patient's water retention disorder, and gradual elevation in his plasma sodium and the level of mental function can be expected. Given the significant cerebral pathology and surgical intervention, as well as the resolving pneumonia, SIADH may persist for some time, and sometimes an adjunctive measure to assist free water clearance can be used. Depending on local experience, this may take the form of oral demeclocycline (600–900 mg per day), or alternatively oral urea therapy (30–45 g per day) can be instituted under careful supervision. Intravenous infusion of hypertonic (3%) saline should be reserved for situations where hyponatraemia is severe, has developed very abruptly, and is associated with marked neurological complications such as seizures. Overly rapid correction of hyponatraemia which has developed over 2 days or more brings the risk of inducing severe neurological injury due to osmotic demyelination of cerebral neurons.

Global issues

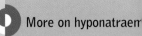 More on hyponatraem

- Hypovolaemic causes of hyponatraemia are encountered in areas where gastroenteritis is common and where water rather than electrolyte-containing rehydration solutions are used.

- Assay of plasma ADH is quite unnecessary to make this diagnosis, given the appropriate clinical context and consistent plasma and urine biochemistry results.

See Chapter 16 of
Davidson's Principles and Practice of Medicine
(20th edn)

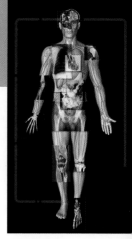

26

A young man found incidentally to have hypokalaemia

M. J. FIELD

Presenting problem

A 26-year-old man is found incidentally to have a plasma potassium of 2.4 mmol/l (meq/l) following an elective hernia repair. He has an apparently healthy diet, is taking no prescribed or illicit drugs, and specifically denies using purgatives or diuretics. He says he has experienced occasional tingling in his fingertips and a few episodes of spasm in the hands over the previous 10 years. The initial blood tests results are shown in Box 26.1.

What would your differential diagnosis include before examining the patient?

The association of hypokalaemia with a high plasma bicarbonate is a common one. It is possible that the high bicarbonate is associated with a primary metabolic alkalosis and is contributing to the hypokalaemia by causing shift of potassium into cells. However, in this case, the very low potassium concentration suggests that there is some factor causing excessive potassium loss from the body, although this might also be associated with loss of acid.

Both gastrointestinal and renal causes for such potassium loss should be considered. In the case of gastrointestinal losses, the association with alkalosis would particularly suggest vomiting, but there is no report of this here

BOX 26.1	
Initial investigations	
Sodium	148 mmol/l (meq/l)
Potassium	2.4 mmol/l (meq/l)
Chloride	98 mmol/l (meq/l)
Bicarbonate	34 mmol/l (meq/l)
Urea	6.5 mmol/l (18.21 mg/dl)
Creatinine	140 µmol/l (1.58 mg/dl)
Calcium	2.21 mmol/l (8.86 mg/dl)
Magnesium	0.78 mmol/l (1.9 mg/dl)
Albumin	41 g/l (4.1 g/dl)

(although the possibility of surreptitious self-induced vomiting has to be kept in mind, especially if there were a psychosocial setting suggestive of anorexia nervosa). Renal losses of potassium are a more likely underlying cause in this patient. A useful distinction is between renal potassium loss caused by primary mineralocorticoid excess, which is associated with renal sodium retention and hypertension, and other causes which are associated with normal or low volume states and in which blood pressure is normal or low.

The neuromuscular symptoms are suggestive of episodes of low ionised calcium concentration in the extracellular fluid, probably due to alkalosis causing increased binding of calcium to plasma albumin.

Examination

The patient is a normally built young man in apparent good health. There is no obvious evidence of frank hypovolaemia, and the blood pressure is 115/75 mmHg lying and 110/80 mmHg standing. Neurological examination is normal, and tests for muscular irritability associated with hypocalcaemia (Chvostek's and Trousseau's signs) are negative.

Has examination narrowed down your differential diagnosis?

The absence of hypertension argues against primary mineralocorticoid excess. A renal tubular disorder associated with potassium wasting, and possibly also acid wasting, is now more likely, although covert diuretic use still needs to be excluded.

BOX 26.2

24-hour urine results

Volume	3.2 l
Osmolality	350 mmol/kg
Sodium	44 mmol/l (meq/l)
Potassium	38 mmol/l (meq/l)
Chloride	29 mmol/l (meq/l)

Further investigations

A set of arterial blood gases is useful to define more precisely the disorder of acid–base balance. This shows H^+ 31 nmol/l (pH 7.51), PO_2 11.9 kPa (89 mmHg), PCO_2 6.9 kPa (52 mmHg), base excess + 5 mmol/l (meq/l). Plasma renin activity is 25 ng/ml/hr (normal range 4–8), and plasma aldosterone is 480 pmol/l (17.3 ng/dl) (normal range 100–500 pmol/l (3.6–18 ng/dl)). A 24-hour urine collection is also performed and the results are shown in Box 26.2. A urine drug screen is negative for diuretics and all other drugs.

Does this narrow down your differential diagnosis?

The blood gases confirm that the hypokalaemic state is associated with a significant metabolic alkalosis, with some compensatory hypoventilation. The plasma renin and aldosterone results indicate secondary hyperaldosteronism, consistent with an acute or chronic hypovolaemic stimulus, i.e. the aldosterone concentration is in the high normal range and is associated with an increased plasma renin activity.

The urine results show that the patient is polyuric and has a relatively dilute urine, especially taken in the context of a high-range plasma sodium (and thus a high plasma osmolality). This is consistent with a partial defect of the urinary concentrating mechanism (i.e. partial nephrogenic diabetes insipidus). The appearance of significant quantities of sodium and chloride in the urine, in the face of this patient's low blood pressure and activated renin system, suggests that there is a primary renal tubular leak of sodium chloride, while the high urine potassium level in the setting of hypokalaemia suggests that there is a simultaneous tubular leak of potassium. The high urine chloride effectively excludes surreptitious vomiting, as this is associated with marked renal chloride conservation. The negative drug screen excludes surreptitious diuretic abuse.

While the plasma magnesium is in the low normal range, this suggests some parallel loss of magnesium as part of the primary problem, rather than profound magnesium depletion itself being the cause of the hypokalaemia.

All of these results are consistent with Bartter's syndrome. This condition mimics loop diuretic therapy in virtually every way, in that there is an inherited defect of the carrier mechanism mediating reabsorption of sodium, potassium and chloride in the thick ascending limb of the loop of Henle. The consequences are:

1. sodium wasting leading to hypovolaemia and activation of the renin–angiotensin–aldosterone system
2. potassium wasting, both from the loop of Henle itself and also because of enhanced potassium secretion in the late distal/cortical collecting duct segment, due to high sodium delivery and high aldosterone levels
3. an impaired urinary concentration mechanism (nephrogenic diabetes insipidus). This is partly caused by the failure to build up a medullary concentration gradient, due to faulty loop of Henle action. In addition, there is resistance to the action of antidiuretic hormone (ADH) associated with the hypokalaemia and also increased medullary prostaglandin synthesis (which is also stimulated by hypokalaemia).

The metabolic alkalosis is due to increased urinary excretion of acid, provoked in part by aldosterone-stimulated distal acid secretion. The low-range plasma magnesium is a direct result of the impaired thick ascending limb reabsorptive mechanisms.

How will you treat this patient?

While the underlying tubular transport defect in this condition cannot be reversed, much can be done to alleviate the high rates of urinary loss of potassium and acid, which bring about many of the most troublesome consequences of this disorder. Therapy usually involves three elements:

1. Oral supplements of potassium chloride (e.g. slow-release KCl) are generally required, although even in high doses they are not adequate by themselves to correct the hypokalaemia, due to continuation of tubular mechanisms driving high potassium excretion rates. Typically, 6–12 slow-release KCl tablets are needed per day.
2. Much can be gained by interfering with aldosterone action in the late distal/cortical collecting duct segment. This can be achieved using either spironolactone (50–100 mg per day) or amiloride (10–20 mg per day), both of which serve to inhibit the secretion of potassium and acid in exchange for reabsorbed sodium in this tubular segment.
3. In some cases it can be beneficial to prescribe an inhibitor of prostaglandin synthesis, such as a non-steroidal anti-inflammatory drug (NSAID, e.g. indometacin), since increased renal prostaglandin synthesis amplifies urinary losses of sodium and potassium, while inhibiting ADH action. However, once potassium balance is restored by the above two measures, continued prostaglandin inhibition may not be necessary.

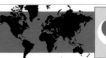

- In many parts of the developing world, hypokalaemia will be most commonly associated with malnutrition and/or gastroenteritis. In such cases, especially where diarrhoea is the predominant symptom, the hypokalaemia will typically be associated with metabolic acidosis.

- Chronic diuretic therapy in patients with chronic valvular heart disease secondary to rheumatic heart disease is frequently associated with hypokalaemia in the developing world. Where digoxin is also administered to control the heart rate, careful monitoring for hypokalaemia is required, as serious arrhythmias can occur when diuretics and digoxin are administered concomitantly. Potassium supplementation should be provided on a regular basis to these patients.

- Diuretic and laxative abuse should always be considered in the differential diagnosis of hypokalaemia.

- Hypokalaemia may increase the difficulty in weaning patients from mechanical ventilation.

See Chapter 16 of

Davidson's Principles and Practice of Medicine

(20th edn)

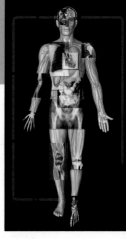

27

A 72-year-old man with breathlessness

A. CUMMING

Presenting problem

A 72-year-old man is referred to the Accident and Emergency department with a 3-week history of breathlessness. The symptoms began following an episode of diarrhoea lasting 3 days; other members of the family also suffered a febrile diarrhoeal illness at that time.

Further enquiry reveals symptoms of increasing tiredness for several months, nocturia for 3 years (which has recently increased in frequency to 3–4 times per night) and a poor urinary stream, hesitancy and post-micturition dribbling for several years. He was diagnosed with hypertension 5 years ago and is currently treated with bendroflumethiazide 5 mg daily and atenolol 50 mg daily.

What would your differential diagnosis include before examining the patient?

The differential diagnosis includes all causes of progressively worsening breathlessness. Given the history of hypertension, this would include heart failure, either due to hypertensive heart disease or ischaemic heart disease. The pointers in the history to chronic urinary tract disease might indicate a degree of renal failure, which in some patients is associated with fluid retention and development of pulmonary oedema. Respiratory causes, such as asthma, would also have to be considered (possibly aggravated by his β-blocker therapy). Anaemia is also a possibility, and this may or may not be related to chronic kidney disease.

Examination and initial investigations

On examination, there are signs of extracellular fluid depletion (reduced tissue turgor and eyeball tone). Blood pressure is 95/50 mmHg, with a 10 mmHg postural drop. Pulse is 55/min and regular. Respiratory rate is increased at 25 breaths/min, with a deep, sighing quality to the respiration.

Heart sounds are normal and the chest is clear. There is no oedema and the jugular venous pressure is not elevated. Peripheral pulses are present with no bruits. The patient's bladder is palpably enlarged up to the umbilicus. Abdominal examination is otherwise unremarkable. Urinalysis shows proteinuria +.

Initial venous blood test results are shown in Box 27.1.

BOX 27.1

Initial investigations

Urea	53 mmol/l (148.5 mg/dl)
Sodium	128 mmol/l (meq/l)
Potassium	7.4 mmol/l (meq/l)
Bicarbonate	9 mmol/l (meq/l)
Creatinine	874 µmol/l (9.88 mg/dl)
Calcium	1.25 mmol/l (5.0 mg/dl)
Phosphate	3.86 mmol/l (11.97 mg/dl)
Albumin	36 g/l (3.6 g/dl)
Haemoglobin	84 g/l (8.4 g/dl)
WCC	$11.3 \times 10^9/l$ ($10^3/mm^3$)

Have examination and initial investigations narrowed down your differential diagnosis?

Physical examination shows no signs of fluid overload or cardiac failure, and indeed there is evidence of fluid depletion, hypotension and bradycardia. The respiratory pattern is typical of that seen in severe metabolic acidosis. The blood analysis shows a very low venous bicarbonate, in keeping with that diagnosis. Blood tests also confirm severe renal failure, with associated hyperkalaemia, hypocalcaemia and hyperphosphataemia. The calcium and phosphate abnormalities, together with the low haemoglobin, suggest at least some degree of chronic renal impairment. The prostatic symptoms and bladder distension are compatible with obstructive uropathy as the underlying diagnosis.

Further investigations

An arterial blood gas (on room air) and further venous blood analyses are performed (Box 27.2).

An urgent ultrasound of the renal tract is carried out and demonstrates that both kidneys are reduced in size, at 8.2 cm and 8.4 cm respectively, with markedly reduced cortical thickness. There is dilatation of the renal pelvis and ureters down to the level of the bladder. The bladder is thick-walled and contains a residual urine volume of approximately 500 ml after micturition. The prostate gland is markedly enlarged.

A 12-lead electrocardiogram (ECG) shows tall, peaked T waves consistent with hyperkalaemia.

BOX 27.2

Arterial blood gas analysis

Arterial blood

Hydrogen ion	70 nmol/l (pH 7.16)
$PaCO_2$	3.2 kpa (24 mmHg)
Bicarbonate	7 mmol/l (meq/l)
PaO_2	11.4 kpa (85.5 mmHg)

Venous blood

Lactate	0.9 mmol/l (8.10 mg/dl)
Chloride	103 mmol/l (meq/1)

Does this narrow down your differential diagnosis?

This patient has severe renal failure, with a history strongly suggestive of long-term bladder outlet obstruction causing chronic renal impairment. However, the admission biochemistry is not compatible with long-term survival; therefore there must be an acute element, i.e. acute on chronic renal failure. The likely precipitating factor is salt and water depletion secondary to his diarrhoeal illness. Impaired renal tubular reabsorptive capacity due to chronic obstruction and the ongoing intake of a diuretic mean that the kidneys cannot conserve salt and water as normal. The very high urea also acts as an osmotic diuretic.

The metabolic acidosis is primarily due to the reduced renal function and tubular damage. There is impaired tubular generation of bicarbonate in the proximal and distal tubules and reduced distal secretion of hydrogen ions. The diarrhoea, which initiated the acute decompensation, will have promoted additional loss of bicarbonate in the stools, for which the diseased kidneys are unable to compensate.

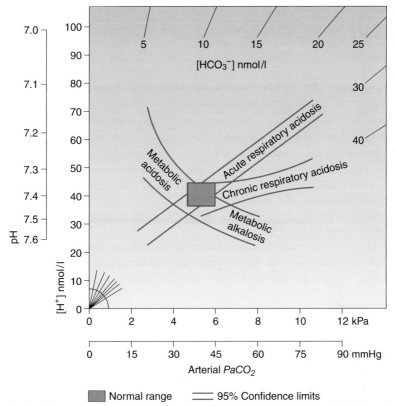

Fig. 27.1 Changes in blood [H+], $PaCO_2$ and plasma [HCO_3^-] in stable compensated acid–base disorders. The rectangle indicates limits of normal reference ranges for [H+] and $PaCO_2$. The bands represent 95% confidence limits of single disturbances in human blood in vivo. When the point obtained by plotting [H+] against $PaCO_2$ does not fall within one of the labelled bands, compensation is incomplete or a mixed disorder is present.

The concomitant salt and water depletion reduces the delivery of filtered sodium to nephron sites of Na^+/H^+ exchange. The end result is extreme metabolic acidosis, with only partial respiratory compensation in the form of increased ventilation (Kussmaul's respiration) and the resultant low $PaCO_2$ (Fig. 27.1).

While some degree of metabolic acidosis is commonly seen in any patient with renal failure, the degree of acidosis here is extreme. Some patients with chronic renal failure, typically those who are elderly and with diabetic nephropathy, have a type 4 renal tubular acidosis (hyporeninaemic hypoaldosteronism) and associated hyperkalaemia. This can be aggravated by β-blocker therapy, which lowers renin activity. Other factors may influence the severity of acidosis, including addition of hydrogen ion to the circulation, e.g. over-production of lactic acid (lactic acidosis) or ketoacids (diabetic ketoacidosis). Another source of additional hydrogen ions is cell lysis — as in rhabdomyolysis, in gastrointestinal blood loss or after extreme hypoxia (e.g. protracted cardiac arrest). These conditions are associated with an elevated anion gap (see below). In the UK, the most common source of *exogenous* additional hydrogen ion would be poisoning (accidental or deliberate), including aspirin, polyethylene glycol (antifreeze) or methanol. These can be measured in the laboratory. Other factors influencing the severity of acidosis involve loss of bicarbonate from the body, i.e. from the kidney or gastrointestinal tract.

The anion gap — $[Na^+] - [Cl^- + HCO_3^-]$ — is calculated here as 18 mmol/l (normal 8–16 mmol/l). This is typical of renal failure, where there is some accumulation of exogenous acidic compounds such as sulphate, phosphate and urate, but also reduced renal tubular function and an inability to compensate for loss of bicarbonate from the gastrointestinal tract (as in this case).

How will you treat this patient?

The patient has very advanced renal failure, but the immediate life-threatening factors are his hyperkalaemia and metabolic acidosis. These will be most effectively controlled by haemodialysis, but there may be a delay in instituting this. Immediate therapy would therefore include:

1. 10 ml of 10% calcium gluconate i.v. to counteract the effect of the hyperkalaemia on the myocardium
2. 50 ml of 50% dextrose i.v. to lower the plasma potassium acutely
3. fluid resuscitation, which could include 1.26% sodium bicarbonate and 0.9% sodium chloride given alternately at a rate of 500 ml/hr.

The patient requires frequent biochemical monitoring since correcting his acidosis too rapidly may lead to cerebral oedema and convulsions. Correcting the acidosis will also lower the ionised calcium further, and may cause tetany and laryngeal spasm.

The patient requires renal replacement therapy (haemofiltration or haemodialysis) as soon as possible. Continuous venous haemofiltration may well be preferable in offering gradual control of the acidosis and uraemia. If haemodialysis is chosen, the bicarbonate concentration in the dialysis fluid should be set as low as possible (e.g. 15 mmol/l) to avoid disequilibration, and treatment time should be limited to one hour initially.

The patient is likely to need 4–5 litres of isotonic volume expansion over the next 48 hours to restore extracellular fluid volume and optimise renal function. If he recovers useful renal function, he will probably need long-term oral sodium bicarbonate supplements.

Clearly, the cause of his renal failure must be corrected by bladder catheterisation and eventual bladder neck surgery.

Global issues

More on metabolic acidosis?

- By far the most common cause of established metabolic acidosis is chronic renal failure. The most common underlying causes vary in different parts of the world, although diabetic nephropathy and renal vascular disease are common everywhere.

- Obstructive uropathy is more commonly due to schistosomiasis and tuberculosis in the developing world.

See Chapter 16 of
Davidson's Principles and Practice of Medicine (20th edn)

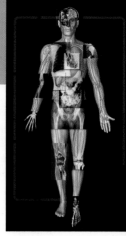

28

A young man with muscle cramps and weakness

A. N. TURNER

Presenting problem

A 28-year-old male pharmacy worker is admitted to hospital complaining of muscular cramps over several weeks, worsening over the last few days, during which time he has developed progressively more severe weakness so that he now cannot stand. He has no significant past medical history, is a non-smoker who describes moderate alcohol intake, and is not on any medication. Initial investigations show potassium 2.4 mmol/l (meq/l) and the patient is given intravenous potassium, which raises it to 3.0 mmol/l (meq/l); his symptoms continue, however. Further tests show that plasma calcium is normal but magnesium concentration is very low (Box 28.1).

What would your differential diagnosis include before examining the patient?

Hypomagnesaemia rarely occurs as an isolated biochemical abnormality, and hypokalaemia is the most commonly associated abnormality, as in this patient; the symptoms may be attributable to both. Deficient magnesium intake and major shifts in magnesium balance, as may occur in 'hungry bones' syndrome, are exceptionally rare. Thus, hypomagnesaemia is invariably a consequence of magnesium loss and the initial diagnostic question is whether the losses are occurring through the gastrointestinal tract or the kidneys. In the absence of any history, renal loss is more likely, although patients may sometimes be reluctant

BOX 28.1	
Further investigations	
Sodium	136 mmol/l (136 meq/l)
Potassium	2.4 mmol/l (2.4 meq/l)
Bicarbonate	33 mmol/l (33 meq/l)
Urea	4.2 mmol/l (25 mg/dl)
Creatinine	90 μmol/l (1 mg/dl)
Calcium	2.35 mmol/l (9.4 mg/dl)
Phosphate	0.8 mmol/l (2.48 mg/dl)
Magnesium	0.45 mmol/l (1.1 mg/dl) (0.75–1.05)

to admit to gastrointestinal disease. Alcohol abuse is an occasional cause of both dietary deficiency and gastrointestinal loss. The patient is slightly alkalotic (raised bicarbonate) and has a normal phosphate, which rules out renal tubular acidosis and generalised proximal tubular disorders.

Examination

Routine examination is essentially normal, apart from global weakness. Pulse is 72/min and supine blood pressure is 110/64 mmHg. There are no signs of malnutrition, liver disease, thyroid disease or any other disorder. Prolonged inflation of the blood pressure cuff leads to spasm of the muscles of the forearm (Trousseau's sign).

Has examination narrowed down your differential diagnosis?

The absence of signs of liver disease or undernutrition makes gastrointestinal loss still less likely as an explanation. Although Trousseau's sign is typically associated with hypocalcaemia, it may also occur in hypomagnesaemia and does not help with the differential diagnosis.

Further investigations

A 24-hour urine collection was performed and the following electrolyte results were obtained: potassium 240 mmol (meq)/24 hours (normal range ~40–100 mmol (meq)/24hours); chloride 390 mmol (meq)/24 hours (normal range ~110–250 mmol (meq)/24 hours); magnesium 8 mmol (19.4 mg)/24 hours (normal range ~3.3–4.9 mmol (8.0–11.8 mg)/24hours).

Has the diagnosis been clinched?

High urinary magnesium loss at a time of hypomagnesaemia confirms that the primary problem is renal. The elevated 24-hour urinary chloride helps to exclude concealed vomiting as a cause of magnesium losses. Of the list of conditions that can cause renal hypomagnesaemia, the normal phosphate and lack of acidosis (phosphate loss and acidosis are common in tubular disorders) rule out several possibilities. The most likely cause is Gitelman's syndrome, in which there is a mutation in the sodium chloride co-transporter in the distal tubule. This is the target of thiazide diuretics, and patients with Gitelman's syndrome have many characteristics of patients overtreated with diuretics, showing modest sodium wasting and hypokalaemia. It is not clear why hypomagnesaemia is such a prominent feature of Gitelman's syndrome (more severe than in patients on diuretics), but it is diagnostically helpful. Bartter's syndrome is an analogous condition in which the abnormality is in the loop of Henle, similar to the target of loop diuretics. Sodium losses are usually much more severe, leading to presentation in childhood. Hypomagnesaemia is not a feature but hypercalciuria is common.

The patient's job in a pharmacy raises the important question of whether the abnormalities could be due to undeclared exposure to diuretics. This is very difficult to exclude altogether, although the degree of hypomagnesaemia makes this less likely. Diuretic exposure may have worsened the abnormality in a patient with another underlying cause. Diuretic abuse is associated with disorders of body image such as anorexia nervosa and bulimia. There are some rarer causes of renal magnesium wasting, and confirmation of Gitelman's requires investigation.

How will you treat this patient?

Initially, treatment involves replacement of potassium and magnesium intravenously. Magnesium is not easy to supplement orally, as magnesium salts may cause diarrhoea. Magnesium glycerophosphate tablets may be useful.

Supplementation of potassium is easier and large amounts may be required. Potassium-sparing diuretics (spironolactone, amiloride) may be useful for the hypokalaemia and help to conserve magnesium too.

Although it may be difficult to identify precipitating causes for some attacks, gastrointestinal upset is a common cause and alcoholic binges may increase magnesium excretion, so the patient should be warned to temper his alcohol intake.

Global issues

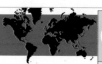

 More on hypomagnesaemia?

- After sodium, potassium and calcium, magnesium is the fourth most abundant cation in the human body. It is the second most abundant intracellular cation.

- Magnesium deficiency is frequent in hospitalised patients (about 65% in intensive care units and 12% in general wards). Diabetes mellitus and alcohol consumption are commonly associated with magnesium deficiency.

See Chapter 16 of
Davidson's Principles and Practice of Medicine (20th edn)

- Symptoms of magnesium deficiency are non-specific and the deficiency frequently coexists with other abnormalities such as hypokalaemia, hypocalcaemia and metabolic alkalosis.

- Monitoring for magnesium deficiency is important in emergency rooms and intensive care units in critically ill patients. Access to facilities for laboratory monitoring of magnesium may be limited in the developing world.

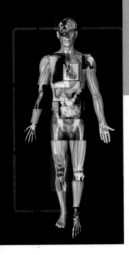

29

Haematuria and facial puffiness in a young man

S. JAIN

Presenting problem

A 20-year-old man presents to the outpatient department with a 3-day history of facial puffiness and passing red-coloured urine. There is no associated loin or abdominal pain. He had a sore throat and fever 10 days ago. He has no previous history of note and does not take any regular medication.

What would your differential diagnosis include before examining the patient?

The red urine in this young patient suggests haematuria, indicating bleeding in the urinary tract, anywhere from the glomerulus to the urethra. Haematuria can present in various ways. It can be intermittent or persistent; painful or painless; microscopic or macroscopic. It must be emphasised, however, that none of these variations in itself is enough to diagnose the cause of bleeding. All patients with haematuria will eventually require investigations. It must also be remembered that a very small amount of blood (as little as 1 ml) can change the colour of 1 litre of urine.

Red urine is not always due to haematuria; it may be caused by haemoglobinuria, myoglobinuria, porphyria, the ingestion of beetroot, and certain drugs such as furadantin and pyridium. Urine dipsticks can detect 1–2 red blood cells (RBCs) per high-power field but can also give false-positive results. Discoloured urine, not due to haematuria, and a false positive dipstick result can be distinguished from haematuria by the absence of RBCs on urine microscopy. Isolated haematuria (absence of proteinuria with no other cells or cellular casts on microscopy) indicates bleeding from the urinary tract, and common causes include stones, tumours, tuberculosis and prostatitis.

Haematuria in an adult is of either glomerular or extraglomerular origin. The glomerular causes of haematuria include post-streptococcal glomerulonephritis (PSGN), IgA nephropathy and Henoch–Schönlein purpura, mesangioproliferative glomerulonephritis and Alport's syndrome (hereditary nephritis with haematuria, sensorineural deafness and ocular abnormalities). Gross haematuria with blood clots is most unlikely to have a glomerular cause and suggests a post-renal source in the urinary collecting system. Extraglomerular causes of haematuria include renal stones, renal tumours, cysts, renal infarction, bladder tumours, acute urinary tract infection, chronic infections such as tuberculosis and schistosomiasis, and the use of anticoagulants.

In this case some of the causes of haematuria can be ruled out straightaway. Acute urinary tract infection typically presents with fever, shaking chills and rigors, dysuria, pyuria, haematuria and increased frequency of micturition. Acute cystitis and urethritis in women can produce gross haematuria. Renal stones usually produce painful haematuria, whereas tuberculosis classically presents with painless haematuria along with fever. About 90% of renal stones can be demonstrated confidently on plain X-ray of the abdomen. Urogenital tumours should be suspected in older patients presenting with isolated painless haematuria.

The facial puffiness in this patient is most likely to be due to a decline in glomerular filtration (due to inflammation of glomeruli), with subsequent fluid and salt retention.

Examination

This man has facial puffiness, most prominent below the eyes, and pitting oedema of both lower legs. His blood pressure is 150/96 mmHg. The remainder of the physical examination is normal. The results of initial investigations are detailed in Box 29.1.

Have examination and initial investigations narrowed down your differential diagnosis?

The most important test in the evaluation of haematuria is urinalysis. The presence of RBC casts in this patient's urine is characteristic of glomerular pathology. Although this finding is specific, the absence of RBC casts does not exclude glomerular disease. An associated proteinuria of more than 500 mg per day also favours a glomerular cause for the haematuria. RBC morphology can help to differentiate a glomerular from a non-glomerular origin of haematuria. Glomerular haematuria is characterised by the presence of dysmorphic (altered shape) RBCs, while they are round or oval in non-glomerular haematuria when examined by phase-contrast microscopy. The raised blood urea and serum creatinine in this patient suggest renal insufficiency.

The presence of hypertension, oedema, haematuria and renal insufficiency suggests an acute nephritic syndrome; this is the clinical correlate of acute glomerular inflammation, characterised by gross haematuria (red or 'smoky' urine) and 'nephritic urinary sediment' (dysmorphic RBCs, RBC casts, leucocytes and subnephrotic proteinuria (< 3 g/day) on urinalysis). Important causes of acute nephritic syndrome include PSGN, membranoproliferative glomerulonephritis,

BOX 29.1	
Initial investigations	
Haemoglobin	145 g/l (14.5 g/dl)
Serum sodium	140 mmol/l (meq/l)
Serum potassium	4.6 mmol/l (meq/l)
Urea	14.2 mmol/l (40 mg/dl)
Serum creatinine	266 µmol/l (1.8 mg/dl)
Urine examination	
Albumin	++
Microscopy	50–60 RBCs per high-power field, with occasional RBC casts

rapidly progressive glomerulonephritis (RPGN) and vasculitis. The absence of skin nodules, ulcers and nasal or ear discharge argues against a diagnosis of vasculitis in this patient. The history of a recent upper respiratory tract or skin infection clearly favours a diagnosis of PSGN or IgA nephropathy. Characteristically, the latent period between the preceding infection and the onset of nephritis is shorter in IgA nephropathy (24–48 hours) compared with acute post-infectious glomerulonephritis (about 10 days). IgA nephropathy derives its name from the IgA deposits in the mesangium that are detected by immunofluorescence. Several episodes of occult or overt exacerbations of nephropathy following pharyngeal infections culminate in end-stage renal disease (ESRD). As renal and serological abnormalities in IgA nephropathy (a renal-limited form of glomerulonephritis) and Henoch–Schönlein purpura (a systemic disease) are similar, both conditions are considered in the spectrum of a single disease.

Further investigations

Throat culture for streptococci is negative. The antistreptolysin O (ASO) titre is high and the serum complement (C3) level is low. Tests for antineutrophilic cytoplasmic antibody (ANCA), antinuclear and anti-glomerular basement membrane (GBM) antibodies, and circulating cryoglobulins are negative. Hepatitis B and C serologies and human immunodeficiency virus (HIV) enzyme-linked immunosorbent assay (ELISA) are negative. A percutaneous renal biopsy is performed and this shows an acute diffuse proliferative glomerulonephritis. There is diffuse hypercellularity of glomeruli due to endocapillary proliferation of mesangial and endothelial cells and to an influx of neutrophils (Fig. 29.1).

Does this narrow down your differential diagnosis?

Yes. The presence of a raised ASO titre and low complement (C3) and the renal biopsy findings confirm PSGN, i.e. glomerulonephritis following a throat infection with a nephritogenic strain of a group A β-haemolytic streptococcus. The complement levels usually return to normal within 8 weeks. If the serum

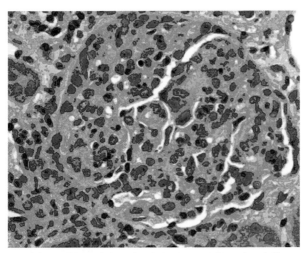

Fig. 29.1 Renal histopathology of post-streptococcal glomerulonephritis. Note the diffuse hypercellularity of glomeruli due to endocapillary proliferation of mesangial and endothelial cells and to an influx of neutrophils.

C3 levels were to be persistently depressed, one should think of membranoprolif-erative glomerulonephritis, occult sepsis, systemic lupus erythematosus or endo-carditis as the cause of this patient's glomerulonephritis.

How will you treat this patient?

Treatment should be largely supportive. He needs bed rest and the administra-tion of a loop diuretic (furosemide) and antihypertensive drugs (calcium channel blocker or angiotensin-converting enzyme (ACE) inhibitors). Potassium-sparing diuretics should be avoided, as they might produce hyperkalaemia. A low-salt diet with fluid restriction should be recommended. Penicillin therapy is usually given for 10 days. The majority of patients with PSGN usually undergo sponta-neous remission within 7–10 days of the onset of the disease. However, a few adult patients with PSGN may have persistent proteinuria and deranged renal functions on long-term follow-up.

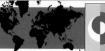

Global issues

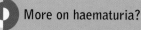 More on haematuria?

- Acute PSGN is becoming rare in developed countries.

- In developing countries, PSGN is a common cause of acute nephritic syndrome, especially among children. The prognosis is excellent and spontaneous recovery occurs in most cases.

- IgA nephropathy is also common in southern Europe and Asia. It is more common in blacks than in whites.

See Chapter 17 of
Davidson's Principles and Practice of Medicine
(20th edn)

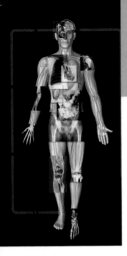

30

A man with chest pain, haemoptysis and leg swelling

J. GODDARD

Presenting problem

A 43-year-old man presents to the Accident and Emergency department with left pleuritic chest pain and minor haemoptysis. He gives a 3-month history of increasing bilateral leg swelling that is now up to his thighs. He has gained 10 kg in weight over this time. His wife has noticed that his eyes are puffy. He has previously been well, except for what he describes as arthritis. He has not sought medical advice about this.

What would your differential diagnosis include before examining the patient?

In addition to the usual differential diagnoses for the respiratory symptoms, with pulmonary embolism and pneumonia at the top of the list, the oedema raises the possibility of an underlying aetiology. Increased hydrostatic pressure will cause dependent oedema. The patient could have bilateral leg deep venous thromboses (DVTs) but this would be unlikely to be associated with increasing swelling up to the thighs. It is possible that this patient has had multiple thromboembolic events with consequent raised right heart pressure and right heart failure. Oedema may also be a consequence of liver disease and malnutrition, both of which could be associated with infection. However, both infection and thromboembolism are recognised complications of nephrotic syndrome, which typically presents as increasing oedema.

Examination and initial investigations

Blood pressure is 160/105 mmHg. The patient has pitting oedema to the mid-thighs. Heart sounds are normal and the jugular venous pulse (JVP) is elevated at +7 cm. On abdominal examination there is no organomegaly or ascites. Chest auscultation reveals a pleural rub heard over the left lateral chest. Oxygen saturation is 98% on air.

The chest X-ray is normal but the electrocardiogram (ECG) shows a sinus tachycardia. A computed tomography pulmonary angiogram (CTPA) demonstrates a left subsegmental pulmonary embolism but no other abnormality. Doppler ultrasound demonstrates a DVT in the right calf. The left leg venous system appears normal. Initial blood tests are shown in Box 30.1. Urinalysis shows 4+ proteinuria but no haematuria.

Have examination and initial investigations narrowed down your differential diagnosis?

The cause for the pleuritic chest pain is revealed as a pulmonary embolism secondary to a right leg DVT. The normal chest X-ray and otherwise normal CTPA (aside from the pulmonary embolism) go against chronic lung disease and secondary right heart failure (cor pulmonale) as a cause for his bilateral leg oedema. The depressed serum albumin could suggest either liver disease or malnutrition. However, the strongly positive urinalysis for protein suggests nephrotic syndrome is the underlying cause of the low serum albumin. The peripheral oedema is a consequence of low oncotic pressure and avid sodium retention.

BOX 30.1	
Initial investigations	
Urea	6.3 mmol/l (17.7 mg/dl)
Creatinine	96 μmol/l (1.1 mg/dl)
Sodium	135 mmol/l (meq/l)
Potassium	3.7 mmol/l (meq/l)
Glucose	8.2 mmol/l (148 mg/dl)
Albumin	21 g/l (2.1 g/dl)
LFTs	Normal

Further investigations

Twenty-four-hour urine protein excretion is 9.6 g. Serum cholesterol is 12.5 mmol/l (483 mg/dl).

Does this narrow down your differential diagnosis?

The abnormally high urinary protein excretion, associated with the low serum albumin, confirms nephrotic syndrome. Low oncotic pressure stimulates the liver to increase lipoprotein synthesis, resulting in hypercholesterolaemia.

Over 50% of cases of nephrotic syndrome are due to primary renal disease. The three major non-inflammatory glomerular conditions are minimal change nephropathy, focal and segmental glomerulosclerosis (FSGS) and membranous nephropathy. If a primary renal cause for this man's nephrotic syndrome is suspected, it may be appropriate to treat with empirical steroids, as these would be used initially for both minimal change nephropathy and FSGS.

While these renal conditions are usually idiopathic, this patient should be screened for conditions known to be associated with them, or other causes of nephrotic syndrome: for example, the use of non-steroidal anti-inflammatory drugs (NSAIDs). Hodgkin's lymphoma and other haematological malignancies have also been implicated in minimal change disease. Membranous nephropathy can also be associated with NSAIDs, which this patient might have bought at a pharmacy and taken for his arthritis. It is also one form of renal involvement in systemic lupus erythematosus (which could also link to this patient's arthritis). Additionally, malignancy, hepatitis B, syphilis and rarely hepatitis C may underlie this condition. Primary FSGS is, by definition, idiopathic (Fig. 30.1). It may be familial. Secondary FSGS, which is the consequence of glomerular hypertrophy or scarring due to another condition, causes proteinuria but rarely nephrotic syndrome. Inflammatory or proliferative glomerulonephritides will usually also be associated with haematuria, so are less likely in this case. A monoclonal band on serum or urine electrophoresis might point towards amyloidosis as a cause for this patient's nephrotic syndrome and should be excluded. Proteinuria as a consequence of diabetic nephropathy can be severe enough to cause nephrotic syndrome, but diabetes has usually been present for at least 10 years for involvement to progress to this stage.

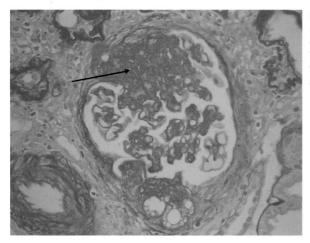

Fig. 30.1 Focal and segmental glomerulosclerosis. The glomerulus in the centre shows a segmental scar (arrow).

How will you treat this patient?

Ideally, he should have a renal biopsy to establish the cause for his nephrotic syndrome, as some are treated with immunosuppression. However, he also needs anticoagulation for his thromboembolic disease; a renal biopsy must either be performed under tightly controlled conditions with intravenous heparin which can be rapidly discontinued if post-biopsy bleeding occurs, or be postponed. His blood pressure will also need to be lowered before biopsy to reduce the risk of bleeding.

With regard to his volume overload, loop diuretics will increase natriuresis and help reduce oedema. Daily measurement of weight will help establish whether this measure is successful. The patient should also be advised about taking a low-salt diet. He may need a combination of loop diuretics and a thiazide, but care must be taken not to achieve over-diuresis, as intravascular volume depletion may cause worsening of renal function. Angiotensin-converting enzyme (ACE) inhibitors may also be used to reduce proteinuria with regular careful monitoring of renal function and again care to avoid volume depletion. His hypercholesterolaemia should also be treated with a statin, but should resolve as his proteinuria reduces. His risk of thrombotic complications will continue as long as the nephrotic syndrome persists, and he should be anticoagulated accordingly. If his nephrotic syndrome persists for a long period, then pneumococcal and meningococcal vaccination should be considered.

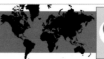

Global issues

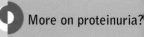 More on proteinuria?

- Human immunodeficiency virus (HIV) can cause a 'collapsing' variant of FSGS that presents with nephrotic syndrome.

- Tuberculosis is a common cause of AA amyloidosis, which can present with nephrotic syndrome.

See Chapter 17 of
Davidson's Principles and Practice of Medicine (20th edn)

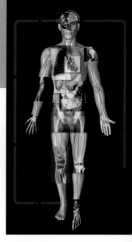

31

A middle-aged farmer with pain and swelling of the lower limb and acute renal failure

H. R. SALKAR

Presenting problem

A 40-year-old farmer presents to the Accident and Emergency department with a 28-hour history of pain and swelling of his left foot and leg. On questioning, the patient says that, while working in the fields the previous day, he was probably bitten by a snake. There is no history of fever or other trauma. He lives in a very remote community and was not able to reach hospital until today. Over the last few hours there has been extension of the swelling to the thigh, and a few ecchymotic patches and blisters have appeared on the left leg; blood has continued to ooze from the bite mark on the dorsum of the foot. The patient has been persistently sick and has developed oliguria, haematuria and puffiness of the face.

What would your differential diagnosis include before examining the patient?

The patient has an acute problem with localisation of the symptoms and signs to the left lower limb. In addition, he has features suggestive of acute renal failure. The possibility of sepsis should be considered, but working against this diagnosis are the absence of fever, the brief duration of the symptoms and the rapid progression to acute renal failure. In view of the sudden pain and swelling of the foot and leg and extension to the thigh, venous thrombosis is another possibility. However, the main clues are obviously the man's occupation and the history of a snake bite; all the ensuing signs and symptoms fit in with this and he has now developed systemic features of envenomation, including acute renal failure.

Examination

The patient is conscious and alert but looks apprehensive. Pulse rate is 94/min regular. Blood pressure is 110/80 mmHg and respiratory rate is 20 breaths/min regular. The dorsum of the left foot has two fang marks from which blood is oozing (Fig. 31.1). There is swelling of the left leg, and this extends up to the knee joint. Systemic examination is within normal limits and there is no evidence of any neurological manifestation.

Has examination narrowed down your differential diagnosis?

Yes, no need for Sherlock Holmes here; even Dr Watson would get this right! The fang marks and all the other signs confirm that this man's problems are due to a snake bite. What we need to know now is what damage has been done and what we can do about it.

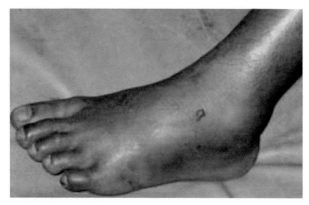

Fig. 31.1 Snake bite of left foot, with associated cellulitis and blistering of the skin.

BOX 31.1	
Initial investigations	
Haemoglobin	132 g/l (13.2 g/dl)
PCV	0.40
WCC	$15 \times 10^9/l$ ($10^3/mm^3$)
Differential	
Neutrophils	78%
Lymphocytes	22%
Platelets	$100 \times 10^9/l$ ($10^3/mm^3$)
Clotting time	> 30 min
Blood urea	10 mmol/l (60 mg/dl)
Serum creatinine	220 µmol/l (2.5 mg/dl)
Sodium	140 mmol/l (meq/l)
Potassium	6 mmol/l (meq/l)
Bicarbonate	12 mmol/l (meq/l)
$PaCO_2$	3.9 kPa (30 mmHg)
Blood glucose	5.4 mmol/l (108 mg/dl)

Investigations

Some investigations are important (Box 31.1). The patient's blood group is O Rhesus positive. Urine examination reveals albumin ++ and no glycosuria. Microscopic examination shows 3–4 red blood cells per high-power field and 1–2 white blood cells per high-power field. An electrocardiogram (ECG) shows tall and tented T waves.

Has the diagnosis been clinched?

The diagnosis was never in doubt but the investigations give us a good measure of the damage caused by the envenomation. There is a mild coagulopathy and the farmer has developed acute renal failure. Progressive increase in the local swelling can also be due to envenoming or, more rarely, secondary bacterial infection. There are no neurological manifestations; therefore the snake probably belongs to the Viperidae family. Vipers like *Echis* and hump-nosed snakes do not produce neurotoxicity; however, Indian Russell's viper can produce neurological features.

Venomous snakes are grouped into following families: Viperidae (vipers), Elapidae (cobras and coral snakes), Hydrophidae (sea snakes), Atractaspididae (the burrowing asps) and Colubridae (the majority of this group are non-poisonous).

Snake venoms are complex mixtures of enzymes, low molecular weight polypeptides, glycoproteins and metal ions. Deleterious components include haemorrhagins, which promote vascular leaking with local and systemic bleeding, and proteolytic enzymes, which cause local tissue necrosis and affect coagulation pathways. Both produce changes concomitantly in one or more systems of the body. Snake venoms also contain nephrotoxins that commonly cause acute tubular necrosis or cortical necrosis resulting in acute renal failure. Other mechanisms of acute renal failure include hypovolaemia, hypotension, haemoglobinuria, myoglobinuria and coagulopathy. Myocardial depressant factors in some venoms reduce cardiac output. Neurotoxins act either pre- or post-synaptically or inhibit peripheral nerve impulses.

In this patient acute renal failure is diagnosed because of oliguria, haematuria and raised levels of serum creatinine and blood urea, together with a metabolic acidosis and hyperkalaemia. It is important to distinguish pre-renal from intrinsic kidney causes of acute renal failure, as both can occur following a snake bite. The presence of proteinuria and haematuria favours the latter, but there may be a concurrent pre-renal element.

How will you treat this patient?

First of all, antivenin must be given. This patient should be informed that effective treatment is available despite the presence of systemic envenomation and that mortality is low with appropriate treatment. The local wound is cleaned and dressed. In order to minimise the spread of venom, the application of a pressure bandage is preferred to tourniquets. Incision/excision at the bite site should not be performed.

Correct identification of the snake is important. The presence of local abnormalities of the left lower limb, prominent bleeding manifestations and acute renal failure, and the absence of neurotoxicity in our patient are highly suggestive of envenomation by a viper. Ideally, a species-specific antivenin should be administered; however, this is not available in most resource-limited countries. Specific treatment with polyvalent anti-snake venom is given intravenously, after a test dose, at the earliest opportunity; 100 ml (10 vials) of anti-snake venom is given as a stat dose, followed by 50 ml (5 vials) 6-hourly until progression of swelling stops and coagulopathy improves. Coagulopathy is assessed by bedside measurement of clotting time. Anti-snake venom administration may result in early (anaphylactic; 10 minutes–3 hours), pyrogenic (1–2 hours later) or late (serum sickness-type; after many days) reactions.

Second, treatment must be given for renal failure. In people with acute renal failure, it is usually worth giving intravenous fluids to ensure that they are adequately rehydrated. Clearly, in an oliguric individual, fluid resuscitation has to be monitored closely to avoid over-hydration. Since this patient has developed acute renal failure with metabolic acidosis, intravenous sodium bicarbonate (500 ml of 1.26% solution) will help correct the acidosis and reverse the hyperkalaemia. Given the ECG changes, 10 ml of 10% calcium gluconate should be administered, and a glucose and insulin infusion commenced. If the metabolic acidosis and hyperkalaemia persist and there is a progressive rise of the blood urea and serum creatinine, the patient may require dialysis. The choice of method employed will depend on the resources available. Haemofiltration is the method of choice but requires expensive equipment; peritoneal dialysis can be performed in low-resource settings, but there is a risk of peritonitis and severe bleeding associated with the dialysis catheter. In both forms, correction of the coagulopathy will be required beforehand. Whether or not dialysis is required, renal function should start to improve after a few days and should eventually return to normal.

With regard to other treatment, tetanus toxoid is given. Routine administration of antibiotics is not necessary, but as this patient has progressive increase in limb swelling, along with leucocytosis, broad-spectrum antibiotics and metronidazole are appropriate. A surgical consultation will help to rule out muscle compartment syndrome or, if muscle oedema impedes tissue perfusion despite adequate antivenin administration, the surgeon should proceed to a fasciotomy. This procedure should be carried out only after normalisation of the coagulation profile. In severe coagulopathy with thrombocytopenia, large quantities of fresh frozen plasma, cryoprecipitate and platelets should be administered.

Global issues

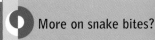

More on snake bites?

- Snake bite is a common life-threatening condition in many tropical countries.
- Farmers, hunters and rice-pickers are at particular risk.
- Worldwide estimates reveal 3–5 million victims per year, with nearly 50 000 deaths and 400 000 amputations.
- All patients with suspected envenomation should be observed for 12–24 hours, as the initial manifestations may be delayed.
- Prompt medical treatment is vital.
- Early immobilisation, hospitalisation and administration of polyvalent anti-snake venom are important.
- Antivenin reactions should be carefully observed in the intensive care unit.

See Chapter 9 of
Davidson's Principles and Practice of Medicine
(20th edn)

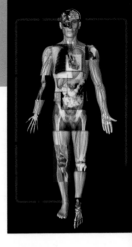

32

A young man with generalised oedema

V. SAKHUJA

Presenting problem

A 22-year-old man from northern India presents with a history of diarrhoea for 2 days. He has been treated with intravenous fluids at a peripheral clinic. Although the diarrhoea has settled, there has been a decrease in his urine output and he has become breathless. Consequently, he has been transferred to a referral hospital. For the last 6 months, the patient has noticed puffiness of his face in the mornings and tiredness, but has not sought medical attention. He denies nocturia. At the age of 7 years, he developed swelling of his feet and face, and reported to his parents that he was passing blood in his urine. He remembers that he had a kidney biopsy but cannot recall any further details.

What would your differential diagnosis include before examining the patient?

Oliguria and breathlessness, in the setting of likely dehydration following diarrhoea, are suggestive of acute renal failure with fluid overload. However, this would be unusual in a young adult, unless the diarrhoea has caused severe dehydration. Tiredness is a non-specific symptom and could be due to a host of conditions. However, coupled with a history of facial puffiness in the mornings, it should suggest pre-existing chronic renal failure (CRF). The fact that this man had a probable nephritic illness in childhood, warranting kidney biopsy, should further strengthen the suspicion that he has chronic rather than acute renal failure.

Examination

The patient is pale, tachypnoeic and unable to lie down. Puffiness of the face is evident and he has bilateral pitting pedal oedema. He is hypertensive, with a blood pressure of 180/100 mmHg and a pulse rate of 110/min. Auscultation of the lungs reveals bilateral coarse crepitations. The heart sounds are normal and there are no murmurs or pericardial rub. The results of initial investigations are provided in Box 32.1.

Have examination and initial investigations narrowed down your differential diagnosis?

Based on the clinical findings of crepitations in the lungs in an orthopnoeic patient, a diagnosis of pulmonary oedema is appropriate. Excessive intravenous fluid therapy in a setting of oliguric renal failure can precipitate a fluid overload

Initial investigations

Haemoglobin	80 g/1 (8.0 g/dl)
Blood urea	39.6 mmol/1 (240 mg/dl)
Serum creatinine	720 µmol/1 (8.2 mg/dl)
Serum sodium	135 mmol/1 (meq/l)
Serum potassium	7.8 mmol/l (meq/l)
Serum calcium	2.1 mmol/l (8.4 mg/dl)
Serum phosphate	2.8 mmol/l (8.7mg/dl)
Serum albumin	32 g/l (3.2 g/dl)
Urine examination	
Albumin	++ (by dipstick)
Microscopy	1–2 granular casts per high-power field, no erythrocytes or pus cells seen
Chest X-ray	Typical bat-wing appearance of pulmonary oedema
Ultrasound	Right kidney length 8.0 cm, left kidney 8.2 cm, kidney outlines smooth

state. However, probable anaemia and hypertension are two important clinical findings in this patient that once again point towards underlying CRF. A diagnosis of CRF is usually suspected in the setting of a constellation of signs and symptoms including oedema, hypertension, anaemia and the uraemic syndrome. Pulmonary oedema can be the result of a cardiac pathology too, but the setting of oliguria after diarrhoea, history of early morning facial puffiness and essentially normal cardiac auscultation makes this unlikely.

The blood results clearly indicate that this man has renal failure. Bilaterally shrunken kidneys on ultrasound establish that there is at least a chronic element to this. Hyperkalaemia is another life-threatening complication of CRF in this patient and warrants urgent intervention.

Establishing an underlying diagnosis may have important implications for this man when considering renal transplantation in the future. Diabetes mellitus and glomerular disease are the most common causes of chronic kidney disease. He has no history of the former, but the history of a nephritic illness in childhood indicates that the most likely aetiology of his CRF is chronic glomerulonephritis. A history of polyuria and nocturia, in the absence of significant hypertension or oedema, might have suggested chronic interstitial nephritis. However, these differences become blurred in end-stage renal disease. The renal ultrasound has excluded polycystic kidney disease. Other rarer causes of CRF to be considered would include renovascular disease and systemic inflammatory diseases, such as systemic lupus erythematosus and vasculitis.

Further investigations

The patient's previous biopsy slides are reviewed and reveal membranoproliferative glomerulonephritis (Fig. 32.1). Hepatitis (B and C) and human immunodeficiency virus (HIV) serology are negative. Serial blood cultures are also negative.

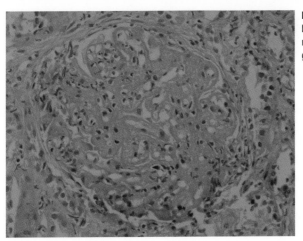

Fig. 32.1 Renal biopsy showing membranoproliferative glomerulonephritis.

How will you treat this patient?

He needs immediate dialysis in view of fluid overload and hyperkalaemia. A trial of high-dose intravenous furosemide and conservative measures for hyperkalaemia (injection of calcium gluconate, glucose–insulin infusion and potassium-binding resins) may be used to buy time. Box 32.2 lists the indications for dialysis in CRF.

If the acute insult of diarrhoea and consequent dehydration is significant, this young man's renal function may improve partially and there may be no further need for dialysis. In such a non-dialysis-dependent patient with CRF, there are many facets to therapy. Anaemia can be improved by recombinant human erythropoietin and parenteral iron therapy. Hyperphosphataemia and hypoc-

BOX 32.2
Indications for dialysis in chronic renal failure
• Clinical symptoms and signs of uraemic syndrome
• Fluid overload
• Hyperkalaemia
• Uraemic pericarditis
• Severe metabolic acidosis

alcaemia, as seen in this patient, can be corrected by the use of phosphate binders and 1-α-hydroxylated analogues of vitamin D. This will also prevent, or at least control, renal osteodystrophy. However, these drugs should be judiciously used, with frequent monitoring of calcium, phosphate and parathyroid hormone levels, for fear of precipitating hypercalcaemia and bone disease. It is possible to retard progression of CRF by tight control of blood pressure (target < 130/85 mmHg, and < 125/75 mmHg if proteinuria >1 g/day) using a combination of angiotensin-converting enzyme (ACE) inhibitors and angiotensin receptor blockers, which also reduce proteinuria. Restriction of dietary sodium and diuretics will help in control of oedema.

Membranoproliferative (or mesangiocapillary) glomerulonephritis can be associated with chronic infections such as hepatitis B and bacterial endocarditis, but often no underlying cause is found. Immunosuppressive therapy is of no proven benefit. Our patient is likely to progress to end-stage renal disease over a period of time and will eventually require long-term renal replacement therapy. The options at that stage would be renal transplant, maintenance haemodialysis or continuous ambulatory peritoneal dialysis. Given his young age, 5-year survival on haemodialysis would be in excess of 80%, but this treatment is associated with a poor quality of life. His best option for long-term survival and quality of life would be a renal transplant.

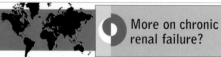

More on chronic
renal failure?

See Chapter 17 of
**Davidson's
Principles and
Practice of
Medicine**
(20th edn)

- The most common cause of CRF in the Western world is diabetic nephropathy. In the developing world, chronic glomerulonephritis remains the most frequently found cause, but the incidence of diabetic nephropathy is on the increase.

- Long-term renal replacement therapy is very expensive and financial constraints often preclude such treatment in the majority of patients in resource-poor countries.

- Cadaveric renal transplant programmes are well established in the Western world. In the developing world, transplants from live relatives are much more common than cadaveric transplants.

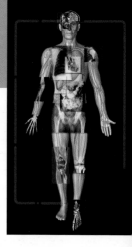

33

A man with sudden and severe chest pain

P. BLOOMFIELD

Presenting problem

A 55-year-old man of Asian origin presents to hospital with a new onset of chest pain. The pain is severe, is located in the centre of his chest and radiates into his left arm. The pain has come on suddenly and the man reports feeling very sick and sweaty. It has lasted more than an hour and at one point the man thought he was going to die. He gives a history of breathlessness and some chest discomfort when moving heavy boxes in his shop over the last few months. He admits to taking little exercise outside his work, and has gained weight in recent years. He has smoked 15 cigarettes a day since he left school. He had his blood pressure taken once at a visit to his doctor a year or so ago, was told it was high but has been too busy to go back and have it measured again. There is a strong family history of diabetes mellitus and his older brother has had a heart attack.

What would your differential diagnosis include before examining the patient?

The most common cause of chest pain with characteristic features of myocardial ischaemia is an acute coronary syndrome. This is particularly so in any patient, including this man, with risk factors for the development of ischaemic heart disease, e.g. hypertension, smoking and family history. The features of autonomic upset here — sweating and nausea — suggest possible myocardial infarction. The sudden onset of pain in a patient with a history of hypertension should also raise the suspicion of aortic dissection.

Examination

The patient looks unwell and sweaty. He is overweight (98 kg) with significant central obesity. Pulse is 104/min and blood pressure is 190/105 mmHg in both arms. All peripheral pulses are present and equal. The heart sounds are normal and there are no murmurs or added sounds. His respiratory rate is 17/min and there are bilateral crepitations in both lung bases.

Has examination narrowed down your differential diagnosis?

The physical examination has revealed signs of pulmonary oedema. Heart failure is a common accompaniment of myocardial infarction and reflects a significant degree of myocardial damage; hence it is associated with a worse

Urea	5.2 mmol/l (mg/dl)
Creatinine	50 µmol/l (0.56 mg/dl)
Sodium	138 mmol/l (14.6 mg/dl)
Potassium	3.6 mmol/l (meq/l)
Glucose	14.3 mmol/l (258 mg/dl)

prognosis. Rarely, acute pulmonary oedema may be a consequence of rupture of a papillary muscle (of the mitral valve) or of rupture of the interventricular septum. Both would tend to be associated with a murmur and with significant haemodynamic compromise, which is not the case here. Acute coronary syndrome is often not accompanied by any physical signs; pallor and sweating are part of the autonomic upset that may be a feature of myocardial infarction. The presence of all peripheral pulses does not exclude aortic dissection, which is commonly accompanied on presentation by hypertension.

Further investigations

Initial blood test results are shown in Box 33.1. A 12-lead electrocardiogram (ECG) is performed and shows features diagnostic of an acute anterior myocardial infarction (Fig. 33.1).

Does this narrow down your differential diagnosis?

The ECG is diagnostic of an acute anterior wall myocardial infarction. The ECG is the most important bedside investigation in patients presenting with chest pain. The high blood glucose indicates probable undiagnosed diabetes mellitus, a powerful risk factor for the development of coronary disease. The blood glucose results could also be a consequence of 'stress hyperglycaemia', i.e. a consequence of the autonomic and catecholamine response to severe illness. An elevated glycated haemoglobin concentration (HbA$_{1c}$) would support the former, but a normal level would be compatible with both possible diagnoses.

How will you treat this patient?

The patient needs treatment for pain with morphine and an antiemetic. He should be given aspirin (300 mg) and clopidogrel (300 mg) to swallow. Intravenous access should be promptly established and high-flow oxygen given. The patient should be monitored (ECG), as ventricular fibrillation may occur. Treatment should be given to lower blood pressure before thrombolytic drugs are given, and this can usually be achieved with sublingual or intravenous nitrates. He should be treated as an emergency for reperfusion therapy with primary percutaneous coronary intervention (PCI) if facilities are available; if not, he should be treated with thrombolytic drugs. All patients, except those with a bradycardia (< 65/min), hypotension (systolic blood pressure < 105 mmHg) or pulmonary oedema, should be given intravenous β-blockade (metoprolol 5–15 mg); in this patient pulmonary oedema would preclude the use of a β-blocker. The elevated blood glucose should be controlled with intravenous insulin. If PCI is not performed, coronary angiography should be carried out in the days following the event to determine the need for revascularisation therapy.

After the acute episode has settled, attention should turn to interventions that might improve this gentleman's prognosis and reduce the morbidity associated with the myocardial infarction. Aspirin therapy should be continued long-term. Clopidogrel should be continued for at least 1 month, or 3 months if PCI with coronary stenting was performed. Angiotensin-converting enzyme (ACE) inhibitors reduce ventricular remodelling and should be commenced in all patients, and

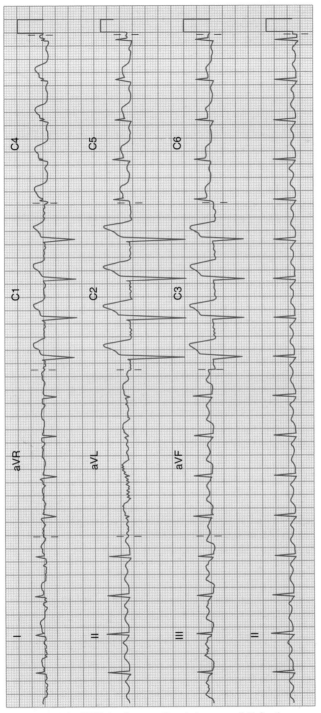

Fig. 33.1 A 12-lead ECG showing an acute anterior myocardial infarction.

especially if there is evidence of left ventricular impairment at echocardiography, which should be carried out before this man leaves hospital. Patients with acute myocardial infarction complicated by heart failure and left ventricular dysfunction appear to benefit from additional aldosterone receptor antagonism (e.g. eplerenone 25–50 mg daily). Beta-blockade reduces mortality in the weeks following a myocardial infarction, and again should be instituted in the absence of any contraindications.

Modification of risk factors is also crucial. The patient should be advised to stop smoking in the strongest possible terms, to lose weight and to take regular exercise. Statin therapy reduces the risk of further cardiovascular events by 25% over a 10-year period and should be commenced in all patients following a myocardial infarction, irrespective of total cholesterol concentration, unless there is a significant contraindication. Blood pressure should be treated aggressively, and if the patient's blood glucose levels remain elevated (i.e. he has true diabetes rather than stress hyperglycaemia), then oral hypoglycaemic therapy should be started. Metformin would be the first-line antidiabetic agent, providing that the patient does not have persistent overt heart failure or renal impairment.

Finally, the psychological morbidity of this event should not be overlooked. This gentleman has had a life-threatening illness that is likely to reduce his life expectancy and may affect his ability to work and perform other activities of daily living. Psychological support should be offered and often patients find value from attending rehabilitation classes where they can receive advice on lifestyle and exercise from trained practitioners.

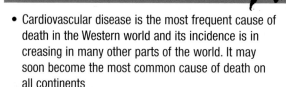

Global issues

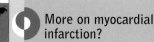
More on myocardial infarction?

- Cardiovascular disease is the most frequent cause of death in the Western world and its incidence is increasing in many other parts of the world. It may soon become the most common cause of death on all continents

- Ischaemic heart disease commonly affects those with diabetes, the incidence of which is increasing throughout the world, especially as obesity becomes more common.

See Chapter 18 of
Davidson's Principles and Practice of Medicine (20th edn)

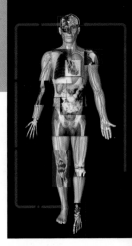

34

A 56-year-old man with breathlessness on exertion

D. E. NEWBY

Presenting problem

A 56-year-old man presents with a 6-month history of exertional breathlessness and fatigue. There is no associated chest pain or chest tightness. Over the last 2 months, he has noticed progressive swelling of his ankles and recently describes three-pillow orthopnoea and abdominal bloating. He is now limited to walking 200–300 metres on the flat.

He has no history of hypertension, diabetes mellitus or hypercholesterolaemia. He admits to drinking 40 units of alcohol per week and smokes 20 cigarettes per day. He had tuberculosis and rheumatic fever as a child. He also reports a cough productive of sputum for 2 months during the winter.

What would your differential diagnosis include before examining the patient?

Breathlessness as a symptom is predominantly caused by cardiac or respiratory disease, although occasionally metabolic acidosis or anaemia may present in this way. The most likely differential diagnoses here are congestive cardiac failure (with many potential causes), progressive chronic obstructive pulmonary disease or a combination of the two factors (cor pulmonale). The differential diagnosis would also include chronic pulmonary thromboembolism, interstitial lung disease, chronic bronchial asthma, angina equivalent and bronchogenic carcinoma.

Examination

The patient is mildly dyspnoeic on moving to the examination couch. He is pink with no evidence of central cyanosis. The pulse is weak and fast with a blood pressure 95/60 mmHg. The jugular venous pressure is markedly elevated up to the level of the ear lobes. Heart sounds reveal an added sound. The lung bases have reduced breath sounds and there is marked pitting peripheral oedema up to the knees. On abdominal examination there is shifting dullness and hepatomegaly.

Has examination narrowed down your differential diagnosis?

The clinical features are more suggestive of congestive cardiac failure with predominantly right-sided signs of fluid retention. Cor pulmonale remains a possibility. However, it must be remembered that congestive heart failure is not a diagnosis in itself. The underlying cause should be identified; coronary heart disease is a common aetiological factor.

Investigations

Serum biochemistry demonstrates a marginally elevated serum urea and creatinine concentration, normal serum bicarbonate concentration and deranged liver function tests.

The electrocardiogram (ECG) shows no evidence of myocardial ischaemia or prior infarction. There is a sinus tachycardia, low-voltage QRS complexes and T wave flattening.

The chest X-ray shows small bilateral pleural effusions and upper lobe venous diversion. The cardiothoracic ratio is at the upper limit of normal.

Echocardiography demonstrates good left ventricular function with no left ventricular dilatation, hypertrophy or regional wall motion abnormality. The heart valves function normally and there is a trivial pericardial effusion. The motion of the septum appears unusual and the Doppler velocities across the aortic valve are reduced. The right ventricle is not dilated and there is no evidence of pulmonary hypertension.

Spirometry demonstrates a forced expiratory volume in 1 second (FEV_1) of 2.0 l/min and forced vital capacity (FVC) of 3.0 l/min. Pulse oximetry records an oxygen saturation of 97% on air.

Have examination and initial investigations narrowed down your differential diagnosis?

The clinical features demonstrate a patient with symptomatic congestive cardiac failure and the associated examination findings of a raised jugular venous pressure and peripheral oedema. The three most common causes of heart failure are coronary artery disease, hypertension and valvular heart disease. These are unlikely, given the clinical findings and investigations. Although mild airways obstruction is present, the patient has no cyanosis and is well oxygenated on room air; there is no suggestion of cor pulmonale or pulmonary artery hypertension. This makes a respiratory cause for the patient's breathlessness unlikely.

Although alcoholic and viral cardiomyopathies are potential causes, echocardiography has demonstrated a normal-sized left ventricle with good systolic function. Further investigation of the patient's diagnosis should therefore focus on the causes of heart failure in the presence of good left ventricular function and including diastolic dysfunction and high-output cardiac failure. The latter is usually associated with a hyperdynamic circulation and is unlikely, given the low-volume pulse and hypotension.

Definitive investigations

Causes of diastolic heart failure include restrictive cardiomyopathies (including amyloidosis, myocardial fibrosis and left ventricular hypertrophy), constrictive pericarditis and pericardial effusions. Given the echocardiographic appearances, the differential diagnosis focuses on the presence of a restrictive cardiomyopathy or constrictive pericarditis. Causes of restrictive cardiomyopathy include amyloidosis and sarcoidosis. The former can be confirmed by histological examination of a fat, rectal or myocardial biopsy. Such patients should also be investigated for the presence of multiple myeloma.

Severe constrictive pericarditis can sometimes be detected on the chest X-ray by the presence of pericardial calcification. The patient therefore undergoes computed tomography (CT) of the chest. This demonstrates marked pericardial thickening and calcification (Fig. 34.1). Pericardial calcification can occur in the absence of constrictive pericarditis and the diagnosis is made at cardiac catheterisation.

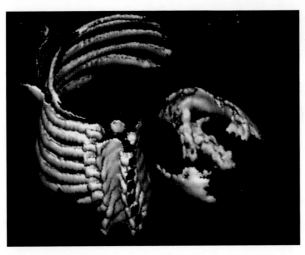

Fig. 34.1 Three-dimensional reconstruction of CT of a patient with constrictive pericarditis. Ribs and spine are to the left and the calcified shell of pericardium to the right.

34

BOX 34.1

Causes of constrictive pericarditis

- Tuberculous pericarditis
- Haemopericardium
- Viral pericarditis
- Rheumatoid arthritis and systemic lupus erythematosus
- Post-pericardotomy syndrome
- Purulent pericarditis, such as is caused by *Staphylococcus aureus*
- Neoplastic infiltration
- Polyserositis
- Idiopathic

The final, definitive investigation is cardiac catheterisation and this shows high filling pressures as well as equalisation of the diastolic pressures in all chambers of the heart.

How will you treat this patient?

Breathlessness and peripheral oedema are treated with loop diuretic therapy. This will reduce the fluid retention and filling pressures of the heart. However, over-vigorous diuresis may lead to hypotension and pre-renal failure, and this limits the ability to relieve the symptoms completely.

Patients with constrictive pericarditis should undergo surgical removal of the pericardium–pericardiectomy. This removes not only the parietal, but also the visceral pericardium and can cause considerable cardiac damage, especially to the right ventricle. Although symptoms are improved, patients are often left with significant peripheral oedema, breathlessness and right heart failure post-operatively. This limits their symptomatic recovery and they often remain chronically disabled by their condition.

Global issues

 More on constrictive pericarditis?

- Although it is often impossible to identify the original insult, causes of constrictive pericarditis (Box 34.1) have marked geographical variability.

- Tuberculous pericarditis is the most common cause in Asia and Africa, and arises as a complication of pulmonary tuberculosis.

- In Africa, a tuberculous pericardial effusion is a common feature of the acquired immunodeficiency syndrome (AIDS).

See Chapter 18 of

Davidson's Principles and Practice of Medicine (20th edn)

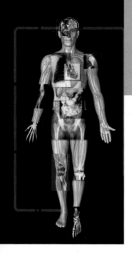

35

A young adult with hypertension

P. L. PADFIELD

Presenting problem

A 28-year-old man with no previous health problems decides to join a local health club. As part of his initial assessment for a fitness programme, he has his blood pressure (BP) measured. The reading is 182/106 mmHg and he is advised to call and see his general practitioner, who discovers that the young man's father is on drug treatment for hypertension, which was picked up when he was in his fifties. There is no other relevant family history. The young man is well, although anxious about the implications of having hypertension. He is a non-smoker, drinks 18 units of alcohol per week, takes no prescribed or self-administered medications, and admits to enjoying salt on his food. He has no knowledge of any childhood illnesses such as urinary infections. On direct questioning he describes no headaches, palpitations or sweating attacks, and appears truly asymptomatic.

What would your differential diagnosis include before examining the patient?

Hypertension is relatively uncommon in young people. Systolic BP increases with age in Western society and individuals destined to become hypertensive in later life tend to have BPs in the higher centiles at all ages. It is worth considering 'white coat hypertension' (high BP in a clinic setting with normal BP at home or outside hospital) in all apparently hypertensive individuals; there is no reliable way of identifying this without some form of 'out of office' measurement (ambulatory or self-monitored BP) and possible causes of secondary hypertension should be on every physician's mind (Box 35.1). It is difficult to know the true prevalence of secondary hypertension, but the younger the patient, the more likely a specific disorder will be present. Most guidelines suggest investigation for a cause if hypertension is detected before the age of 30 years, but the pick-up rate of correctable conditions is small above the age of 20 years.

Examination

There is no obvious suggestion of an endocrine disease such as Cushing's syndrome or acromegaly (both of which can cause hypertension), although the patient is a little overweight with a body mass index of 27. All peripheral pulses are present and synchronous, there are no abdominal bruits and the kidneys are not palpable. Auscultation of the heart is normal and funduscopy is

BOX 35.1

Causes of hypertension

- Renal
  Any chronic renal
  disease
  Polycystic kidneys
  Renovascular disease
- Adrenal
  Phaeochromocytoma
  Primary hyperaldo-
  steronism
  Cushing's syndrome
  Some congenital adrenal
  enzyme defects
- Coarctation of the aorta
- Takayasu's
  aorto-arteritis
- Drug effects
  NSAIDs
  Liquorice
  Combined oral
  contraceptive pill
  (women)

also unremarkable. BP is recorded as 168/100 mmHg (mean of two readings after 5 minutes' rest).

Initial investigations

Urinalysis is negative and reveals no overt proteinuria or microalbuminuria. Renal function is normal, as are plasma electrolytes. The full blood count and erythrocyte sedimentation rate are likewise unremarkable. An electrocardiogram shows no evidence of left ventricular hypertrophy (best assessed by adding up the depth of the S wave in chest lead V2 and the height of the R wave in chest lead V5, which should come to < 35 mm).

Have examination and initial investigations narrowed down your differential diagnosis?

Coarctation of the aorta and polycystic kidney disease might have been picked up if present. In someone of this age an abdominal bruit would have suggested renal artery stenosis (less discriminatory in older people with an increased likelihood of aortic turbulence), but the absence of a bruit means nothing. A normal level of plasma potassium makes primary aldosteronism less likely, though not impossible. Funduscopy is a poorly practised art, but the presence of haemorrhages and 'exudates' (with or without papilloedema) would have increased the likelihood of renovascular disease (a prevalence rate of 40% in some series with grade III retinopathy). It remains most likely that this young man has primary hypertension.

Further investigations

There is no generally agreed list of investigations but it would be prudent to perform a 24-hour urine collection for metadrenaline and normetadrenaline (to exclude a phaeochromocytoma), and to obtain blood in the supine or seated position for plasma renin activity (PRA) and aldosterone. (A low renin with a high aldosterone means primary hyperaldosteronism, whereas a high PRA might suggest renovascular disease.) How far one should go to exclude a diagnosis of renovascular disease is debatable. A renal ultrasound will pick up a disparity in kidney size (and would also diagnose polycystic kidneys) and might be carried out in such a person. Doppler ultrasound to measure renal blood flow is very observer-dependent and magnetic resonance imagining (MRI) of the renal arteries is expensive, but either may be indicated if a high index of suspicion arises from other tests. Before life-long medication is decided on, either ambulatory BP monitoring (Fig. 35.1) might be performed or, more cost-effectively, the patient might be given an electronic self-monitoring device to use for several days (Fig. 35.2).

The young man is fitted with an ambulatory monitor and the day-time average BP is recorded as 158/96 mmHg. A 24-hour urine collection shows no evidence of catecholamine excess, and supine PRA and aldosterone are within the normal range. An MR angiogram shows no evidence of renal artery stenosis.

Does this narrow down your differential diagnosis?

The ambulatory monitor confirms that the young man has sustained hypertension and investigations have revealed no evidence of a secondary cause. Therefore, he has primary hypertension.

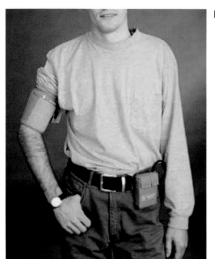

Fig. 35.1 An ambulatory BP monitor.

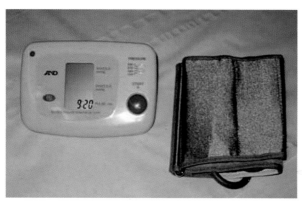

Fig. 35.2 A home BP monitor. Data can be downloaded directly to a PC.

How will you treat this patient?

Hypertension is an undeniable risk factor for cardiovascular disease but is not an illness in its own right. People should be discouraged from considering themselves unwell. There is good evidence that salt restriction will lower BP, and weight reduction with exercise should also help. If BP remains in excess of 160/100 mmHg, then British guidelines recommend drug therapy. If BP is lower, then treatment decisions are guided by whether or not the 10-year cardiovascular risk is in excess of 20%. One of the difficulties in interpreting such guidance is that 10-year risks are vanishingly low in young people, but many take the view that treatment is needed to prevent the long-term damage to blood vessels that may become less reversible by the time someone reaches 40 or 50 years of age.

Assuming the young man accepts the need to take life-long medication that will not make him feel better (a great deal of skill in communication is needed for such discussions), then current advice would recommend starting him on an angiotensin-converting enzyme (ACE) inhibitor (or an angiotensin receptor antagonist if he develops a cough with the ACE inhibitor, of which there is a 10%

chance); these classes of drug are most suited to young people. Goal BP would be 140/90 mmHg and it is unlikely that a single agent will achieve this; the second stage would be to add a calcium channel blocker or thiazide diuretic. The best third drug (if necessary) is uncertain, but most likely one would add a thiazide or a calcium channel blocker (depending upon the second choice).

Global issues

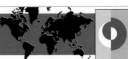

- Hypertension is amongst the most common disorders recognised by the World Health Organization as a cause of premature deaths — both in the developed and developing worlds.

- Many countries cannot afford the cost of drugs to treat hypertension effectively.

- Takayasu's aorto-arteritis is a rare but an important cause of hypertension, especially in young Asian females.

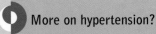 More on hypertension?

See Chapter 18 of
**Davidson's
Principles and
Practice of
Medicine**
(20th edn)

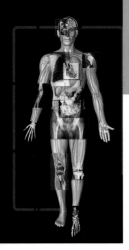

36

A young man with a sudden transient loss of consciousness

P. S. SHANKAR

Presenting problem

A 25-year-old man presents with a history of lightheadedness, giddiness and a transient loss of consciousness. There is a history of prior physical exertion and fatigue. The episode is preceded by a feeling of warmth, with a dry mouth and a desire for fresh air. He mentions a similar episode 2 months earlier when he was in a crowded place watching a festival procession. He is fit and well and does not take any regular medication.

What would your differential diagnosis include before examining the patient?

Is this a faint (syncope) or a fit (seizure)? Any episode of 'blackout' should be reviewed with special reference to the manifestations preceding the attack and features noted during the period of loss of consciousness and after regaining consciousness and orientation. Though the patient can narrate the events prior to the attack, an eye-witness account is essential to gain information about the loss of consciousness and its subsequent course. Distinguishing features of syncope and seizures are shown in Box 36.1.

Syncope is a transient sudden loss of consciousness, with loss of postural tone due to reduced cerebral blood flow. Causes include disorders of vascular tone or blood volume, cardiovascular disorders, including cardiac arrhythmias, and cerebrovascular disease.

BOX 36.1

Distinguishing features of syncope and seizure

Features	Vasovagal syncope	Seizure
Posture at the time of attack	Upright	Any posture
Onset	Gradual	Sudden
Pallor	Present	Uncommon
Unconsciousness	Seconds	Minutes
Recovery	Rapid	Often slow
Post-ictal confusion, amnesia, headache	Uncommon	Common
Injury	Uncommon	Occasionally
Tongue-biting	Never	Common

Vasovagal syncope is a common disorder accounting for nearly 50% of all episodes of syncope. Before the attack, the patient may experience symptoms of cerebral hypoperfusion, such as lightheadedness, dizziness, tinnitus, nausea, weakness, salivation, pallor and dimness of vision. Vasovagal syncope is usually precipitated by stimuli such as a crowded environment, extreme fatigue, severe pain, hunger, prolonged standing and emotional disturbances or stressful situations. The loss of consciousness is gradual and brief, and the individual recovers quickly, without confusion, after assuming the horizontal position. Sufferers often feel nauseated and unwell for several minutes before and after the episode.

Cardiac syncope has a sudden onset and is independent of body position. It may be a consequence of an arrhythmia (profound bradycardia or ventricular tachyarrhythmia) or structural cardiac disease, including severe aortic stenosis, critical coronary artery disease or hypertrophic obstructive cardiomyopathy (HOCM). There may not be any prior warning or symptoms may be related to exercise.

Hypersensitivity of carotid baroreceptors to external pressure may also cause altered consciousness by promoting inappropriate bradycardia and vasodilatation. Syncope may also occur during micturition and during prolonged coughing. Postural hypotension can cause transient lightheadedness on standing and, rarely, individuals can black out.

A seizure is any clinical event caused by an abnormal electrical discharge in the brain, whilst epilepsy is the tendency to have recurrent seizures. In epilepsy consciousness is lost instantaneously. It may develop regardless of the position of the patient. (Syncope is very unusual when the individual is recumbent.) Often there are distinct prodromal symptoms and, at the onset of an epileptic attack, tonic spasm of muscles with upturning of the eyes may be noted. The patient regains consciousness slowly, whereas recovery is quick following syncope. Drowsiness, mental confusion, amnesia and headache are common sequelae, and urinary incontinence, tongue biting and other forms of injury may occur.

Examination

Examination is essentially unremarkable. The patient's pulse is 62/min and blood pressure is 90/50 mmHg, with no postural drop; there are no murmurs. There is no injury or evidence of tongue-biting. He has fully regained consciousness and now feels well, if a little shaky. Neurological examination does not reveal any untoward findings.

Fortunately, a friend has accompanied the young man to the hospital and he witnessed the event. He reports that the patient had just finished playing a game of football. The patient was not feeling well beforehand and had apparently been suffering from a coryzal illness. The patient was sitting down at the end of the match, feeling very tired, when he vomited. He then went very pale and passed out. One of his fellow players had just completed a first aid course and placed the patient in the recovery position. He noted the patient's pulse to be 40/min. After a few seconds in this position, the patient regained consciousness and was able to sit up. He quickly regained orientation. At no stage during the episode was there any jerking of the limbs.

Has examination narrowed down your differential diagnosis?

Examination, as is often the case in syncope, has not helped, but the collateral history has provided crucial information. We are clearly dealing with a syncopal episode rather than a seizure. The key question now is, what is the underlying cause of the syncope? The relationship to exercise is a concern. Could this man have a serious underlying cardiac disorder, such as HOCM; has he had an exercise-induced arrhythmia? The fact that he had not been feeling well and vomited beforehand raises the possibility that this was a simple vasovagal disorder, and we know that the prior episode occurred at rest. However, it would be a brave doctor who would make this diagnosis without further investigation.

Further investigations

Routine blood tests are normal. A 12-lead electrocardiogram (ECG) shows no abnormality and an echocardiogram is also normal. A 24-hour (Holter) monitor shows no underling rhythm disturbance, although no symptoms occur during the period of the recording. Carotid sinus massage does not induce any symptoms or any change in heart rate.

Does this narrow down your differential diagnosis?

The echocardiogram provides reassurance that this man does not have a major structural cardiac abnormality. A 24-hour tape is at its most useful when an individual has the offending symptom (in this case, syncope) during the period of the recording. More often than not, the individual is asymptomatic. More prolonged periods of recording can be undertaken but the yield from these remains low. This man is probably too young for carotid sinus hypersensitivity and the lack of effect of carotid sinus massage supports this. The decision as to whether to pursue more investigations or to adopt an expectant approach really depends on the feelings of the patient, the confidence of the doctor in being able to make a positive diagnosis of vasovagal syncope, and the facilities at hand for further investigation.

The typical symptoms of vasovagal syncope may be provoked during head-up tilt table testing and may sometimes be diagnostically useful. The patient is secured to a table and is tilted to 70° head-up for 45 minutes. Blood pressure and ECG are monitored throughout. A positive test requires typical symptoms and profound bradycardia (cardio-inhibitory response) and/or hypotension (vasodepressor response).

To explore the possibility of cardiac syncope further, other investigations are also possible. A Cardiomemo device is a hand-held monitor that can be placed on the chest during an event and which will record the heart rhythm. It is only useful, though, when there is a clear warning of the onset of symptoms and is of no benefit to people who black out suddenly! *It is now* also possible to fit a tiny continuous heart monitor subcutaneously. It can remain *in situ* for up to 2 years and can be retrospectively interrogated if an event occurs; this is ideal for people who have very infrequent events.

How will you treat this patient?

This patient can be reassured that he has had a simple fainting spell; he should be given advice on potential precipitants, so that these might be avoided if possible. If he were to have further episodes on a regular basis, then tilt testing and implantation of an ECG monitor should be considered. Dual chamber pacing can be useful in patients with severe vasovagal syncope or carotid sinus hypersensitivity where symptoms are due to bradycardia. Beta-blocker therapy may also be of benefit in patients with severe vasovagal syncope, as they inhibit the initial sympathetic activation.

Global issues

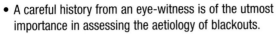

 More on syncope?

- A careful history from an eye-witness is of the utmost importance in assessing the aetiology of blackouts.

- Crowded environments, extreme fatigue, severe pain, hunger, prolonged standing and emotional conditions may provoke vasovagal syncope.

See Chapter 26 of
Davidson's
Principles and
Practice of
Medicine
(20th edn)

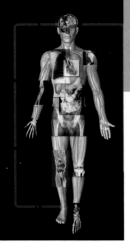

37

A student with intermittent palpitation

N. GRUBB

Presenting problem

A 19-year-old student with no prior medical history is referred to a cardiology clinic with a history of intermittent palpitation. Since the age of 16 she has been aware of sudden episodes of a rapid, regular, forceful heart rhythm but these always stopped within 15 minutes. Sometimes she was able to terminate the palpitation by holding her breath. She has not identified any specific triggers for episodes, although they are more likely to occur when she is tired. In between episodes she feels completely well. In the past few months, prior to university examinations, she has had two episodes of dizziness associated with very rapid and irregular palpitation and during one of these she blacked out. Her general practitioner ordered some blood tests, which are unremarkable (Box 37.1).

BOX 37.1

Initial investigations

Haemoglobin	125 g/l (12.5 g/dl)
TSH	1.4 mU/l
Free T$_4$	16 pmol/l (800 pg/dl)

What would your differential diagnosis include before examining the patient?

Palpitation is a common symptom in young people. Sinus tachycardia can cause palpitation, and may be triggered by anxiety or by external factors such as alcohol, caffeine or some recreational drugs (e.g. amphetamines, ecstasy). Thyrotoxicosis and anaemia can also cause a sinus tachycardia, but have been excluded here. In this case the sudden onset and recurring pattern would be unusual for sinus tachycardia, and suggests a paroxysmal tachyarrhythmia. Supraventricular tachycardia (SVT) is the most likely diagnosis in a young patient with no cardiac history, whereas ventricular tachycardia would be more likely in an older patient with a history of cardiovascular disease. The history of syncope is worrying and suggests that this patient requires urgent investigation.

Examination

The patient appears well and relaxed. Radial pulse is 65/min and regular. The young woman is normotensive and there is no clinical evidence of cardiac failure. Precordial examination is normal and she has no added heart sounds or murmurs. There are no abnormal cardiorespiratory findings.

Has examination narrowed down your differential diagnosis?

Examination is done principally to identify structural heart disease and heart failure. Palpitation and syncope occurring in the presence of cardiomyopathy, heart failure or valve disease may signal a tendency to malignant ventricular arrhythmia. The normal examination findings here are reassuring, but do not help to discriminate the underlying cause of the patient's palpitation.

Further investigations

A 12-lead ECG shows sinus rhythm, with a short PR interval and abnormal QRS complexes (Fig. 37.1). The upstroke of the QRS complex is slurred and there are associated T-wave abnormalities. An ambulatory electrocardiogram (ECG) recording shows sinus rhythm and, during symptoms of regular palpitation, a narrow-complex tachycardia, rate 190/min, suggestive of SVT. There is one episode during which she felt dizzy, associated with an extremely rapid, broad-complex tachycardia. Transthoracic echocardiography shows a structurally normal heart.

Does this narrow down the differential diagnosis?

The combination of a short PR interval and a 'delta wave' (slurred upstroke to the QRS complex) is diagnostic of the presence of an accessory atrioventricular pathway. If this is associated with palpitation, the condition is known as the Wolff–Parkinson–White (WPW) syndrome. Usually, WPW syndrome causes paroxysms of SVT characterised by regular, rapid palpitation. These episodes are caused by atrioventricular re-entry, in which anterograde conduction usually proceeds via the atrioventricular node and retrograde conduction proceeds via the accessory pathway. The ECG typically shows a regular tachycardia with narrow QRS complexes. The occurrence of syncope in a patient with WPW syndrome should immediately raise suspicion of pre-excited atrial fibrillation, in which atrial fibrillation waves conduct extremely rapidly to the ventricles via the accessory pathway, producing a very fast, irregular, broad-complex tachycardia. In some cases the ventricles are stimulated so rapidly that ventricular fibrillation and sudden death occur. Ambulatory ECG monitoring is used to confirm the nature of the rhythm during symptom episodes. This is important in directing treatment, since patients with WPW syndrome may experience palpitation unrelated to their accessory pathway (e.g. from extrasystoles or sinus tachycardia).

How will you treat this patient?

Episodes of SVT can be terminated by triggering vagal reflexes, which inhibit the tachycardia by causing transient atrioventricular nodal block. Patients can be taught the Valsalva manœuvre and carotid sinus pressure, although these are not always effective. Persistent episodes may require hospital treatment. For patients known to have WPW syndrome, an intravenous flecainide infusion is probably the safest way to terminate the SVT. Flecainide blocks sodium channel conduction in accessory pathway tissue. Intravenous adenosine, whilst indicated for SVT management in general, should be avoided in known WPW syndrome because there is a small risk of it precipitating pre-excited atrial fibrillation. Digoxin is contraindicated because it promotes accessory pathway conduction.

First-line treatment for patients with WPW syndrome is catheter ablation therapy. This involves a procedure carried out under light sedation, in which catheter electrodes are introduced into the heart via the femoral vein. These are used to help locate the accessory pathway, which is then ablated using radiofrequency energy. Success rates exceed 95% and the risk of major complication is very small. Rarely, the accessory pathway is located close to the atrioventricular node; if damaged, permanent pacing may be required. Catheter ablation therapy eliminates the risk of death from pre-excited atrial fibrillation.

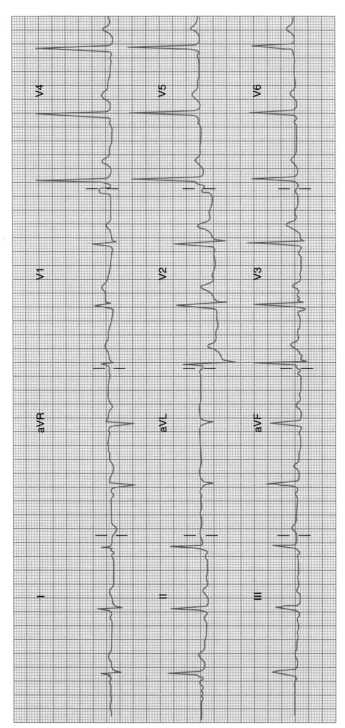

Fig. 37.1 A 12-lead ECG showing classical features of pre-excitation. The PR interval is short and the onset of the QRS complex is characterised by a 'delta wave' or slurred upstroke.

Long-term drug therapy tends to be used only in patients awaiting catheter ablation or in rare cases where the accessory pathway cannot be eliminated by catheter ablation. Sodium channel blockers such as flecainide or propafenone reduce the risk of SVT and pre-excited atrial fibrillation but do not eliminate it. The small procedural risk associated with catheter ablation is, for most patients, offset by eliminating the risk of pre-excited atrial fibrillation and the need for life-long drug prophylaxis.

Global issues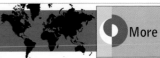

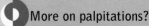 More on palpitations?

- Wolff–Parkinson–White syndrome is associated with some structural cardiac diseases, e.g. hypertrophic cardiomyopathy, mitral valve prolapse and Ebstein's anomaly. An echocardiogram should be performed in all cases.

- Catheter ablation facilities are not available in all centres. Where catheter ablation is not feasible, patients should be referred to an electrophysiology centre or, less ideally, treated with a class Ic anti-arrhythmic drug, such as flecainide.

See Chapter 18 of
Davidson's Principles and Practice of Medicine
(20th edn)

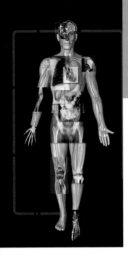

38

A prolonged fever in a young boy with acyanotic congenital heart disease

M. E. YEOLEKAR

Presenting problem

A 14-year-old boy is admitted to a tertiary care hospital for evaluation of a prolonged fever. The history is given by his mother, who says that his symptoms began at the age of 6 weeks, when he started having difficulty in breastfeeding, with increased sweating and frequent crying episodes. He has never appeared blue. The boy has required frequent hospitalisations for repeated respiratory infections and one of these admissions prompted referral to a cardiac specialist. After initial evaluation, a transthoracic echocardiogram demonstrated a large ventricular septal defect (VSD) and early surgery was advised. Due to financial constraints, surgery was deferred and the boy continued with conservative medical treatment, avoiding any form of exertion. For the last 3 months he has had a low-grade fever, increasing breathlessness, exertional palpitations, a poor appetite, muscle pains and weight loss (about 5 kg). He also has vague pains involving all joints of his hands and feet, although there is no joint swelling or restriction of movements. He denies having paroxysmal nocturnal dyspnoea (PND) or orthopnoea. There is no history of any chest pain, syncope or pedal swelling.

What would your differential diagnosis include before examining the patient?

This young boy has a large VSD. Difficulty in breastfeeding with increased sweating and frequent crying episodes are suggestive of congestive cardiac failure during infancy. His current symptoms of prolonged fever, weight loss, anorexia and polyarthralgia, on the background of congenital heart disease, would put infective endocarditis (IE) at the top of the differential diagnosis list. IE is a well-known precipitating factor for worsening of stable congenital heart disease, and VSD is the most common congenital heart disease to be complicated by IE.

Other causes of such a prolonged fever include infections (tuberculosis, fungal infections, occult abscess), malignancy (lymphomas, leukaemias), connective tissue disorders and sarcoidosis, but they all seem unlikely. Fever is the most common symptom of IE and is present in 85–90% of patients, although rarely it may be absent in elderly patients, immunocompromised individuals and those with cardiac or renal failure. Fever with polyarthralgia, dyspnoea and palpitations would also raise the possibility of acute rheumatic fever in this age group, but a duration of 3 months and the absence of a preceding sore throat make this unlikely.

38

Examination

This patient is thin and febrile. He is pale and has clubbing of all fingernails and toenails. His vital signs are stable, except for a pulse rate of 110/min. All peripheral pulses are felt equally. There are subconjunctival haemorrhages in his right eye, and splinter haemorrhages (dark red linear streaks) are noted in the nail beds of many fingers. His oral hygiene is poor and he has caries in a left upper molar.

Examination of the cardiovascular system reveals a grade 3/6 high-pitched pansystolic murmur, best heard in the third and fourth left intercostal spaces close to the sternum; these are consistent with a large VSD. The spleen is palpable 2 cm below the left costal margin and is non-tender. The remainder of the examination is normal.

Has examination narrowed down your differential diagnosis?

The presence of a prolonged history of pyrexia, pallor, clubbing, subconjunctival and splinter haemorrhages, and splenomegaly is highly suggestive of IE. The other peripheral manifestations of IE that may be encountered include petechiae (the most common one), Osler's nodes (painful, pea-sized, purplish nodules on the pulp of the fingers), Janeway lesions (non-tender erythematous macules over palms and soles), Roth's spots (oval retinal haemorrhages with a pale centre) and arthritis. Most of these signs are seen after 6 weeks and are characteristic of subacute bacterial endocarditis caused by *Streptococcus viridans.* Poor orodental hygiene in this patient has probably predisposed to the development of IE by causing intermittent bacteraemia.

Investigations

The patient's haemoglobin is 100g/l (10g/dl), with a peripheral smear showing normocytic normochromic anaemia. The total white cell count is 15 × 10^9/l (15 × 10^3/mm^3) with 80% polymorphs. The erythrocyte sedimentation rate (ESR) is 60 mm/1st hour and the platelet count is normal. Urinary examination reveals numerous red blood cells and casts. Renal and liver function tests are normal. The chest X-ray shows cardiomegaly and a prominent pulmonary vasculature. A 12-lead ECG reveals evidence of biventricular hypertrophy (large equiphasic QRS in the mid-precordial leads).

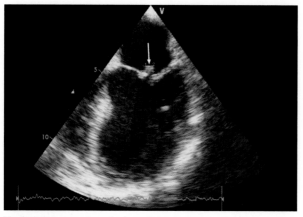

Fig. 38.1 Transoesophageal echocardiography reveals a vegetation on the anterior mitral leaflet (arrow).

Blood cultures result in a significant growth of Strep. viridans after 48 hours of incubation, and the growth is sent for sensitivity testing. Two-dimensional transthoracic and transoesophageal echocardiography (Fig. 38.1) reveals a large VSD with a 6 × 10 mm vegetation attached to the anterior mitral valve leaflet.

Has the diagnosis been clinched?

Yes. The positive blood culture for *Strep. viridans* and the echocardiographic evidence of a vegetation confirm infective endocarditis. The presence of a mild normocytic normochromic anaemia, poly-morphonuclear leucocytosis, a raised ESR and an active urinary sediment (due to the immune com-plex glomerulonephritis) all support the diagnosis. A VSD increases the risk of IE on both right- and left-sided valves; in this patient the vegetation is present on the mitral valve due to increased blood flow across the valve. Blood culture is a crucial investigation (even though it is negative in about 14% of all cases — Box 38.1), which helps not only in diagnosis but also in guiding antibiotic therapy. Therefore, in all suspected cases of IE, three sets of blood cultures must be drawn 1 hour apart under strict aseptic precautions before starting antibiotic treatment. The most common organism identified, as in this case, is *Strep. viridans*.

How will you treat this patient?

If left untreated, IE has a high mortality (20–40%) due to its inherent complications (Box 38.2). Therefore, empirical treatment must be started with a synergistic combination of bactericidal antibiotics effective against *Strep. viridans* (pend-ing the sensitivity report). Typically, this would involve intravenous benzyl penicillin and gen-tamicin for 2 weeks, with intravenous benzyl penicil-lin continued for a further 2 weeks. Vancomycin may be substituted for benzyl penicillin in penicil-lin-allergic patients or when staphylococcal infec-tion is suspected. Improvement usually follows 3–7 days of successful antimicrobial therapy. A shorter course of treatment may be considered in 'low-risk' patients, including those with a rapid clinical response, small vegetations and infection of a native valve with a sensitive organism (low minimum inhibitory concentration). Persistent or recurrent fever may be a manifestation of treatment failure, drug fever, secondary nosocomial infection or abscess (intracardiac or extracardiac) formation. Surgery for IE (needed in 30–50% patients) is potentially life-saving and should never be delayed in an unstable patient. After treatment of this patient's IE, the VSD should be surgically closed.

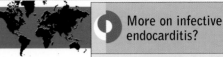

Global issues

More on infective endocarditis?

See Chapter 18 of
Davidson's
Principles and
Practice of
Medicine
(20th edn)

- Despite improvements in health care, the global incidence of IE has not decreased over the past decades. This apparent paradox is due to emerging risk factors like intravenous drug use, an increasing incidence of degenerative valve disease in the elderly, an increasing use of prosthetic valves and occurrence of nosocomial infections.

- The most common causative organism of IE in intravenous drug abusers is *Staphylococcus aureus*. It causes right-sided endocarditis with recurrent pulmonary emboli, manifesting as lung abscesses.

- The most common predisposing condition for IE in developing countries continues to be rheumatic heart disease, while in the Western world degenerative valve disease, mitral valve prolapse, intravenous drug abuse and prosthetic valves top the list. The most common organisms implicated in early endocarditis of a prosthetic valve is coagulase-negative staphylococci (*Staph. epidermidis*).

- Newly identified pathogens which are difficult to culture (e.g. *Bartonella* species) and multidrug-resistant organisms (*Staph. aureus*, *Enterococcus*) challenge conventional antimicrobial therapy. Newer serological and molecular techniques (which assist in blood culture-negative IE), novel antimicrobials and potential vaccines are emerging to meet this challenge.

- Antibiotic prophylaxis should be given to all patients with cardiac conditions, in whom the risk of IE is significant, to cover invasive procedures that may cause transient bacteraemia.

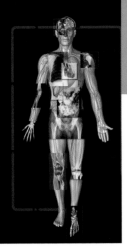

39

A young man with joint pains and fever

P. S. PAIS

Presenting problem

A 20-year-old carpenter's apprentice presents to his local hospital in India complaining of pain and swelling of his joints, together with fever, for the previous week. The pain and swelling first started in his knee joints. For the last 3 days, although the pain in the knees has eased, pain and swelling have appeared in his right elbow and left wrist. He has been unable to work since the onset of symptoms. A neighbouring physician prescribed diclofenac, which has given some temporary relief, and advised the young man to go to hospital. Together with the joint pain, he has been running a fever associated with sweating. He does not recall any preceding sore throat or fever. On questioning, he recalls that 8 years ago he had a similar episode of fever, pain and swelling of his knees, which was severe enough to keep him off school for a few weeks. He was not investigated at that time and, other than analgesics, took no medicines. He denies any history of shortness of breath or chest pain at the present or in the past.

What would your differential diagnosis include before examining the patient?

When a young man presents in India with arthritis involving a few large joints and fever, with a similar episode some years earlier, rheumatic fever (rheumatic arthritis) will be close to the top of the list of potential diagnoses. The absence of a history of preceding tonsillitis does not weaken this possibility; only about 40% of subjects will give this 'typical' history. If the previous episode was due to rheumatic fever, the patient could already have developed rheumatic valvular disease, as a proportion of patients with acute rheumatic fever subsequently develop rheumatic heart disease. If this is so, bacterial endocarditis, which at times causes arthritis, must also be considered, especially as it is a potentially life-threatening yet treatable condition. Also crippling yet treatable is septic arthritis, but the sequential involvement of four joints makes this unlikely. Another condition to be considered is reactive arthritis. Here again, a preceding episode of diarrhoeal infection would be typical but is not essential. In reactive arthritis there is usually involvement of the axial skeleton and often the joints of the fingers or toes; tendonitis, urethritis and uveitis may also occur. Finally, juvenile-onset spondyloarthropathy may present in young males with oligo-articular involvement of lower limb joints, and this is often associated with tendonitis.

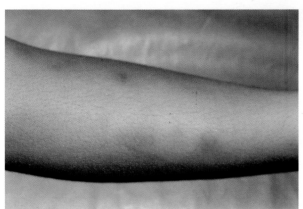

Fig. 39.1 Classic lesions of erythema nodosum.

39

Examination

The patient weighs 60 kg and is febrile with a temperature of 38°C. His blood pressure is 110/76 mmHg and pulse rate 112/min, with a regular rhythm and normal character. Both knee joints and the right elbow are swollen, red and tender, and their movements are restricted because of pain. The left elbow is also tender, swollen and painful on movement. The young man has no subconjunctival haemorrhages; neither are Roth's spots seen on examination of the optic fundi. There is no erythema marginatum, but lesions typical of erythema nodosum are found on the shins (Fig. 39.1). On examination of the precordium, the apical impulse is normal and there is no sternal lift. Auscultation at the cardiac apex reveals a loud first heart sound and a mid-diastolic rumbling murmur, with a pre-systolic accentuation and a soft systolic murmur. There is no accentuation of the pulmonary component of the second heart sound. There is no pericardial rub. The lungs are clear and neither liver nor spleen is palpable.

Has examination narrowed down your differential diagnosis?

The clinical findings suggest that this man has mitral stenosis, and this makes the present cluster of symptoms and signs most likely due to a recurrent episode of rheumatic fever. Erythema marginatum is a major criterion for the diagnosis of acute rheumatic fever but is seen in less than 5% of patients. Erythema nodosum is found much more often than erythema marginatum or rheumatic nodules, but is not specific for rheumatic fever. In the context of acute rheumatic fever it represents a reaction to recent streptococcal infection. There remains the possibility of infective endocarditis.

Investigations

Haemoglobin is 107 g/l (10.7 g/dl) and total white blood cell count is 14 600 × 10⁹/l (10³/mm³), with 84% neutrophils, 15% lymphocytes and 1% eosinophils. The erythrocyte sedimentation rate (ESR) is 90 mm/1st hr. The C-reactive protein (CRP) is increased at 87 mg/l and antistreptolysin O (ASO) antibody titre is positive (600 U), while rheumatoid factor is negative. Three blood cultures are negative and urinalysis is normal. A 12-lead ECG shows a sinus rhythm at 110/min and a PR interval of 0.22 sec. A chest X-ray reveals cardiomegaly. A transthoracic echocardiogram shows thickened mitral valve cusps and an abnormal opening pattern of the mitral valve suggestive of

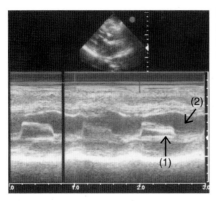

Fig. 39.2 An M mode echo showing typical mitral stenosis (1) with paradoxical movement of the posterior leaflet and thickening of the mitral valve leaflets (2).

mitral valvular stenosis (Fig. 39.2), with a mitral valve area of 1.6 cm². The left ventricle appears dilated but left ventricular systolic function is preserved; there is moderate mitral regurgitation but no vegetations are seen.

Does this narrow down your differential diagnosis?

The investigations suggest that the patient has rheumatic fever with carditis, superadded to pre-existing chronic valvular heart disease. Carditis is suggested because of the tachycardia, a possible new onset of mitral valve regurgitation and a dilated left ventricle on echocardiography. With regard to the diagnosis of rheumatic fever, this young man has two major Jones criteria (Box 39.1), polyarthritis and carditis, and a number of minor criteria, i.e. fever, raised ESR and CRP, leucocytosis and first-degree heart block. He also has evidence of a preceding streptococcal infection — namely, a raised ASO antibody titre. The three negative blood cultures make infective endocarditis unlikely, although endocarditis caused by fastidious organisms cannot be excluded.

How will you treat this patient?

The patient should be treated as a case of rheumatic fever with carditis. If infective endocarditis is suspected, in most cases it would be best to await the results of blood culture before starting antibiotics. In sick patients it is reasonable to begin antibiotic treatment for endocarditis once the blood cultures have been drawn and, if necessary, change the antibiotics after the blood culture results become available. This patient should be kept in bed and given 1.2 million units of benzyl penicillin intramuscularly. He should also be commenced on oral aspirin, three tablets of 325 mg each 6-hourly — a total of 3.8 g daily (60 mg/kg). This should be continued until his ESR has fallen and then gradually tailed off. Given the high-dose aspirin therapy, it is usually prudent to prescribe a proton pump inhibitor too. Since the carditis is not symptomatic, he does not require treatment with diuretics or corticosteroids.

With this therapy, the patient improves rapidly. Within 10 days, his ESR comes down to 25 mm/hr and the left ventricular dilatation on echo screening almost completely regresses. He is discharged but advised not to return to his job, at least until his next review in 2 weeks. He is also advised to take 1.2 million units of benzathine penicillin i.m. once every 3–4 weeks, at least until he is 40 years old. The importance of this prophylaxis is explained to both the patient and his parents. Although oral antibiotics are often used as prophylaxis (phenoxymethylpenicillin, sulfadiazine or erythromycin), it is easier to track the patient's compliance with intramuscular penicillin. In addition, he is warned to tell any doctor or dentist that he consults that he has valvular heart disease, so that precautions could be taken to prevent 'infection in his heart'. He is also advised that, should he develop a fever persisting for over a week, it would be important for him to consult a doctor. At present the mitral stenosis does not require any active intervention, but this may well be required in the years ahead. The young man is told about this and warned of the importance of coming for review at least once a year.

Global issues

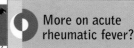

More on acute rheumatic fever?

See Chapter 18 of
Davidson's Principles and Practice of Medicine (20th edn)

- Although acute rheumatic fever (ARF) and its chronic sequela, rheumatic heart disease (RHD), have become rare in the most affluent populations, they continue to be a daily challenge to doctors who work in developing countries, where ARF is still the most common cause of acquired heart disease in childhood and adolescence.

- Poor living conditions with overcrowding and limited access to health care are responsible for the continuing high rate of this eminently preventable disease.

- While ARF peaks in childhood (5–15 years) and adolescence, the prevalence of RHD peaks in adulthood. RHD is responsible for a significant economic burden in developing countries, as sadly it commonly affects the young and the most productive members of society.

- Primary prevention of ARF (which involves providing antibiotic treatment for all symptomatic pharyngitis caused by group A streptococcus) has been unsuccessful because the majority of patients with ARF do not have a sore throat and therefore do not seek medical attention.

- Secondary prevention of ARF (which involves long-term administration of antibiotics to patients with a history of ARF or RHD, to prevent the recurrence of rheumatic fever) is the only proven cost-effective intervention available to date.

- An effective group A streptococcal vaccine (based on M-protein) is not yet on the horizon, and even if the obstacles of serotype coverage and safety were overcome, the cost of the vaccine would make it inaccessible to the populations that need it most.

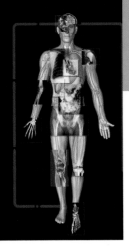

40

A young man with sudden onset of chest pain and breathlessness

M. K. DAGA

Presenting problem

A 26-year-old man, who is tall and thin, presents with a history of sudden-onset pain on the right side of the chest and breathlessness of 1 hour's duration. At the time of onset of his symptoms, he was not carrying out any physical activity and was resting at home. The breathlessness has worsened rapidly over the intervening hour. He has smoked cigarettes for the last 8–9 years. He has never suffered from any significant illness in the past. There is no history of episodic breathlessness or incessant dry cough in the past. He has never been hospitalised for any other illness. He has no history of trauma to the chest and has not undergone any surgical intervention.

BOX 40.1

Differential diagnosis

- Pneumothorax
- Lobar pneumonia
- Acute severe asthma
- Acute pulmonary thromboembolism
- Pleuropericarditis
- Angina or myocardial infarction
- Severe anxiety

What would your differential diagnosis include before examining the patient?

This is a tall, lanky individual with no history of any significant illness in the past. The possible diagnoses are shown in Box 40.1. Pneumothorax would be the most likely diagnosis, given his age and body habitus. The absence of fever and a productive cough makes a community-acquired pneumonia unlikely. Acute asthma must be excluded, but there is no preceding history and he does not report wheeze. If these causes can be excluded, then thromboembolic disease should be considered next. Severe anxiety is very much a diagnosis of exclusion.

Examination

On clinical examination this person has Marfanoid features in the form of arachnodactyly (long, thin 'spider' fingers) and a high arched palate. He has a tachycardia (110/min) with an increased respiratory rate (24 breaths/min); blood pressure is normal. The trachea is central. There are decreased movements on the whole of the right side of the chest and vocal fremitus is decreased. The percussion note is hyper-resonant and breath sounds are absent on the right side of the chest.

Has examination narrowed down your differential diagnosis?

Physical examination reveals signs of disease on the right side of the chest. There is decreased movement of the chest wall, which can occur with either collapse of the lung, pleural effusion or pneumothorax. The combination of absent breath sounds and a resonant percussion note is virtually diagnostic of pneumothorax.

Investigations

A chest X-ray shows a right-sided pneumothorax with a sharply defined edge to the deflated lung and complete translucency (absence of lung markings) between this and the chest wall (Fig. 40.1). The left lung is absolutely normal.

Has the diagnosis been clinched?

A simple chest X-ray confirms the clinical suspicion of pneumothorax. This patient has primary spontaneous pneumothorax. There is rarely a need in such a case for any further investigations. In an older person with pre-existing chronic obstructive pulmonary disease care must be taken to distinguish between a large pre-existing emphysematous bulla and a pneumothorax. In such circumstances, a computed tomography (CT) of the thorax is useful, but this is not required here.

The chest X-ray is important not only to confirm the diagnosis, but also to give a clue to any other underlying pulmonary disease or pleural fluid. It also helps in the planning of treatment of the pneumothorax; if the lung edge is less than 2 cm from the chest wall and the patient is not significantly breathless, then the pneumothorax will resolve without intervention.

How will you treat this patient?

Primary spontaneous pneumothorax in this young man, which seems to occupy more than 15% volume of the hemithorax, cannot be left alone for spontaneous absorption. A 16-gauge needle for percutaneous aspiration should be inserted into the second intercostal space anteriorly and the air should be aspirated. This should lead to a marked improvement in symptoms. If a repeat chest X-ray confirms re-expansion of the lung, the man may be discharged after observation in hospital for 6 hours. However, there remains the possibility that he could have

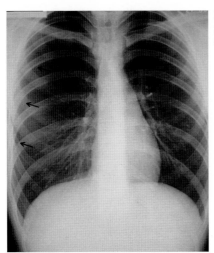

Fig. 40.1 Chest X-ray showing a right pneumothorax. The lung edge is marked by the arrows.

a persistent pleural leak and so he should be advised to return to hospital if his symptoms recur.

If the expansion of the lung is inadequate with simple aspiration or if an underlying chronic lung disease is present, the treatment of choice is intercostal tube drainage. Patients with recurrent pneumothoraces or secondary pneumothorax should be considered for surgical pleurodesis by instilling a sclerosing agent such as tetracycline or doxycycline.

The other issue to consider in this case is the Marfanoid habitus of the individual. Marfan's syndrome is a rare autosomal dominant disorder caused by mutations in the fibrillin gene. The fact that this man has a high arched palate and arachnodactyly does not mean he definitely has Marfan's syndrome, but it should certainly be considered, because the morbidity from cardiovascular disease (aortic disease and mitral incompetence) is substantial. He should, therefore, be referred to a clinical geneticist for further evaluation.

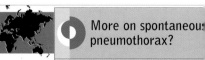

Global issues

More on spontaneous pneumothorax?

- Primary spontaneous pneumothorax is known to occur universally.

- In the majority of cases no definitive aetiology is established, although smokers have an increased risk of developing primary spontaneous pneumothorax.

- Patients should be advised to avoid air travel for 2 weeks after complete expansion of the lung.

- Recurrence of pneumothorax within 1 year occurs in approximately 25% of patients.

See Chapter 19 of
Davidson's Principles and Practice of Medicine
(20th edn)

41

An elderly man with progressive breathlessness and a cough

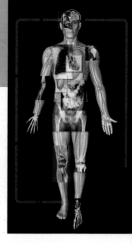

A. T. HILL

Presenting problem

A 62-year-old man is referred by his general practitioner to a respiratory outpatient clinic with a history of cough, sputum production and breathlessness. He has had a persistent cough for the past 12 years and produces a teaspoonful of mucopurulent phlegm on a daily basis. The breathlessness started 1 year previously and has progressively worsened, such that he is now breathless on climbing 12 stairs at a normal pace. He has no nocturnal chest symptoms and has received one course of antibiotics from his GP in the last year. His only past medical history is hypertension, which has been suboptimally controlled due to poor compliance with antihypertensive therapy. His current therapy is atenolol 50 mg once daily. He is a current smoker and has a 44-pack year history. He used to work in the demolition industry but took voluntary redundancy and retired at the age of 55.

What would your differential diagnosis include before examining the patient?

Cough and sputum production for more than 3 months of the year over 2 consecutive years meets the UK Medical Research Council definition of chronic bronchitis. The differential diagnosis should also include bronchiectasis, although patients with bronchiectasis normally have higher volumes of sputum production and suffer recurrent chest infections (this patient expectorates only a teaspoonful of mucopurulent phlegm a day and has had only one exacerbation in the past year).

The cause of the breathlessness is not clear at this stage. In view of the smoking history and the history of chronic bronchitis, he may be suffering from chronic obstructive pulmonary disease (COPD). Asthma should be considered, as the patient is on a β-blocker, but the lack of nocturnal symptoms and the development of progressive breathlessness over the last year is more in keeping with COPD.

He was employed in the demolition industry and thus would have worked with asbestos. The differential diagnosis should include occupational lung disease — asbestos-related pleural thickening or asbestosis (interstitial pulmonary fibrosis due to asbestos).

In view of his non-compliance with the antihypertensive medication, hypertensive left ventricular failure should be excluded, although the lack of nocturnal breathlessness also goes against this diagnosis.

Examination

The patient is breathless on exertion but there is no cyanosis. He has obvious finger clubbing. Respiratory rate is 22 breaths/min, blood pressure is 160/90 mmHg, heart rate is regular at 96/min and oxygen saturations are 94% breathing room air. His jugular venous pulse (JVP) is not elevated. Chest expansion and percussion are normal, but there are mid- to late fine inspiratory crackles on chest auscultation. Both heart sounds are normal and there is no peripheral oedema.

Initial investigations

Initial investigations are shown in Box 41.1.

Have examination and initial investigations narrowed down your differential diagnosis?

The clinical examination has been helpful in this circumstance. The findings are not typical of COPD. With COPD one would have expected hyper-inflated lung fields, reduced chest expansion, hyper-resonance on percussion and reduced breath sounds. The initial investigations confirm that he has poorly controlled hypertension, which has led to left ventricular hypertrophy identified on the electrocardiogram (ECG).

The examination findings of mid- to late inspiratory crackles and finger clubbing point to a diagnosis of pulmonary fibrosis. In view of this man's occupation, the possibility that the pulmonary fibrosis is due to heavy asbestos exposure, i.e. asbestosis, should be considered. Left ventricular failure could also cause the inspiratory crackles

---

BOX 41.1

Initial investigations

ECG	Voltage criteria for left ventricular hypertrophy
Chest radiograph	Indistinct cardiac borders and bilateral reticulonodular shadowing suggestive of pulmonary fibrosis (Fig. 41.1)
Forced expiratory volume in 1 second (FEV$_1$)	1.3 l (46% of predicted)
Forced vital capacity (FVC)	1.6 l (42% of predicted)
FEV$_1$/FVC	81% (normal 73%)

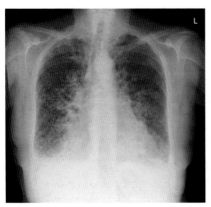

Fig. 41.1 Chest X-ray showing indistinct cardiac borders and bilateral reticulonodular shadowing suggestive of pulmonary fibrosis.

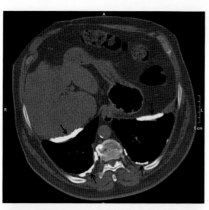

Fig. 41.2 High-resolution CT of the chest (mediastinal windows). There are bilateral pleural plaques (arrows).

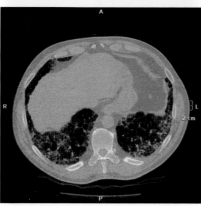

Fig. 41.3 High-resolution CT of the chest (lung windows). There is interlobular and intralobular septal thickening with honeycombing, consistent with pulmonary fibrosis.

but would not be associated with finger clubbing. The typical chest X-ray findings in this type of case are often incorrectly interpreted as left ventricular failure.

Spirometry reveals a moderate to severe restrictive defect. This is the typical pattern seen in pulmonary fibrosis (in patients with COPD an obstructive ventilatory defect would be expected).

Further investigations

An echocardiogram confirms left ventricular hypertrophy, with normal left ventricular function. More detailed lung function tests reveal that total lung capacity is reduced to 53% of predicted. Gas transfer for carbon monoxide is reduced to 50% of predicted. A high-resolution computed tomogram (CT) of the chest (mediastinal windows) reveals bilateral pleural plaques (Fig. 41.2); on the lung windows there is interlobular and intralobular septal thickening with honeycombing, particularly in the lower lobes and in a subpleural position (Fig. 41.3).

Does this narrow down your differential diagnosis?

To diagnose asbestosis, patients should have:

1. Significant asbestos exposure.
2. Suitable lag time (usually 20+ years) between exposure and presentation of illness.
3. Mid- to late inspiratory crackles on examination.
4. Finger clubbing (present in about 40% of cases).
5. A high-resolution CT of the chest showing pulmonary fibrosis predominantly in the lower lobes and in a subpleural distribution. There is usually

interlobular and intralobular septal thickening, and in more advanced cases there is honeycombing. There may be subpleural lines and parenchymal bands. There may be accompanying bilateral pleural thickening and plaques.

6. Lung function tests showing a restrictive defect; in more advanced cases a reduction in carbon monoxide gas transfer is seen.

7. Bronchoalveolar lavage revealing asbestos bodies. This reflects a substantial lung burden with asbestos, but it only establishes the exposure, not the disease.

8. Final confirmation is by histological examination via thoracoscopic or open lung biopsy. This will help differentiate from other causes of pulmonary fibrosis. The Helsinki criteria for the histological diagnosis of asbestosis require at least two asbestos bodies per 5 micron thick tissue section measuring 1 cm^2. There remains controversy about the value of asbestos fibre counts and this is not routinely carried out.

This man is likely to have had significant asbestos exposure while working in the demolition industry, and meets the first six of the above criteria. There is no histological confirmation, but the overall clinical impression is that he has asbestosis.

How will you treat this patient?

Unfortunately, there is no treatment that will reverse the asbestosis. Smoking cessation is critical to reduce the risk of development of both lung cancer and mesothelioma. Supportive treatment is available. Oxygen therapy is helpful in advanced cases. Ambulatory oxygen can help patients leave the house and remain mobile. Long-term oxygen therapy is given when patients' PaO_2 is < 7.3 kPa (55 mmHg). Diuretics are used once cor pulmonale with right ventricular failure develops. Both opiates and benzodiazepines may be useful in the terminal phase of the illness for palliation.

In the UK, asbestosis is an occupational lung disease and is compensatable. Claimants can receive a pension from the Department of Social Security but can also make a civil claim against their former employers. To pursue a civil claim, the claimants have to make a claim within 3 years of knowing the diagnosis.

Global issues

 More on asbestosis?

- Internationally, asbestosis is an important occupational industrial disease. Prevention of asbestos-related disease should be a global priority.

- Chrysotile (a serpentine white asbestos that shears into smaller fibrils) is the most widely used form of asbestos. Straight asbestos fibres (amphiboles) include crocidolite (blue asbestos), amosite (brown asbestos) and tremolite. Russia and Quebec Province in Canada are major producers of chrysotile, while South Africa produces crocidolite and amosite.

See Chapter 19 of
Davidson's Principles and Practice of Medicine (20th edn)

- All forms of asbestos are carcinogenic and can cause lung cancer, mesothelioma and other asbestos-related diseases. Although crocidolite appears to be more potent than others in inducing mesothelioma, all forms have an equal potential to cause bronchogenic carcinoma.

- A detailed occupational history enquiring about asbestos exposure should be sought in all individuals with respiratory disease. Such patients should be targeted for smoking cessation.

42

A businessman with chest pain

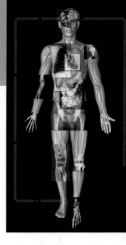

J. A. INNES

Presenting problem

A 65-year-old man, who works for an international hotel group, is referred to the Accident and Emergency department with a 2-week history of intermittent chest pains. He has a history of moderate chronic obstructive pulmonary disease (COPD) and also a 2-year history of prostate cancer, for which he receives androgen-suppressing treatment. Otherwise he was well until 2 weeks prior to admission, when he developed sharp pain on inspiration below the right scapula. This made exercise, coughing and yawning painful. Two days later he developed a mild cough productive of small amounts of yellow sputum. His symptoms settled within 5 days without specific treatment, but on the day of admission a new sharp pain has developed posteriorly, at the base of the left lung. This time the pain is more severe and even breathing at rest hurts.

What would your differential diagnosis include before examining the patient?

Pleuritic pain limiting breathing is usually due to infection, thromboembolism or inflammatory pleuritis. If unilateral, pneumothorax would be another possibility, but it is unlikely in this patient, who has bilateral pains separated in time. In any patient, but particularly in one with underlying COPD, pain which limits coughing will itself predispose towards infection by limiting airway clearance, so the history of yellow sputum does not really narrow the diagnostic possibilities. Inflammatory pleuritis occurs in connective tissue disease, especially systemic lupus erythematosus (SLE), but onset in a male of this age would be very unusual. Thus, the main possibilities are infection (bacterial or viral) causing pleural inflammation and thromboembolism. From the history the patient may be predisposed to thromboembolism, both by his underlying prostatic malignancy and by his occupation (remember to ask about recent long journeys!). The most important feature of this history is the two sequential episodes of pleuritic pain separated in both time and site. This should raise a high index of suspicion with regard to thromboembolism.

Examination

The patient has a modestly elevated respiratory rate (20/min) and is reluctant to take deep breaths due to pain. His temperature is mildly elevated (38.1°C), but he has no pallor or cyanosis. Pulse is 90/min,

BOX 42.1

Initial investigations

Haemoglobin	137 g/l (13.7 g/dl)
WCC	12.1×10^9/l (10^3/mm³)
Oxygen saturation breathing room air	93%
Chest X-ray	Small patch of shadowing at the left base
D-dimer	1.45 mg/l (1450 ng/ml)
Arterial blood gas breathing air	
PO_2	8.5 kPa (64 mmHg)
PCO_2	4.5 kPa (34 mmHg)
H⁺	39 nmol/l (pH 7.41)

there is sinus rhythm and blood pressure is normal, as is the remainder of the cardiovascular examination. Examination of the chest reveals limited expansion on both sides due to discomfort, and a soft pleural rub on inspiration posteriorly, at the left base. There is no detectable abnormality in the abdomen.

Initial investigations

Results of initial investigations are shown in Box 42.1.

Have examination and initial investigations narrowed your differential diagnosis?

In this common clinical situation, the examination has merely confirmed that the pleura are inflamed at the left base, but it has not helped to distinguish the main causes. Low-grade fever is typical in patients with pulmonary infarcts, as well as in those with pneumonic infection. Small pulmonary emboli (PE) commonly cause pleural pain without causing clinical features of right heart failure (raised jugular venous pulse, right ventricular heave, loud P2); these usually occur only with multiple or very large emboli (e.g. 'saddle emboli') obstructing a large fraction of the pulmonary circulation. It is also common for clinical features of deep venous thrombosis (DVT) to be absent in this situation. The diagnosis remains ambiguous after initial investigations. Both pulmonary infarction and infection can produce X-ray patches, modest elevation of the white cell count and type 1 respiratory failure (hypoxia with normal CO_2). The elevated D-dimer is also unhelpful, as this marker is raised by a number of conditions apart from PE and indeed correlates with clinical outcome in pneumonia. Only a low value (below 0.3 mg/l or 300 ng/ml) would have excluded thromboembolism.

Further investigations

 The choice of further investigations is important here. Radionuclide ventilation/perfusion scanning is likely to be unhelpful in this patient, because he has a past history of COPD. This will typically cause multiple areas of matched ventilation and perfusion abnormality obscuring any unmatched perfusion defects. Computed tomogram (CT) pulmonary angiography (Fig. 42.1) is now the investigation of choice in this area.

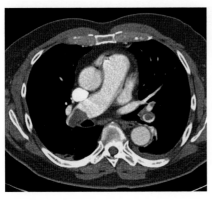

Fig. 42.1 Image from the patient's CT pulmonary angiogram. Thrombus appears as dark filling defects in the right main pulmonary artey and also in the left lower lobe pulmonary artery, with a bright crescent of contrast surrounding. it. There are also small areas of pleural reaction posteriorly on both sides corresponding to the sites of the patient's chest pains.

Does this narrow down your differential diagnosis?

The finding of thrombus, appearing as filling defects in otherwise contrast-filled lobar or segmental pulmonary arteries, is diagnostic of PE.

How will you treat this patient?

The main risk to the patient is of further major PE; therefore, as soon as there is a suspicion of thromboembolism from the history, the correct treatment is immediate formal anticoagulation using subcutaneous low molecular weight heparin (LMWH) pending further investigations. Oxygen should be given to relieve hypoxia, and analgesics to ease pleural pain. There is evidence that continuing LMWH for at least 5 days while commencing oral anticoagulation leads to improved clearance of thrombus. If purulent sputum persists, it may be prudent to add antibiotics such as amoxicillin, as pulmonary infarcts easily become infected. In this patient it would also be appropriate to reassess the prostatic carcinoma, in case it has spread to involve pelvic veins, precipitating his thromboembolism. More commonly, however, thrombosis with malignancy arises due to systemic activation of coagulation by the tumour.

Global issues

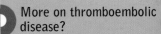

More on thromboembolic disease?

- PE and DVT are different manifestations of the same disease process, which is collectively known as venous thromboembolism (VTE).

- The diagnosis of PE is frequently missed and is difficult to confirm in resource-limited settings, due to non-availability of most of the diagnostic tools. Untreated PE is associated with a high mortality.

See Chapter 19 of
Davidson's Principles and Practice of Medicine
(20th edn)

- When compared with unfractionated heparin (UFH), LMWH preparations are safe, efficacious and cost-effective for the treatment of acute VTE. However, at present, the evidence to support the use of LMWH in the management of massive PE is limited.

- Anticoagulant prophylaxis significantly reduces the risk for VTE in at-risk hospitalised medical patients.

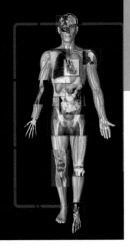

43

A middle-aged woman with haemoptysis and a previous history of tuberculosis

S. K. SHARMA

Presenting problem

A 45-year-old lady presents with a 3-month history of cough, expectoration and haemoptysis. She also complains of low-grade fever in the evenings. She has anorexia and has lost about 10 kg in weight during the last 2 months. She is a heavy cigarette smoker. Four years ago she received treatment for sputum smear-positive fibrocavitary pulmonary tuberculosis involving the left lower lobe. This involved directly observed thrice-weekly intermittent treatment with rifampicin, isoniazid, pyrazinamide and ethambutol for 2 months, and rifampicin and isoniazid for the subsequent 4 months.

BOX 43.1
Causes of haemoptysis in a patient with past history of tuberculosis
Reactivation tuberculosis
Reinfection tuberculosis
Post-tuberculosis bronchiectasis
Aspergilloma
Scar carcinoma

What would your differential diagnosis include before examining the patient?

This patient had sputum smear-positive pulmonary tuberculosis 4 years ago and received a full course of antituberculosis treatment. She now presents again with a history of fever, toxaemic symptoms, haemoptysis, loss of appetite and weight loss. Bleeding from the cavity wall, rupture of Rasmussen's aneurysm (i.e. the dilatation of a small to medium-sized pulmonary artery in a tuberculosis cavity), direct erosion of capillaries/arteries by granulomatous inflammation, tuberculosis, endobronchiolitis, broncholith and cavernolith have all been postulated to be the mechanisms responsible for haemoptysis in patients with pulmonary tuberculosis. The causes of haemoptysis in a patient with a past history of tuberculosis are listed in Box 43.1.

Examination

Physical examination reveals mild pallor and crepitations in the infra-mammary and infra-axillary areas on the left side. There is no evidence of peripheral lymphadenopathy. Physical examination is otherwise unremarkable.

Has examination narrowed down your differential diagnosis?

Physical examination points to a lesion in the left lower lobe. There is no other localisation clue. Physical examination can sometimes be unremarkable in patients with reactivation/reinfection tuberculosis, and several other conditions should be considered under the differential diagnosis. Further investigations are needed.

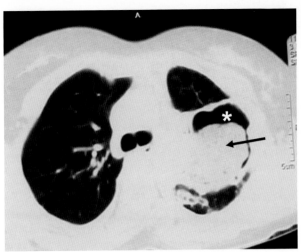

Fig. 43.1 CT of the chest (lung window) showing a fungus ball (arrow) in a cavity in the left lower lobe. A semicircular, crescentic air shadow (asterisk) can also be seen around the radio-opaque fungus ball (air-crescent sign).

Further investigations

The patient is human immunodeficiency virus (HIV)-seronegative. Full blood count, serum biochemistry, urine examination and abdominal ultrasonography are normal. An oral glucose tolerance test rules out a diagnosis of diabetes mellitus. Sputum smear examination does not reveal acid-fast bacilli or malignant cells, and sputum culture does not grow mycobacteria. Sputum examination does, however, reveal fragments of fungal hyphae and sputum culture grows Aspergillus fumigatus. A chest X-ray reveals a left lower zone fibrocavitary lesion. Computed tomography (CT) of the chest (Fig. 43.1) reveals a cavity in the left lower lobe containing a radio-opaque shadow with a semicircular air crescent around it. The differential diagnosis for this radiographic presentation is shown in Box 43.2. When the CT is repeated with the patient in the prone position, the fungal ball is observed to have changed its position. An intradermal skin test with extracts of Aspergillus fumigatus is positive. Serum precipitins (double diffusion in gel method) and immunoglobulin G (IgG) against Aspergillus fumigatus are positive.

Does this narrow down the differential diagnosis?

Though lower lobe involvement is uncommon in immuno-competent individuals, the patient has had left lower lobe sputum smear-positive pulmonary tuberculosis in the past for which she received adequate standard treatment. Since she has been sputum smear-negative on three occasions, reactivation/reinfection pulmonary tuberculosis appears unlikely. The radiological evidence of the cavity in the left lower lobe, the positive skin test and the mycological and serological results strongly favour the diagnosis of aspergilloma in a tuberculosis cavity.

BOX 43.2
Differential diagnosis of a radio-opaque shadow in the lungs with a semicircular air crescent shadow ('air-crescent sign')
Fungus ball
Organised haematoma or pus inside a cavity
Hydatid cyst
Lung cancer

A fungus ball may be present for a long period without producing any clinical symptoms and may be incidentally detected. Most patients develop haemoptysis, which can sometimes be life-threatening, due to various causes such as mechanical friction, secretion of endotoxin with haemolytic properties, an anticoagulant factor derived from *Aspergillus*, local vasculitis and direct invasion of the blood vessels in the cavity by the fungal ball. Other clinical features include cough, weight loss, anorexia, fever and dyspnoea.

How will you treat this patient?

There is no consensus regarding the ideal treatment for aspergilloma. Systemic antifungal treatment is ineffective. Local instillation of antifungal agents using a bronchoscope has been used with varying results. Bronchial artery embolisation has been used for the management of recurrent haemoptysis in some patients. Some authorities have advocated surgery because of the potential for haemoptysis, which can sometimes be massive. Surgery is indicated if the haemoptysis is repetitive, severe or life-threatening. Asymptomatic patients and those with mild infrequent haemoptysis should be carefully monitored.

Global issues

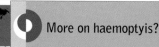 More on haemoptyis?

- Fungus balls are particularly common in areas of endemic tuberculosis, e.g. India, sub-Saharan Africa.

- HIV infection has contributed to an increasing prevalence of tuberculosis.

- In Western countries, fungal balls have been described in cystic fibrosis, sarcoidosis, bronchiectasis, asbestosis, histoplasmosis and bronchial cysts.

- The 'air-crescent sign' can be identified by plain film chest tomography, as well as by CT.

See Chapter 19 of
Davidson's Principles and Practice of Medicine
(20th edn)

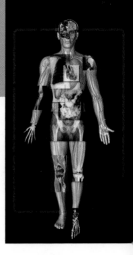

44

A solitary radiographic pulmonary lesion in a middle-aged man

S. K. SHARMA

Presenting problem

A 55-year-old asymptomatic man is referred to the chest clinic because a solitary lesion has been detected in the left lower hemithorax on a chest X-ray taken as part of pre-operative evaluation for hernia surgery about 2 months ago. He is a heavy cigarette smoker who is healthy, but for left-sided indirect inguinal hernia. Otherwise, his general health has been good in the past and he is not taking any form of medication. There is no history of contact with animals or international travel.

What would your differential diagnosis include before examining the patient?

The evaluation of a solitary pulmonary radiographic lesion in an asymptomatic patient is a common diagnostic dilemma. The goal in evaluating such a lesion is to distinguish a benign from a potentially malignant lesion. Considering the age of this patient and his smoking habit, malignant conditions like bronchogenic carcinoma and solitary metastasis would top the list of possibilities (Box 44.1), but benign conditions such as tuberculosis, fungal infections, hydatid disease and Wegener's granulomatosis, among others, must be ruled out.

Examination

The patient is apyrexial, and there is no evidence of Horner's syndrome, cutaneous lesions or peripheral lymphadenopathy. No abnormal masses are noted on palpation of the abdomen and examination of the respiratory system is normal. In short, the physical examination is unremarkable.

Has examination narrowed down your differential diagnosis?

The physical examination is not infrequently unremarkable in patients with a solitary pulmonary radiographic lesion. Narrowing down of the differential diagnosis requires more investigations.

Further investigations

Full blood count, serum biochemistry, urine examination and abdominal ultrasonography are normal. Sputum smear does not reveal acid-fast bacilli or malignant cells, and sputum culture does not grow mycobacteria or fungi. This man is human immunodeficiency virus (HIV)-seronegative. A tuberculin skin test (5 tuberculin units), complement fixation and enzyme-linked immunosorbent assay (ELISA) tests for hydatid disease, a serological panel for coccidioidomycosis, antineutrophil cytoplasmic antibodies (ANCA) and rheumatoid factor (RF) are all negative. A repeat chest X-ray (Fig. 44.1) confirms a solitary pulmonary radiographic lesion in the left lower zone. There is no evidence of calcification.

Does this narrow down the differential diagnosis?

The patient has been asymptomatic and apyrexial throughout and there is no evidence of immunosuppression. Therefore, a lung abscess, pneumonia or septic embolism is unlikely. The negative serological panel for fungal infections, together with no history of travel to areas where fungal infections such as coccidiodomycosis are endemic, argues against possible fungal causes. The absence of eye- and kidney-related symptoms and arthralgias, normal urinalysis and negative ANCA and RF tests rule out Wegener's granulomatosis and rheumatoid arthritis as possible causes. As the patient is a heavy smoker and the available investigations are inconclusive, a further diagnostic evaluation is required.

Definitive investigations

Fibreoptic bronchoscopy is unremarkable. The bronchoscopic aspirate does not reveal acid-fast bacilli or malignant cells.

A contrast-enhanced computed tomographic (CT) scan of the chest (Fig. 44.2) verifies a solitary, smooth, round lesion in the lung, with no evidence of calcification. The lesion shows an attenuation value of 18 Hounsfield units (HU) after the administration of intravenous contrast. There is no evidence of mediastinal lymphadenopathy. The attenuation value of 18 HU argues against cystic lesions such as hydatid cyst or lung abscess and suggests a high probability of a malignant lesion. (Normal lung has attenuation values between −400 and −600; cystic lesions are close to zero.) The CT findings in patients with benign and malignant solitary pulmonary nodules are contrasted in Box 44.2. In a patient with a solitary radiographic pulmonary lesion, round margins, the presence of central, laminated, diffuse or 'popcorn' calcification, the presence of fat within the lesion, homogeneous attenuation, the presence of satellite nodules and a CT density value of less than 15 HU all favour a benign aetiology. In the present patient, the lesion has a smooth round margin without spiculation. However, about 20% of malignant lesions can have a round margin. Positron emission tomography (which has high sensitivity and specificity in evaluating lung lesions) is not available at the centre where the patient is being evaluated, as is the case in most developing countries.

A CT-guided percutaneous needle biopsy reveals a well-differentiated squamous cell carcinoma. Abdominal ultrasonography, CT of the brain and a radionuclide

---

BOX 44.1

Common aetiological causes of a solitary radiographic pulmonary lesion

Malignant causes

- Bronchogenic carcinoma
- Lymphoma
- Carcinoid tumour
- Metastasis

Benign causes

- Congenital
  Bronchogenic cyst
  Bronchial atresia
- Infections
  Granulomatous infections, e.g. mycobacterial (tuberculosis), fungal (coccidioidomycosis)
  Lung abscess
  Round pneumonia
  Septic embolisation
  Nocardiosis
  Parasitic, e.g. hydatid disease, *Dirofilaria* (dog heart worm)
  Infected bulla
- Connective tissue disorders
  Wegener's granulomatosis
  Rheumatoid arthritis (necrobiotic nodule)
- Vascular
  Arteriovenous malformation
  Pulmonary infarction
  Pulmonary artery aneurysm
  Pulmonary venous varix
  Haematoma
- Airway diseases
  Mucocoele
- Neoplasms
  Hamartoma
  Inflammatory pseudotumour
- Unknown aetiology
  Sarcoidosis

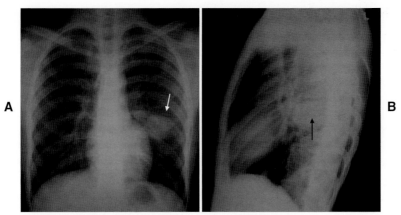

Fig. 44.1 Chest radiograph showing a solitary pulmonary radiographic lesion (arrows) in the left lower zone. A. Postero-anterior view. B. Lateral view.

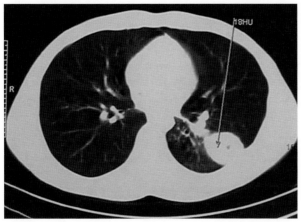

Fig. 44.2 Contrast-enhanced spiral CT of the chest showing an enhancing (18 HU) solitary pulmonary lesion. There is no evidence of mediastinal lymphadenopathy.

bone scan do not reveal any evidence of metastatic disease. In view of the patient's age and smoking history, pre-operative pulmonary function tests are carried out and found to be normal. Cardiac status evaluation, including an electrocardiogram and echocardiography, are normal.

How will you treat this patient?

Unfortunately, the majority of patients with bronchogenic carcinoma of squamous cell histology are inoperable by the time the diagnosis is made. This patient is lucky in that his solitary radiographic pulmonary lesion has been identified incidentally and confirmed to be a primary bronchogenic carcinoma. There is no evidence of involvement of central mediastinal structures or tumour spread to distant sites. Thus, the patient has stage I disease (N0, M0, tumour confined within visceral pleura). He does not have any significant comorbid condition and his cardiac status and respiratory reserve are adequate to allow a surgical resection.

Though the overall prognosis in bronchogenic carcinoma is very poor, with around 80% of patients dying within 1 year of diagnosis, patients with a well-differentiated squamous cell carcinoma which has not metastasised are amenable to surgical treatment and have the best prognosis. This patient should be advised to have surgical resection of the tumour, as this carries the best hope of long-term survival; the 5-year survival rate in stage I disease is over 75%. Many patients

CT findings in solitary benign and malignant lesions

Variable	Benign more likely	Malignant more likely
Size	< 3 cm	> 3 cm
	80% of benign nodules are < 2 cm in size	42% of malignant nodules are < 2 cm in size
Growth (defined as ≥ 26% increase in diameter)	Doubling time < 1 month or > 18 months	Doubling time 1–18 months
Margins	Smooth, well-defined	Spiculated, lobulated margins
Satellite lesions	Frequent	Rare
Calcification	Frequently present	Rare
Presence of fat	50% hamartomas will have fat detectable on thin section CT	Seldom seen
Cavitation	Frequent in tuberculosis, Wegener's granulomatosis, pulmonary infarction and lung abscess	Rare, although squamous cell carcinoma can cavitate
Air bronchograms or bubbly low attenuation	May be rarely seen in organising pneumonia, sarcoidosis, pulmonary infarcts	Frequently seen in adenocarcinoma, especially localised bronchoalveolar carcinoma

with squamous cell carcinoma have undetectable microscopic metastases at diagnosis. After surgery, this patient should also receive adjuvant chemotherapy with carboplatin- or cisplatin-based regimens.

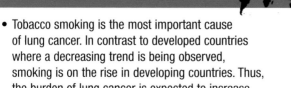

Global issues

More on the solitary radiographic pulmona lesion?

See Chapter 19 of
Davidson's Principles and Practice of Medicine
(20th edn)

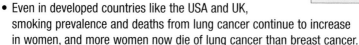

- Tobacco smoking is the most important cause of lung cancer. In contrast to developed countries where a decreasing trend is being observed, smoking is on the rise in developing countries. Thus, the burden of lung cancer is expected to increase in the developing world in the years to come.

- Even in developed countries like the USA and UK, smoking prevalence and deaths from lung cancer continue to increase in women, and more women now die of lung cancer than breast cancer.

- In spite of the advent of CT imaging, the widespread availability of fibre-optic bronchoscopy and facilities for histopathological and cytopathological diagnosis, even in developed countries patients with lung cancer too often present late in the disease, when it is inoperable and only palliative treatment is possible. These facilities are not widely available in developing countries; given that tobacco smoking is increasing there, lung cancer, detected at a stage where nothing other than palliative care will be possible, is likely to emerge as a major public health problem.

45

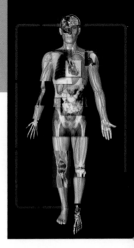

An obese middle-aged man with snoring and day-time sleepiness

P. T. REID

Presenting problem

During the assessment of a 40-year-old man with hypertension, systematic enquiry reveals a history of excessive day-time sleepiness and poor concentration. He has no other symptoms. However, his wife reports that he snores loudly and that, on occasion, she has noticed he appears to stop breathing and she shakes him to make sure he is alive. He has smoked 20 cigarettes per day for 30 years, drinks 30 units of alcohol per week and is overweight. His high blood pressure is treated with lisinopril and bendroflumethiazide. His work involves periods on night shift and he is concerned that he has fallen asleep behind the wheel of the car when sitting at traffic lights. He lives at home with his wife; they have two young children aged 6 months and 3 years.

What would your differential diagnosis include before examining this patient?

Enquiry into the sleep history is good practice during any assessment. This man may be experiencing fragmentation of normal sleep through shift working or is having poor-quality sleep while he raises his young family. However, one of the most important and treatable causes of excessive day-time sleepiness is obstructive sleep apnoea hypopnoea syndrome (OSAHS) and this should be at the forefront of any clinician's mind. Other causes of excessive day-time tiredness include depression, hypothyroidism, certain drugs such as β-blockers or selective serotonin re-uptake inhibitors, and excessive use of sedatives or stimulants. Periodic limb movement disorder, narcolepsy and idiopathic hypersomnolence should also be considered.

Examination and initial investigations

The patient is 1.63 m tall, weighs 110 kg and has marked central obesity. His mandible and tongue appear normal and inspection of the upper airway reveals no evidence of nasal or pharyngeal obstruction. He is in sinus rhythm and his blood pressure is 180/110 mmHg. No abnormal findings are noted on examination of the respiratory, cardiovascular or neurological systems.

Simple spirometry reveals a mild obstructive ventilatory defect with no significant reversibility (Box 45.1) and the Epworth Sleepiness Scale (ESS) is 17/24. Thyroid function tests are normal.

Have examination and initial investigations narrowed down your differential diagnosis?

The most likely diagnosis remains OSAHS. In this condition, the upper airway collapses intermittently and repeatedly during sleep. Partial obstruction results in snoring; complete collapse requires an increased respiratory effort to overcome the obstruction, resulting in a transient wakening of the patient. This pattern occurs repeatedly throughout the night, resulting in poor-quality sleep, excessive day-time sleepiness and poor concentration. The condition is more common in men, particularly if they are obese (this patient has a body mass index of 41.4) and have a collar size > 17 inches (42.5 cm). Abnormalities in the anatomy of the upper airway may increase the likelihood of obstruction, such as an abnormally small mandible, macroglossia, large tonsils or uvula. Examination should also consider whether there are any features of hypothyroidism, acromegaly or Marfan's syndrome.

The ESS is a validated questionnaire for assessing the likelihood of falling asleep in a variety of situations. The maximum score is 24. All patients, and their partners, should complete an Epworth questionnaire; an ESS > 10 suggests significant day-time sleepiness and should prompt referral to a sleep service.

Further investigations

The patient undergoes a formal sleep study. Figure 45.1 details the polsomography (PSG) and shows multiple apnoeic and hypopnoeic events (apnoea being a 10-second breath hold, and hypopnoea being a 10-second event where there is continued breathing, but ventilation is reduced by at least 50% from the previous baseline during sleep). The apnoea/hypopnoea index (AHI) is 63.4. The oximetry trace shows multiple episodes of desaturation, with the lowest oxygen saturation being 57%. There is no evidence of periodic leg movements. A diagnosis of obstructive sleep apnoea (OSA) is made when the AHI score is more than 5 events/hour, while the diagnosis of OSAHS requires the additional presence of day-time sleepiness.

Does this narrow down your differential diagnosis?

Sleep studies confirm the diagnostic suspicion and provide an indication of the severity. The study demonstrates that this patient has OSAHS and the AHI of 63.4 indicates severe disease. PSG is expensive and more limited sleep studies (e.g. a measure of

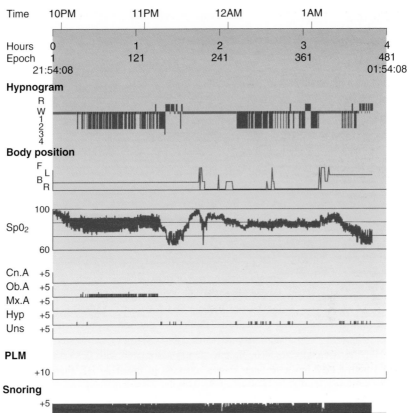

Fig. 45.1 The use of polsomography (PSG) allows the simultaneous recording of breathing and sleep pattern over a period of time (in this example, over 4 hours). Typical recordings include an electroencephalogram (not shown here), a measure of respiratory airflow, thoraco-abdominal movement (allowing identification of hypopnoeas and apnoeas) and oxygen saturation (allowing the identification of significant desaturation events). Some centres also record body position (front, back, left and right) and the occurrence of snoring. In this case, the patient experiences multiple apnoeic and hypopnoeic events; the apnoea/hypopnoea index (AHI) is 63.4 (Box 45.2). The oximetry trace shows multiple episodes of desaturation, with the lowest $SaO2$ being 57% (Box 45.3). There is no evidence of periodic leg movements (PLM).

airflow, thoraco-abdominal movement, oximetry and heart rate) are often sufficient for first-line investigation. Oximetry alone is rarely adequate.

How will you treat this patient?

The AHI provides an indication of the severity of OSAHS and current evidence suggests that patients with an AHI ≥ 15 or a 4% oxygen saturation dip rate at the level of > 10 per hour benefit from treatment. This man should be advised to lose weight (although this is rarely successful) and avoid alcohol, which exacerbates the condition. He should be referred for establishment of continuous positive airways pressure (CPAP), which functions as a pneumatic splint preventing upper airway collapse during sleep. Treatment with CPAP has been shown to improve day-time sleepiness, cognitive function, vigilance, mood and quality of life. The main problem with CPAP therapy is adherence and it is important to review the

Respiratory events (REM and non-REM sleep)

Parameter	REM	Non-REM	Sleep
Obstructive apnoeas	0	46	71
Hypopnoeas	9	23	42
AHI (hr)	–	–	63.4

(AHI = apnoea/hypopnoea index; REM = rapid eye movement)

BOX 45.3

SaO₂ summary

SaO₂ awake average	96%
Lowest SaO₂	67%
Average SaO₂ desaturation	9%
Number of desaturations ≥ 4%	75

patient with this in mind. Use for less than 2 hours per night suggests long-term compliance is likely to be poor. Intra-oral devices are often considered for patients with mild OSAHS and those patients unable to tolerate CPAP. Surgery may be considered in carefully selected patients.

Patients with OSAHS and excessive day-time sleepiness are at increased risk of road traffic accidents. In the UK, the law requires that all patients with OSAHS should inform the Driver Vehicle and Licensing Authority (DVLA) of the diagnosis. Driving is permitted, provided the patient demonstrates satisfactory control of symptoms.

Hypertension appears to be independently associated with OSAHS and treatment with CPAP has also been shown to assist in lowering BP, thereby potentially helping to lower the risk of cardiovascular events or stroke.

Global issues

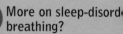 **More on sleep-disorder breathing?**

See Chapter 19 of
Davidson's Principles and Practice of Medicine
(20th edn)

- OSAHS is an emerging public health problem world-wide because of its significant association with obesity, hypertension, insulin resistance and increased cardiovascular morbidity.

- In general, the disease often remains undiagnosed because of a low level of awareness among primary physicians.

- Prevalence of the disease in the Western population is approximately 4% in males and 2% in females.

- Truncal obesity, increased neck circumference (43 cm in males and 40 cm in females), male gender, increasing age (up to 65 years), hypothyroidism, acromegaly and, in the Chinese population, craniofacial features that compromise the upper airway are important risk factors.

- A clinical diagnosis of OSA may be made on the basis of a characteristic history (snoring and day-time sleepiness) and physical examination (anthropometry and neck circumference), but overnight PSG is the gold standard investigation to confirm the diagnosis. Access to PSG may be limited in resource-poor countries.

- Nasal CPAP is the usual first-line treatment but is costly.

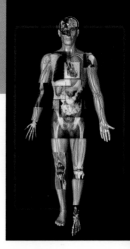

46

A young man with a fever and right-sided chest pain

S. K. SHARMA

Presenting problem

A 25-year-old male presents to the Accident and Emergency department with a high-grade fever, sweating and rapidly worsening breathlessness over the last 24 hours. Over the preceding 2 days, he has developed a cough with scanty sputum, hiccoughs and right-sided chest pain that is stabbing in nature, radiates to the right shoulder and is worse on deep breathing and coughing. He also recollects being tired and having vague discomfort in the right upper abdomen over the last week. He has had no diarrhoea. He is otherwise a healthy bank clerk who does not suffer from any illness. He is a life-long non-smoker and a tee-totaller.

What would your differential diagnosis include before examining the patient?

When an otherwise healthy young male presents with right-sided pleuritic chest pain and a fever, the differential diagnosis includes pleurisy, pneumonia, pulmonary infarction and pneumothorax. When a patient presenting with pleuritic chest pain and fever subsequently develops progressive breathlessness, the possibility of acute pleurisy progressing to pleural effusion is most likely. Radiation of the pain to the right shoulder and a history of hiccoughs indicate involvement of the diaphragm. Considering the preceding history of right-sided upper abdominal discomfort and the subsequent development of right-sided pleurisy, the possibility of an underlying subdiaphragmatic or hepatic lesion with thoracic complications should also be kept in mind.

Examination

Physical examination reveals mild pallor. The patient appears restless and uncomfortable but is alert. His blood pressure is 100/68 mmHg with a pulse of 110/min and a temperature of 38.2°C. He is tachypnoeic, with a respiratory rate of 36 breaths/min and oxygen saturation is 88% while the patient is breathing ambient air. On respiratory examination, the trachea is shifted to the left side and the apical impulse is shifted laterally. The lower intercostal spaces on the right side appear full. The right side of the chest moves less with respiration, and tactile vocal fremitus is reduced on this side. Deep palpation of the chest reveals tenderness of the anterior intercostal spaces on the right side. On percussion, a stony dull note is elicited on the right side and this dullness does not shift with a change in posture. On auscultation, the

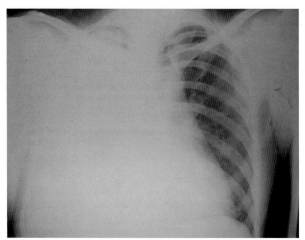

Fig. 46.1 Chest X-ray (postero-anterior view) showing a massive right-sided pleural effusion.

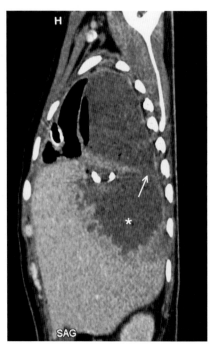

Fig. 46.2 CT scan of the abdomen showing a hypo-intense, large solitary lesion in the right lobe of the liver (asterisk) penetrating the diaphragm and rupturing into the right pleural space (arrow).

breath sounds and the vocal resonance are almost absent on the right side. There is no succussion splash. Abdominal examination reveals an enlarged and markedly tender liver that is 6 cm below the right costal margin. There is no splenomegaly or ascites. Cardiovascular and neurological examination is normal, as is the remainder of the physical examination.

Has examination narrowed down your differential diagnosis?

Physical examination points to a right-sided empyema. It is probably due to the rupture of a pyogenic or an amoebic liver abscess, a hydatid cyst of the liver, a hepatic cold abscess, or a subdiaphragmatic abscess into the right pleural space.

Further investigations

The patient is human immunodeficiency virus (HIV)-seronegative. A full blood count reveals a neutrophilic leucocytosis. Serum biochemistry and urine examination are normal. A sputum smear does not reveal acid-fast bacilli or amoebae. A tuberculin skin test (5 tuberculin units) is negative. Serological tests for antinuclear and rheumatoid factors are negative. A chest X-ray (Fig. 46.1) reveals a massive right-sided pleural effusion. An echocardiogram is normal. Ultrasonography of the abdomen reveals a large non-homogeneous, hypo-echoic, oval mass with well-defined borders in the right lobe of the liver. A computed tomographic (CT) scan (Fig. 46.2) reveals a hypo-intense, large solitary lesion in the right lobe of the liver penetrating the diaphragm and rupturing into the right pleural space. The appropriate site for a thoracocentesis is localised on ultrasonography of the chest and the area is marked.

After securing written informed consent, a diagnostic thoracocentesis is carried out under local anaesthesia and reveals reddish-brown pus. The pus is sterile on culture and does not reveal acid-fast bacilli. On careful microscopic examination of a saline preparation of the empyema pus, an occasional amoebic trophozoite is identified. The immunoglobulin M (IgM) enzyme-linked immunosorbent assay (ELISA) for the detection of Entamoeba histolytica antigens (sensitivity 99% and specificity 95%) and antibody detection by immunofluorescence (sensitivity > 94% and specificity > 95%) tests are positive, confirming a diagnosis of amoebic abscess.

Does this narrow down your differential diagnosis?

Yes; the matter is now settled. The differential diagnosis of empyema thoracis is listed in Box 46.1. The modes of development of pleuropulmonary amoebiasis are shown in Box 46.2 and the thoracic manifestations of an amoebic liver abscess are listed in Box 46.3. Abdominal ultrasonography and a CT indicate a single abscess in the right lobe of the liver. The absence of internal septations or daughter cysts rules out a hydatid cyst. The solitary nature of the lesion, together with its classical location in the right lobe of the liver, points to a diagnosis of amoebic liver abscess. The presence of trophozoites in the empyema pus and serological evidence of infection with *Entamoeba histolytica* confirm that our patient has an amoebic liver abscess that has ruptured through the diaphragm into the right pleural space, resulting in empyema thoracis.

BOX 46.1

Differential diagnosis of empyema thoracis

- Tuberculosis empyema
- Pyogenic empyema
- Lung abscess
- Hydatid disease of the lung
- Malignant disease
  Bronchogenic carcinoma
  Pleural metastasis
  Lymphoma
- Pulmonary infarction
- Subdiaphragmatic causes
  e.g. Rupture of pyogenic
  subdiaphragmatic
  abscess, amoebic liver
  abscess, pyogenic liver
  abscess, pancreatitis
- Connective tissue
  disorders
  e.g. Systemic
  lupus erythematosus
- Post-myocardial infarction

BOX 46.2

Modes of development of pleuropulmonary amoebiasis

Primary (rare)

- Aspiration of cysts/
  trophozoites or inhalation
  of dust containing cysts of
  amoeba

Secondary (rare)

- Haematogenous spread
  from the colon (may spare
  the liver)

Tertiary (most common)

- Extension from the
  amoebic liver abscess by
  contiguous involvement

Thoracic manifestations of an amoebic liver abscess

Pleuropulmonary

- Consolidation
- Lung abscess
- Hepatico-bronchial, hepatico-bronchopulmonary fistula
- Reactive pleural effusion
- Empyema thoracis

Pericardial

- Acute (cardiac tamponade)
- Chronic (Progressive suppurative effusion)

How will you treat this patient?

The patient is treated with metronidazole (800 mg 8-hourly i.v., for 10 days) and an oral luminal amoebicide, diloxanide furoate (500 mg 8-hourly for 10 days). The empyema thoracis is managed with closed-tube thoracostomy, in which an intercostal tube is connected to an underwater seal. By the 10th day, the patient recovers rapidly and repeat ultrasonography of the abdomen shows a significant reduction in the size of the abscess cavity.

Management of an amoebic liver abscess is usually medical. If the liver abscess is large or threatens to burst, if it has ruptured into the pleural or pericardial space (common with left-sided abscess of the liver), or if the response to chemotherapy is not as prompt as expected, then percutaneous aspiration or catheter drainage is required and can be repeated if necessary. Radiographic monitoring of the abdomen by ultrasonography or CT can help in the management. Rarely, surgical intervention is required in some patients. If there is good clinical resolution after instituting appropriate treatment, the mere presence of a lesion in the liver on radiographic monitoring should not prompt hasty intervention, as amoebic liver abscesses may take up to 1 year to heal completely.

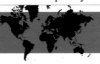

Global issues

More on acute empyer

- Amoebiasis, caused by the protozoan parasite, *Entamoeba histolytica*, is the second leading cause of death from parasitic disease world-wide. Classically, an amoebic liver abscess is solitary and is located in the postero-superior surface of the right lobe of the liver.

- In areas where amoebiasis is highly endemic, the possibility of a right-sided thoracic lesion being due to amoebiasis should be kept in mind, especially as specific curative treatment is available.

- In non-endemic areas, pleuropulmonary amoebiasis should be considered in the differential diagnosis of a patient who develops a right-sided empyema thoracis after travelling to an endemic area. Although a history of previous diarrhoea is usually forthcoming, amoebic liver abscess can develop without a past history of intestinal amoebiasis.

- A left-sided amoebic liver abscess can rarely rupture into the pericardium resulting in severe chest pain, breathlessness and cardiac tamponade with shock. This can be fatal.

- Amoebic liver abscess, especially in patients with thoracic complications, was previously associated with a high mortality rate. The widespread availability of ultrasonography and CT, and effective medical treatment have resulted in a significant decrease in the mortality caused by this condition. However, due to a lack of awareness of the condition, the diagnosis is often missed, resulting in prolonged ill health and death.

See Chapter 19 of

Davidson's Principles and Practice of Medicine
(20th edn)

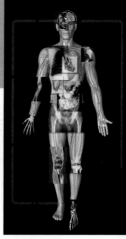

47

A young man with neck swelling, bilateral exophthalmos and proximal myopathy

T. DAS

Presenting problem

A 32-year-old male attends the medical outpatient department with a history of tremor, palpitations, sweating and gradual weight loss for the last 18 months. He also complains of a painless swelling in the front of his neck for 1 year, along with bulging of the eyeballs for the last 6 months. The patient reports difficulty in walking upstairs and in combing his hair for 6 months. He has no significant past history, although his sister is on treatment for what he thinks is an underactive thyroid. He is a non-smoker and is married with two children. There is no recent exposure to any iodine-containing medication.

What would your differential diagnosis include before examining the patient?

Thyrotoxicosis seems a racing certainty here! Other differential diagnoses, such as anxiety neurosis, heart failure due to primary cardiac disease, febrile illnesses, toxic delirium and phaeochromocytoma, can be dismissed.

Examination

The patient is emaciated and his eyes are staring. He is a little pale and has a fine tremor of the hands. A moderate goitre is present. It is diffuse, firm and painless with a bruit. His pulse is 130/min with regular rhythm and blood pressure is 140/70 mmHg. The skin is warm and moist. There is bilateral lid lag and exophthalmos; eye movements are normal and there is no diplopia (Fig. 47.1). He weighs 38 kg. There is mild weakness of the muscles of the hip and shoulder girdles without much wasting. The tendon reflexes are brisk. Other systemic examination is unremarkable.

BOX 47.1

Causes of thyrotoxicosis

- Graves' disease
- Multinodular goiter
- Autonomous thyroid nodule
- Thyroiditis (subacute, post-partum)
- Iodine-induced, e.g. amiodarone
- Factitious thyrotoxicosis (exogenous levothyroxine)
- Thyroid cancer (very rare)

Has examination narrowed down your differential diagnosis?

This patient has clinical features of thyrotoxicosis. The causes are shown in Box 47.1. With bilateral exophthalmos and a diffuse goitre, the diagnosis can only really be Graves' disease. Thyrotoxicosis per se causes lid lag, but

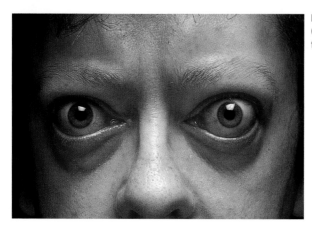

Fig. 47.1 A patient with Graves' disease. Note the exophthalmos.

only Graves' disease is associated with proptosis. Eye disease occurs in about 50% of people with Graves' disease and so determining the cause of thyrotoxicosis may not be as straightforward in someone with absent eye signs. A smooth, diffuse goitre is suggestive of Graves' disease, but again this may not always be present. Toxic multinodular goitre and solitary toxic adenomas are usually palpable but may not be. Individuals with subacute thyroiditis may present with a history of flu-like symptoms and pain in the front of the neck. Factitious thyrotoxicosis should be considered if other causes have been excluded, but is extremely rare.

Investigations

Thyroid function tests are performed (Box 47.2). The serum total triiodothyronine (T_3) and total thyroxine (T_4) are raised but the thyroid-stimulating hormone (TSH) level is suppressed. TSH receptor antibodies are strongly positive. A full blood count, routine biochemical screen and chest X-ray are normal. A 12-lead electrocardiogram (ECG) shows sinus tachycardia. A ^{131}I uptake study of the thyroid gland shows symmetrical increased uptake.

Does this narrow down your differential diagnosis?

The clinical features, along with the high serum T_3 and T_4 with low TSH, confirm the diagnosis of Graves' disease. Graves' disease is usually much more common in females (female:male = 10:1), and is caused by antibodies directed against the TSH receptor. These are often measurable in the serum, as in this case, and provide a diagnostic clue in individuals who do not have obvious eye signs or a typical goitre.

The radioisotope scan could be considered superfluous in this case, but its findings are consistent with Graves' disease. Thyroid scintigraphy is particularly helpful in thyrotoxic individuals who do not have helpful clinical signs and whose TSH receptor antibodies are negative. In multinodular goitre and toxic adenoma, the nodules appear 'hot', due to localised increased uptake of radioactive iodine. Thyroiditis is characterised by a very low uptake of radioisotope.

BOX 47.2	
Thyroid function tests	
Serum TSH	< 0.01 mU/l (0.01 μU/ml)
Serum total T_3	7.9 nmol/l (526 ng/dl)
Serum total T_4	233.5 nmol/l (18.1 μg/dl)

How will you treat this patient?

Graves' disease may be treated with antithyroid drugs, radioactive iodine (^{131}I) or subtotal thyroidectomy. There are advantages and disadvantages to all three therapies. Ideally, this young patient should be put on antithyroid drugs (thionamides), such as carbimazole, methimazole or propylthiouracil. Carbimazole or methimazole is initially started at a daily dose of 10–40 mg; propylthiouracil may be started at 100–200 mg 6–8-hourly. The dosage is gradually reduced as the thyrotoxicosis improves, and dose titration is based on the serum thyroxine level. The patient usually becomes euthyroid after 2–3 months. Following this, the daily maintenance dose of carbimazole or methimazole is 5–10 mg, or propylthiouracil 50–100 mg. The common side-effects of antithyroid drugs include rashes, fever and arthralgia. A rare but an important side-effect is agranulocytosis (< 1%). Hence, a blood count must be checked urgently if a patient develops sore throat, fever or mouth ulcers. Adrenergic features may be controlled with 20–40 mg of propranolol 6-hourly. In patients who have atrial fibrillation, warfarin should be used to prevent thromboembolism. Usually, thionamides are prescribed for 12–18 months. On discontinuation, approximately 50% of patients may be expected to remain in long-term remission, but the other half will relapse and more definitive therapy should be considered.

With regard to radioactive iodine therapy, pregnancy and breastfeeding are absolute contraindications. It can cause exacerbation of thyroid eye disease and so might not be a good first-line choice for this patient. If it is given, a short course of prednisolone may be prescribed simultaneously to reduce the chance of exacerbation. In this young patient, though, if there were a relapse following antithyroid drugs, then subtotal thyroidectomy would be preferred over radioactive iodine therapy. Surgery should also be considered in patients with a large goitre. The risks associated with surgery, including recurrent laryngeal nerve palsy and hypoparathyroidism, should be explained. The patient must be rendered euthyroid with antithyroid medication prior to the operation to reduce the risk of thyroid storm (an acute exacerbation of thyrotoxicosis, which can be life-threatening).

In patients with mild to moderate ophthalmopathy, as in the present case, no active treatment is required. Artificial tears, in the form of 1% methylcellulose eye drops, and dark glasses may be used. In severe ophthalmopathy, prednisolone 40–80 mg/day or pulse therapy with methylprednisolone 1 g i.v. daily for 7 days should be administered, followed by a tapering course of an oral steroid. In refractory cases, surgical orbital decompression and external beam radiotherapy may be used.

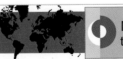

Global issues

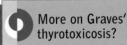

More on Graves' thyrotoxicosis?

- Graves' disease is the most common cause of thyrotoxicosis. Its frequency as the cause of thyrotoxicosis ranges from approximately 60% to 90% in different regions of the world.

- TSH receptor antibodies (TRAb) can be detected in the serum of 80–95% of patients with Graves' disease. Fluctuating levels of serum TRAb correlate with the clinical course of Graves' thyrotoxicosis.

See Chapter 20 of
Davidson's Principles and Practice of Medicine
(20th edn)

- Thyrotoxicosis is sometimes subclinical and this variety has a higher prevalence in black individuals than whites.
- In Caucasians there is an association of Graves' disease with HLA-B8, DR3 and DR2.
- A form of hypokalaemic periodic paralysis may occur in Asian males with thyrotoxicosis.
- Smoking is weakly associated with Graves' thyrotoxicosis, but strongly linked with ophthalmopathy.

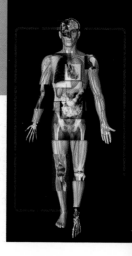

48

A young woman with neck swelling, weight gain and hoarseness of voice

T. DAS

Presenting problem

A 31-year-old lady presents to the medical outpatients department with a history of hoarseness of voice for the last 6 months. She also complains of lethargy, constipation and weight gain of about 5 kg during the same period. She has been aware of a swelling in the front of her neck for the last 3 months. Her menstrual cycles are regular, but she complains of very heavy menstrual bleeding. She is not on an oral contraceptive pill. Her past history has been uneventful without any operative procedure or major illness. She has no history of head and neck irradiation; neither is there any specific drug history. Her two sons, aged 4 years and 2 years, are healthy.

What would your differential diagnosis include before examining the patient?

This young female presenting with hoarseness of voice, lethargy, constipation, weight gain and menorrhagia has all the classic symptoms of hypothyroidism. However, individually, these symptoms are all very non-specific. Other possibilities include simple obesity, Cushing's syndrome, nephrotic syndrome and chronic fatigue syndrome.

Examination

Physical examination reveals a puffy face with oedematous eyelids, mild pallor and non-pitting oedema (myxoedema) (Fig. 48.1). The patient's body weight is 65 kg and her body mass index is 28. Her blood pressure is 150/95 mmHg. There is a diffuse goitre which is firm and non-tender, without any associated bruit. The ankle jerks are delayed bilaterally. There is no other specific finding on physical examination.

Has examination narrowed down your differential diagnosis?

The patient does not have any features of anasarca, i.e. oedema, ascites and pleural effusion, so nephrotic syndrome is ruled out. The patient does not look Cushingoid and has no hirsutism, buffalo hump, centripetal obesity, purple striae or dorsal kyphosis suggestive of Cushing's syndrome. The presence of a goitre, in conjunction with the patient's symptoms, makes hypothyroidism the most likely diagnosis.

Investigations

The serum total triiodothyronine (T_3), total thyroxine (T_4), thyroid-stimulating hormone (TSH) and free thyroxine (fT_4) are measured (Box 48.1). Serum T_3, T_4 and fT_4 are decreased, while serum TSH is increased.

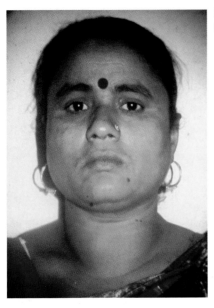

Fig. 48.1 This lady with hypothyroidism has some facial puffiness and a symmetrical goitre.

Thyroid peroxidase antibody (anti-TPO) titre are raised. An ultrasound scan of the thyroid gland shows thyroid enlargement with diffuse hypo-echogenicity.

Haemoglobin level is 105 g/l (10.5 g/dl). Fasting and post-prandial plasma glucose and urine examination are normal. Serum cholesterol is 5.9 mmol/l (225 mg/dl) and serum triglyceride is 1.6 mmol/l (140 mg/dl). Other biochemical reports and a chest X-ray are normal. A 12-lead ECG shows sinus bradycardia, generalised low-voltage complexes and non-specific ST–T wave changes.

Does this narrow down your differential diagnosis?

This patient thus has most of the clinical features of hypothyroidism. As there is a diffuse goitre with raised anti-TPO antibodies, Hashimoto's thyroiditis is most likely. In the absence of goitre, atrophic thyroiditis would have to be considered. Both Hashimoto's thyroiditis and atrophic thyroiditis are variants of autoimmune hypothyroidism.

Because the autoimmune process gradually reduces thyroid function, there is a phase of compensation when normal thyroid hormone levels are maintained by a rise in TSH. As patients are asymptomatic or have minor symptoms, this state is called subclinical hypothyroidism or mild hypothyroidism. In the present case, the patient has many of the classical features of hypothyroidism, along with raised serum TSH and low T$_3$, T$_4$ and fT$_4$ levels. This state is called clinical hypothyroidism or overt hypothyroidism.

Hypothyroidism may also be iatrogenic and result from treatment with ^{131}I radioactive iodine, subtotal or total thyroidectomy, and external irradiation of the neck for lymphoma or cancer. Antithyroid drugs, lithium and amiodarone can also cause hypothyroidism. However, none of these factors is responsible for hypothyroidism in this case. Iodine deficiency is a common world-wide cause of goitrous hypothyroidism, but it typically presents in childhood. Lastly, secondary hypothyroidism is usually diagnosed in the context of other pituitary hormone deficiencies and the serum TSH level is usually low. In this patient, the presence of myxoedema, goitre and the biochemical parameters rule out secondary hypothyroidism.

How will you treat this patient?

This lady requires replacement therapy with levothyroxine at a dose of 1.7 µg/kg of ideal body weight/day (approximately 100–150 µg/day). Adult patients under 60 years with no evidence of heart disease may be started on 100 µg of levothyroxine daily. TSH responses should be measured about 2 months after starting treatment or after any change of dosage. The starting dose in older adults, particularly those with known cardiac disease, should be lower because over-rapid replacement may cause an exacerbation of cardiac disease. Thus the starting dose should be 25–50 µg/day and this may be increased gradually every 14–28 days in 25–50 µg increments until the optimum daily dose is reached. Elderly patients may require up to 20% less levothyroxine than younger patients.

The clinical effects of levothyroxine replacement are usually slow to appear and may even take up to 6 months. After stable TSH levels are achieved with full replacement therapy, TSH levels are measured annually to start with and then 2–3-yearly.

Maternal hypothyroidism may adversely affect fetal neural development. Thyroid function should be evaluated during pregnancy and the dose of levothyroxine may have to be increased, particularly in the third trimester.

Subclinical or mild hypothyroidism may be treated with a low dose of levothyroxine, with the goal of normalising TSH. Opinion differs as to the best time to commence levothyroxine in such individuals. Most authorities treat if the TSH is > 10 mU/l; some will also treat if the TSH concentration is between 5 and 10 mU/l and the patient has positive antithyroid antibodies. If an individual has symptoms of hypothyroidism and the TSH is between 5 and 10 mU/l, then a trial of levothyroxine is also indicated.

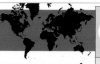

Global issues

 More on hypothyroidism?

- Iodine deficiency remains the most common cause of hypothyroidism world-wide, particularly in South-east Asia.

- For practical purposes, when the prevalence of goitre in children aged 6–12 years in an iodine-deficient population is more than 10%, it is called 'endemic goitre'.

- In Western countries, hypothyroidism is most commonly caused by autoimmune (Hashimoto's thyroiditis and atrophic type) and iatrogenic (following treatment for hyperthyroidism) disorders.

- Fine needle aspiration for cytology or thyroid biopsy will clinch the diagnosis of Hashimoto's thyroiditis, although it is generally not required. Classical findings include diffuse lymphocytic and plasma cell infiltration, with follicular atrophy and fibrosis.

- Myxoedema coma has a very high mortality rate despite intensive treatment.

See Chapter 20 of
Davidson's Principles and Practice of Medicine
(20th edn)

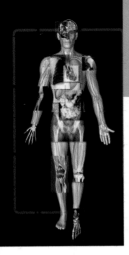

49

A 30-year-old woman with amenorrhoea

G. A. WITTERT

Presenting problem

A 30-year-old nulliparous woman presents with a 6-month history of amenorrhoea since discontinuing the combined oral contraceptive pill. Menarche occurred at the age of 13 and she rapidly established a regular bleeding pattern with no menstrual abnormality. At the age of 18 she commenced a combined oral contraceptive, which she discontinued because she wished to start a family.

There is no history of weight cycling or unusual eating patterns. She is a triathlete and trains daily. She has no unusual stress, but her mood has been somewhat labile and she has not been sleeping well. She has not had any gynaecological procedures at any time. Over the last few months there has been a noticeable reduction in libido, and increasing discomfort during intercourse. She has not had any hot flushes and has not noticed the presence of breast milk. She has no headache or visual disturbance. There are no other symptoms of any sort — in particular, no symptoms of any other hormonal deficiency or excess. She is not taking medication of any kind.

What would your differential diagnosis include before examining the patient?

The scenario, in particular the loss of libido and discomfort during intercourse, suggests oestrogen deficiency, either due to loss of gonadotrophin production or ovarian failure. Galactorrhoea, when present, suggests excess prolactin production as the cause of failure of gonadotrophin production; this will need to be looked for on examination. Depression, weight loss, eating disorders and excessive exercise, particularly if accompanied by caloric restriction, may also cause failure of gonadotrophin secretion. The physical activity undertaken by this patient may be an issue. A careful assessment of nutritional status is required. Loss of gonadotrophin production may be caused by a pituitary or hypothalamic tumour or infiltrative disorder (sarcoidosis, haemochromatosis), but there are no features in the history to suggest either. Autoimmune ovarian failure should be considered. Oestrogen deficiency symptoms would not be typical of pregnancy; nevertheless this should be excluded since it is possible to conceive before the first period occurs after discontinuing the pill.

Examination

The patient's weight is normal (body mass index 21). The skin is normal and there are no signs of acne, hirsutism or dysmorphic features. There is no evidence of pregnancy. Bilateral expressible galactorrhoea is present, along with atrophic vaginitis. There are no clinical features of any hormone excess (e.g. growth hormone, cortisol) or deficiency (e.g. thyroxine). There are no abnormalities of vision or visual fields.

Has examination narrowed down your differential diagnosis?

The presence of galactorrhoea in the setting of oestrogen deficiency symptoms suggests the presence of hyperprolactinaemia. A number of medications (e.g. antiemetics, antipsychotics) can increase prolactin, but she is not taking any of these. A prolactin-secreting microadenoma, or stalk compression from a larger pituitary tumour, or interference of dopamine production as a result of a hypothalamic tumour or infiltrative disorder, are possible causes. The

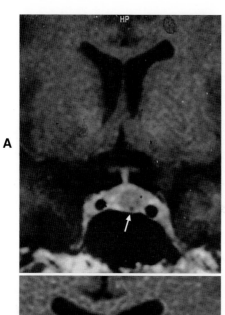

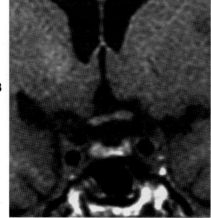

Fig. 49.1 Secondary amenorrhoea. A. An MRI obtained post-gadolinium. The section is a coronal view through the pituitary gland. The optic chiasm and pituitary stalk can be seen as enhancing structures. The internal carotid in each cavernous sinus appears black. A 0.9 cm unenhancing lesion, typical of microadenoma, is visible in the pituitary gland (arrow). B. For comparison, a normal pituitary MRI is also presented.

absence of compressive symptoms or evidence of any other hormone excess or deficiency makes an isolated prolactin-secreting microadenoma the most likely cause.

Investigations

The following hormone results are obtained: follicle-stimulating hormone < 1 U/l (< 0.1 µg/l), luteinising hormone < 1 U/l (< 0.1 µg/l), prolactin 140 µg/l (ng/ml) (normal range 0–25 µg/l (ng/ml) or equivalent), thyroid-stimulating hormone (TSH) 1 mU/l, free T4 13 pmol/l (1000 pg/dl).

A magnetic resonance image (MRI) of the pituitary is obtained. A coronal section through the pituitary, obtained after the administration of gadolinium (Fig. 49.1) shows a 0.9 cm unenhancing tumour typical of a microadenoma.

Does this narrow down your differential diagnosis?

The patient has a prolactin-secreting microadenoma with otherwise normal pituitary function.

How will you treat this patient?

A long-acting dopamine receptor 2 agonist (D2RA) such as cabergoline will normalise prolactin levels, shrink the tumour and restore normal menstrual function and fertility with minimal side-effects. Short-acting D2RAs — for example, bromocriptine — cause significant side-effects (nausea, vomiting, nasal stuffiness and postural hypotension) and the dose needs to be titrated up slowly. Although there is no evidence of harm, D2RAs should be discontinued once pregnancy occurs and need only be reinstated if clinically significant tumour growth occurs (headaches and visual disturbance). In some cases the problem resolves after delivery.

Where appropriate expertise is available, selective microadenomectomy via a trans-sphenoidal approach can be offered.

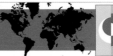

Global issues

More on amenorrhoea

- Amenorrhoea after discontinuing the combined oral contraceptive pill is not due to the use of the pill per se, regardless of how long it has been used. A cause should also be vigorously sought.

- Secondary amenorrhoea, regardless of cause, results in a decrease in bone mineral density and predisposes to significant osteoporosis later in life. Such patients should be specifically targeted for screening and prevention strategies.

- Obesity is now as common as, or perhaps more so than, under-nutrition as a global problem. Particularly when severe and associated with insulin resistance or obstructive sleep apnoea, it may result in secondary amenorrhoea as part of the spectrum of polycystic ovarian syndrome.

- Tuberculosis, as well as being a rare cause of pituitary failure, can cause endometrial adhesions which obliterate the endometrial cavity and result in amenorrhoea.

See Chapter 20 of **Davidson's Principles and Practice of Medicine** (20th edn)

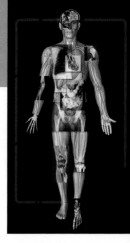

50

An elderly woman with hypercalcaemia

M. W. J. STRACHAN

Presenting problem

A 75-year-old woman is referred to an endocrine clinic with a 4-month history of malaise and increased thirst. Five years ago she had an episode of severe pain in her left loin which settled after a few hours and for which she did not seek medical attention. The lady thinks that she has lost a few inches in height over the last few years and a recent X-ray of her thoracic spine shows several wedge fractures. She does not take any regular medication. Prior to referral, her GP checked some routine blood tests and these identified an elevated serum calcium concentration (Box 50.1).

What would your differential diagnosis include before examining the patient?

The two most common causes of hypercalcaemia are hyperparathyroidism and malignancy. The vertebral fractures are not particularly discriminatory, given the high prevalence of osteoporosis in women of this age; they could be coincidental, or a consequence of hyperparathyroidism or even neoplastic disease (e.g. myeloma). The history suggests that the patient may have had a renal calculus in the past and this would be more in keeping with hyperparathyroidism. Thyrotoxicosis and glucocorticoid insufficiency can cause hypercalcaemia, but it is invariably mild and asymptomatic.

> **BOX 50.1**
>
> **Initial investigations**
>
> Urea 18.3 mmol/l (51.26 mg/dl)
>
> Creatinine 105 µmol/l (1.19 mg/dl)
>
> Sodium 144 mmol/l (meq/l)
>
> Potassium 3.4 mmol/l (meq/l)
>
> Calcium 2.89 mmol/l (11.56 mg/dl)
>
> Phosphate 0.63 mmol/l (1.95 mg/dl)
>
> Albumin 35 g/l (3.5 g/dl)

The lady is not taking lithium or any vitamin D preparations, but vitamin D excess can be caused by sarcoidosis and other granulomatous disorders, and this should certainly be considered if the more common causes are excluded.

Examination

The patient looks a little dry and has a stooped posture. No masses are felt in the breasts or the abdomen.

Has examination narrowed down your differential diagnosis?

As is often the case in endocrinology, if there is no easy spot diagnosis (e.g. a patient with an acromegaloid or Cushingoid appearance), then detailed examination is often unrewarding. There is, though, a general rule of thumb with hypercalcaemia that if the patient is well enough to come to an outpatient clinic, then the likely cause is hyperparathyroidism. However, if the patient requires admission to hospital, then in all probability there is underlying neoplastic disease. All rules of thumb, of course, are there to be broken! If a patient is not already known to have cancer or this is not evident from the initial history, examination and investigations, then the key discriminatory test is measurement of serum parathyroid hormone (PTH).

Further investigations

The serum PTH concentration is 12.6 pmol/l (126 pg/ml) and 24-hour urine calcium is 9.4 mmol/24 hrs (376 mg/24 hrs).

Does this narrow down the differential diagnosis?

The PTH concentration is high and so the diagnosis is almost certainly primary hyperparathyroidism — 'almost certainly' because a rare trap for the unwary is familial hypocalciuric hypercalcaemia. This inherited disorder can cause elevated serum calcium and PTH concentrations, but can usually be diagnosed by the finding of a low 24-hour urinary calcium concentration and the identification of borderline hypercalcaemia in close relatives.

If the PTH had been low, then malignant hypercalcaemia would have been most likely and further investigations, such as protein electrophoresis, urinary Bence Jones protein and a CT of the chest and abdomen, would have been indicated.

BOX 50.2

Indications for surgery in primary hyperparathyroidism

- Complications of hyper-parathyroidism, e.g. renal stones, renal impairment (with no other identifiable cause) and osteoporosis
- Symptoms of hyperpara-thyroidism
- Age < 50 years
- Serum calcium > 2.85 mmol/l (11.4 mg/dl)

How will you treat this patient?

Primary hyperparathyroidism is invariably caused by a solitary parathyroid adenoma and so the definitive therapy is parathyroidectomy. Standard indications for surgery are shown in Box 50.2, but selection of patients is not always straightforward. This lady, providing she is fit enough for a general anaesthetic, should have surgery because of her relatively high serum calcium, thin bones and high urinary calcium excretion. If an ultrasound scan of the kidneys showed evidence of nephrocalcinosis or nephrolithiasis, then the case for surgery would be even stronger.

In some centres, pre-operative localisation of a parathyroid adenoma with ^{99m}technetium-sestamibi scanning (Fig. 50.1) allows targeted resection using

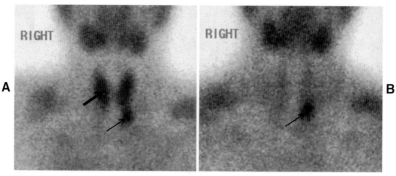

Fig. 50.1 ^{99m}technetium-sestamibi scan. A. Initial uptake into the thyroid (thick arrow) and left inferior parathyroid gland (thin arrow). B. After 3 hours. there is only uptake in the abnormal parathyroid.

minimally invasive techniques. Post-operative hypocalcaemia is not uncommon during the first 2 weeks while residual suppressed parathyroid tissue recovers.

Global issues

More on hypercalcaemia?

- Granulomatous disorders, including tuberculosis, fungal infections and berylliosis, can cause hypercacaemia secondary to vitamin D excess.

- Rarely, human immunodeficiency virus (HIV)-associated *Pneumocystis jirovecii* infection can be associated with severe hypercalcaemia and this is likely to become more common as the prevalence of HIV continues to rise world-wide.

See Chapter 20 of
Davidson's Principles and Practice of Medicine
(20th edn)

- ⁹⁹ᵐtechnetium-sestamibi scanning is not essential, as an experienced surgeon will locate a parathyroid adenoma by careful neck exploration in over 90% of patients.

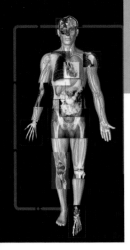

51

A middle-aged man with muscle cramps

G. A. WITTERT

Presenting problem

A 54-year-old male presents with a 3-month history of increasing muscle cramps in the lower back, legs, feet and hands. More recently he has noticed some tingling and burning in the fingers and around the mouth. Four months ago he had a thyroidectomy for a large multinodular goitre. He takes thyroxine and a thiazide diuretic for mild hypertension. He has a sedentary job, works long hours and spends little if any time out of doors. Initial blood tests reveal a low plasma calcium (Box 51.1).

What would your differential diagnosis include before examining the patient?

The patient has symptoms and biochemistry consistent with hypocalcaemia. If the plasma calcium level falls very rapidly, or if the proportion of ionised calcium decreases acutely when the plasma calcium level is already low, laryngospasm, bronchospasm, tetany or seizures may occur.

The most common causes are hypoparathyroidism due to iatrogenic or autoimmune destruction of the parathyroid glands, deficiency or abnormal metabolism of vitamin D, magnesium deficiency and chronic renal failure.

In this patient the parathyroid glands may have been removed or their blood supply damaged during the previous thyroid surgery. Other factors which need to be considered include the possibility of vitamin D deficiency due to lack of

BOX 51.1	
Initial investigations	
Total calcium	1.8 mmol/l (7.2 mg/dl)
Ionised calcium	0.9 mmol/l (3.6 mg/dl)
Phosphate	0.6 mmol/l (1.86 mg/dl)
Albumin	39 g/l (3.9 mg/dl)
Sodium	137 mmol/l (meq/l)
Potassium	3.0 mmol/l (meq/l)
Creatinine	120 µmol/l (1.36 mg/dl)
Urea	7.0 mmol/l (19.6 mg/dl)
TSH	2.5 mU/l

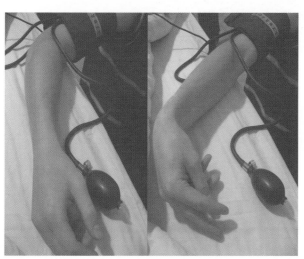

Fig. 51.1 Trousseau's sign. Inflation of the sphygmomanometer cuff causes carpal muscle spasm in an individual with hypocalcaemia.

exposure to sunlight and magnesium deficiency due to the thiazide diuretic. Severe magnesium deficiency results in impaired secretion of parathyroid hormone and resistance to its action. Magnesium deficiency is not infrequent in response to thiazides and, unlike hypokalaemia, is often overlooked.

Hypocalcaemic states are best categorised according to the level of parathyroid hormone (PTH). Ordinarily, PTH secretion is exquisitely sensitive to changes in ionised calcium. In hypoparathyroid states the level of PTH is inappropriately low for the level of calcium. Elevated PTH levels (secondary hyperparathyroidism) suggest normal PTH responsiveness to the low plasma calcium.

Examination

This man is well nourished and there is no evidence of gastrointestinal disease. The scar from the previous thyroid surgery is evident and no thyroid remnant is palpable. There is no vitiligo, mucocutaneous candidiasis or skin lesions of any sort. Twitching of the circumoral muscles occurs in response to tapping the facial nerve just anterior to the ear (Chvostek's sign). Carpal spasm is elicited by inflation of the blood pressure cuff to 20 mmHg above the systolic blood pressure for 3 minutes (Trousseau's sign; Fig. 51.1). There is no obvious ocular calcification, proximal muscle weakness or disorders of movement.

Has examination narrowed down your differential diagnosis?

The examination, together with investigations so far, suggests that the low calcium, which is causing significant neuromuscular irritability, is responsible for this patient's symptoms and that malabsorption, liver or renal disease are unlikely to be factors in the abnormalities of calcium or vitamin D homeostasis. In the absence of evidence of any autoimmune or other system disease process it seems that any abnormality of PTH, if present, is likely to be due to be the result of the previous thyroid surgery.

Further investigations

Further tests reveal magnesium 0.65 mmol/l (1.58 mg/dl), 25 hydroxyvitamin D 45 nmol/l (18 ng/ml) and PTH 1 pmol/l (10 pg/ml).

Does this narrow down your differential diagnosis?

The low PTH level suggests that the primary problem is hypoparathyroidism, most likely as a consequence of damage to the parathyroid glands or their blood supply during surgery. Although the magnesium level is low and may be contributing to the problem, it is usually only when it is very low (0.4 mmol/l (0.97 mg/dl) or less) that it is likely to be the primary cause of hypoparathyroidism. The renal handling of potassium and magnesium is similar, and the low potassium and magnesium are both related to the thiazide diuretic, which induces renal loss of both electrolytes. On the other hand, thiazides decrease renal calcium loss. The low vitamin D is the result of inadequate sun exposure and, while not the primary cause of the problem, will compromise not only the patient's ability to maintain plasma calcium, but also skeletal, muscular and metabolic integrity, and may even increase his cancer risk.

How will you treat this patient?

Commence an oral calcium supplement equivalent to 1–2 g of elemental calcium per day. The thiazide diuretic should be replaced with an angiotensin-converting enzyme (ACE) inhibitor or angiotensin 2 receptor antagonist, and potassium and magnesium should be replaced orally. Sunlight exposure of unprotected skin should be encouraged where feasible for 10 minutes per day in summer and 20 minutes per day in winter. If this is not feasible or if the vitamin D level remains low, an oral supplement should be given. If the plasma calcium remains low, oral 1,25-dihydroxyvitamin D (0.25–1.0 µg) is added. The plasma calcium level should be maintained in the lower part of the normal range.

Global issues

 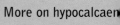 More on hypocalcaen

- The biologically active vitamin D metabolite, $1,25(OH)_2D$, is not exclusively produced in the kidney, but is also synthesised in many other tissues such as the prostate, colon, skin and osteoblasts. There is a relationship between vitamin D deficiency and various types of cancer, bone diseases, autoimmune diseases, hypertension and cardiovascular disease.

  See Chapter 20 of
  Davidson's Principles and Practice of Medicine
  (20th edn)

- Approximately 90% of all requisite vitamin D has to be formed in the skin through the action of the sun. Strict sun protection causes vitamin D deficiency, which is being recognised to be prevalent even in the sunniest countries. The problem can be a particular issue in pregnant women, the institutionalised elderly with dark skin, and other groups where sun exposure does not occur.

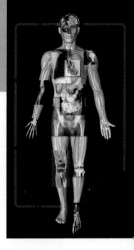

52

Weight gain, amenorrhoea, fatigue and muscle weakness in a young woman

W. F. MOLLENTZE

Presenting problem

A 25-year-old woman presents to an endocrine clinic with a 4-year history of amenorrhoea, progressive weight gain (10 kg during the past year), fatigue and difficulty in climbing stairs and rising from a deep chair. The lady mentions that her body shape has changed with an increase in waist circumference. Her face has become rounder and hairy and she also noticed that she bruises easily. She finds it difficult to concentrate, experiences headaches, and feels depressed and tearful of late. She denies ever having taken any form of glucocorticoid treatment. Her general practitioner has found that her blood pressure was increased on several occasions.

What would your differential diagnosis include before examining the patient?

At least three conditions need to be considered in the differential diagnosis at this stage: polycystic ovarian syndrome (PCOS), primary hypothyroidism and Cushing's syndrome. Although obesity, especially central obesity, is present in most patients with PCOS, it is not recognised as a diagnostic feature of the syndrome. Oligo- or amenorrhoea and hirsutism, however, are both defining features of PCOS but myopathy is not part of this syndrome. Patients with primary hypothyroidism, especially of gradual onset, may complain of weight gain, fatigue and menstrual irregularity. While menorrhagia is the classic menstrual abnormality in female patients with primary hypothyroidism, oligo- and amenorrhoea can also occur. Proximal muscle weakness is an unusual but important feature of primary hypothyroidism. The combination of easy bruising, proximal muscle weakness and hypertension in any obese patient is, however, highly suggestive of Cushing's syndrome.

Examination

The patient weighs 63 kg and her height is 1.56 m (body mass index 25.89). She has an obvious Cushingoid and plethoric appearance (Fig. 52.1) with prominent broad purple striae (Fig. 52.2) over the abdomen and breasts. Ankle oedema is present, as well as mild hirsutism on the upper lip and cheeks. Her supine blood pressure is 170/120 mmHg. The lady is unable to rise from a squatting position (Fig. 52.3). The patient's GP performed some initial investigations before referring the patient (Box 52.1).

Have examination and initial investigations narrowed your differential diagnosis?

The clinical manifestations in this patient, combined with hypokalaemia, increased 24-hour urinary free cortisol secretion and loss of circadian rhythm, are almost diagnostic of Cushing's syndrome. Two more conditions which have overlapping clinical

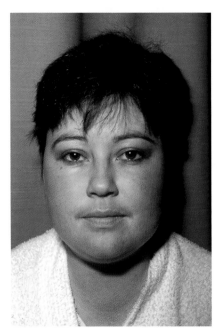

Fig. 52.1 Moon facies with mild hirsutism.

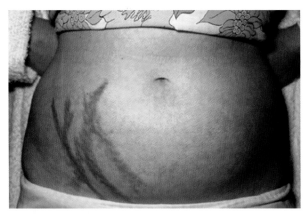

Fig. 52.2 Broad purple striae over the abdomen.

and biochemical features with Cushing's syndrome should now also be considered before embarking on more expensive investigations. Pseudo-Cushing's syndrome caused by alcohol excess may mimic some of the features of Cushing's syndrome, such as central obesity, proximal muscle weakness and overproduction of cortisol. A thorough history, including collateral information, may be useful in this regard. Liver enzymes are frankly abnormal in these patients. Major depressive illness may also be associated with increased 24-hour urinary free cortisol excretion, but proximal muscle weakness, purple striae and severe hypokalaemia argue in favour of an organic illness.

Further investigations

The standard low-dose dexamethasone suppression test, consisting of dexamethasone 0.5 mg every 6 hours taken orally for 48 hours, is now required to confirm the presence of Cushing's syndrome. This is immediately followed by the standard high-dose dexamethasone suppression test, consisting of 2 mg dexamethasone every 6 hours, to establish the cause of

52

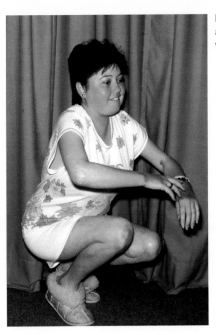

Fig. 52.3 The patient is unable to rise from a squatting position, indicating proximal muscle weakness.

Cushing's syndrome. The reason for performing these two investigations consecutively is, firstly, that the results of the adrenocorticotrophic hormone (ACTH) assays become available only after some time and, secondly, for convenience since the patient is best admitted to hospital to ensure adherence to the test protocol. The results of these tests are shown in Box 52.2.

Does this narrow down your differential diagnosis?

The patient's 0900 hr s-cortisol concentration on day 3, as well as the 24-hour urinary free cortisol during day 2, fails to suppress after 48 hours of low-dose dexamethasone, confirming the presence of Cushing's syndrome. The 'detectable' baseline p-ACTH concentration of 6.61 pmol/l (30 pg/ml) on day 1 in the presence of excess cortisol may point towards a pituitary or ectopic source of this lady's Cushing's syndrome. After 48 hours of high-dose dexamethasone the 0900 hr ACTH concentration, as well as the 0900 hr s-cortisol and 24-hour urinary free cortisol concentrations, fail to suppress. These findings argue against a pituitary tumour. An X-ray of the chest is requested and shows no evidence of a possible source of ectopic ACTH production. A computed tomogram (CT) of the abdomen demonstrates a 2.5 cm tumor in the left adrenal gland. A magnetic resonance image (MRI) of the brain shows some cerebral atrophy and the pituitary gland appears normal. The fact that ACTH was detectable in this patient at baseline, as well as after the high-dose dexamethasone suppression test, is unusual for a cortisol-producing adrenal tumour, as normally the ACTH levels would be undetectable.

BOX 52.1

Initial investigations

Serum sodium	146 mmol/l (meq/l)
Serum potassium	2.1 mmol/l (meq/l)
24-hr urinary free cortisol	3850 nmol (1395 µg) (normal range 30–300 nmol (10–100 µg))
0900 hr s-cortisol	1151 nmol/l (41.72 µg/dl) (normal range 220–660 nmol/l (8–24 µg/dl))
2300 hr s-cortisol	1127 nmol/l (40.85 µg/dl) (normal range 50–410 nmol/l (2–15 µg/dl))
s = serum	

How will you treat this patient?

The patient should be referred for a left adrenalectomy after correcting the hypoka-laemia with intravenous potassium chloride and controlling the elevated blood pressure with an angiotensin-converting enzyme (ACE) inhibitor. Pre-operatively, excess cortisol concentrations can be reduced by treatment with metyrapone. Since the cortex of the contralateral adrenal gland may be atrophic in spite of the measur-able amounts of ACTH, the adrenalectomy must be conducted under full gluco-corticoid cover including intravenous hydrocortisone, followed by full replacement doses of oral hydrocortisone as soon as the patient is allowed to eat. Full recovery of the hypothalamic–pituitary–adrenal axis is expected within 2–12 months, during which period the replacement dose of hydrocortisone can be tapered gradually.

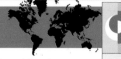

Global issues

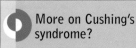

More on Cushing's syndrome?

- Corticotrophin-releasing hormone (CRH) is not freely available in developing countries and even the availa-bility of dexamethasone is under threat in some.

- Although Cushing's syndrome may be fairly obvious clinically, the definitive biochemical diagnosis, including establishing the exact aetiology and often the anatomical localisation of the underlying disorder, may prove to be extremely challenging.

See Chapter 20 of **Davidson's Principles and Practice of Medicine** (20th edn)

- Most, if not all, patients with suspected Cushing's syndrome should preferably be referred to a centre with experience in the management of such patients.

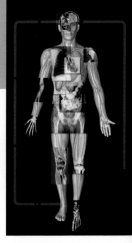

53

A young woman with fatigue, anorexia, weight loss and increased pigmentation

W. F. MOLLENTZE

Presenting problem

A 27-year-old woman is referred by her general practitioner to an endocrine clinic with gradual onset of fatigue, anorexia, weight loss and hyperpigmentation dating back to her second and last pregnancy 5 years ago. She also complains of amenorrhoea of 4 months' duration, intermittent diarrhoea and orthostatic dizziness.

What would your differential diagnosis include before examining the patient?

Fatigue is a frequent complaint in an endocrine clinic. Hypothyroidism is unlikely since the patient lost weight and she also complains of amenorrhoea and not menorrhagia. Rheumatoid arthritis and multiple sclerosis are examples of autoimmune conditions associated with fatigue and could easily be excluded on further enquiry. Chronic fatigue syndrome may follow after a viral infection such as infectious mononucleosis, influenza or hepatitis. Anorexia nervosa should also be considered in the differential diagnosis of weight loss and amenorrhoea. The absence of similar complaints during adolescence would argue against this condition. None of the above conditions is, however, characterised by hyperpigmentation. Primary adrenocortical failure, pellagra and malabsorption (Box 53.1) may also present with hyperpigmentation, weight loss and diarrhoea.

Examination

This young woman's height is 1.69 m and she weighs 52 kg (body mass index 18.2). Generalised hyperpigmentation is present but is more pronounced on the sun-exposed areas (Fig. 53.1). Her hair is dark, and dark freckles are also present over the anterior chest wall. Pressure areas, such as the elbows, the skin over spinous processes and underneath the brassiere straps, are also darker than surrounding skin. The patient's pulse rate is 88/min and blood pressure is 100/70 mmHg

BOX 53.1

Causes of diffuse hyperpigmentation

Endocrinopathies
- Addison's disease
- Nelson's syndrome
- Ectopic ACTH secretion

Metabolic
- Porphyria cutanea tarda
- Haemochromatosis
- Vitamin B_{12} and folate deficiency
- Pellagra
- Malabsorption

Autoimmune
- Hepatic cirrhosis
- Systemic sclerosis

Drug-induced
- Amiodarone
- Busulfan
- Chloroquine
- Minocycline
- Phenothiazines
- Psoralens

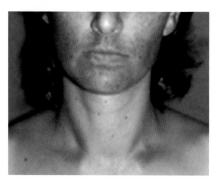

Fig. 53.1 Hyperpigmentation in Addison's disease.

BOX 53.2

Initial investigations

Sodium	131 mmol/l (meq/l)
Potassium	5.4 mmol/l (meq/l)
Urea	7.1 mmol/l (19.9 mg/dl)
Creatinine	106 µmol/l (1.20 mg/dl)
Glucose	3.7 mmol/l (66.65 mg/dl)

lying down and 60/40 mmHg in the erect position. Vitiligo is absent and no abnormal pigmentation is present on the oral mucous membranes. Initial blood test results are shown in Box 53.2.

Have examination and initial investigations narrowed down your differential diagnosis?

Although the hyperpigmentation in this patient is highly suggestive of primary adrenocortical failure (Addison's disease), it is by no means diagnostic. The absence of vitiligo does not exclude Addison's disease since it is seen in only 10–20% of patients with the autoimmune variety. The orthostatic decrease in blood pressure and the raised plasma urea and creatinine are suggestive of primary adrenal insufficiency, but may also be due to hypovolaemia secondary to chronic diarrhoea and malabsorption. Hyponatraemia and hyperkalaemia in the presence of hypovolaemia, however, argue strongly in favour of primary adrenal insufficiency.

Further investigations

The patient's morning (0800 hr) plasma cortisol concentration is 47.1 nmol/l (1.71 µg/dl) and the corresponding plasma corticotrophin (ACTH) concentration is 53.5 pmol/l (243 pg/ml). This lady's thyroid function test results are normal but her thyroid microsomal antibody titre is positive to a titre of 1:6400. A computed tomogram (CT) of the adrenal glands reveals atrophy of both glands, and the serum ferritin concentration is within the normal range.

Does this narrow down your differential diagnosis?

The clinical picture and the finding of low serum cortisol and elevated ACTH concentrations all but clinch the diagnosis of primary adrenocortical failure. In less clear-cut cases, a short Synacthen test should be performed, as the identification of a low stimulated cortisol concentration is a more robust marker of glucocorticoid deficiency than a random or early morning cortisol. In this case, this might be considered superfluous.

Common causes of chronic primary adrenocortical failure include autoimmune adrenalitis (Addison's disease) and infections such as tuberculosis and human immunodeficiency virus-acquired immunodeficiency syndrome (HIV/AIDS). Measurement of antibodies directed against the adrenal cortex is helpful to diagnose autoimmune adrenalitis, but unfortunately this assay is not widely available. The presence of thyroid microsomal antibodies in this patient argues in favour of an underlying autoimmune process. The absence of calcification or evidence of metastatic disease in the adrenal glands rules out tuberculosis and underlying malignancy respectively as aetiological factors.

How will you treat this patient?

Both glucocorticoid and mineralocorticoid replacement therapy should be provided. Hydrocortisone (cortisol) 15 mg orally on waking and 5 mg orally at approximately 1800 hrs constitute the glucocorticoid regimen of choice. This dosage regimen is usually sufficient but may need to be increased to 20 mg and 10 mg respectively in some patients. Unfortunately, measurement of 'trough and peak' cortisol concentrations is not very helpful for determining the optimum dosage of hydrocortisone. Furthermore, the pharmacokinetics of hydrocortisone makes it very hard to mimic circadian cortisol secretion. Therefore, some patients may still experience daily episodes of lassitude and fatigue in spite of an adequate total daily dose of hydrocortisone. In some individuals it may be prudent to advise a small dose after lunch and to postpone the evening dose till bedtime. Cortisol is a powerful appetite stimulant and excessive weight gain usually indicates over-treatment. Hyperpigmentation should improve within several weeks to a few months. Persistent hyperpigmentation indicates insufficient chronic suppression of ACTH secretion.

Fludrocortisone (9α-fluorohydrocortisone) is the mineralocorticoid of choice and can be initiated with 0.05 mg orally on waking. The objective of fludrocortisone treatment is to prevent further sodium loss, to restore intravascular volume and to prevent hyperkalaemia. Adequacy of fludrocortisone replacement can be monitored by routinely measuring blood pressure in the supine as well as the upright position, in addition to the serum sodium and potassium concentrations. Over-treatment with fludrocortisone should be suspected when the blood pressure becomes elevated and oedema and hypokalaemia develop.

Patient education is of the utmost importance in the long-term successful management of primary adrenal insufficiency. Patients should be advised to increase their salt intake during summer in regions known for hot, dry summers. The dose of hydrocortisone must be doubled during periods of emotional and physical stress, e.g. febrile periods, and the GP should be notified if this exceeds 3 days. Parenteral hydrocortisone and intravenous saline must be administered during episodes of vomiting. Patients should also be carefully followed for the development of other autoimmune endocrinopathies such as hypothyroidism and premature ovarian failure.

In known patients, as well as in previously undiagnosed ones, an acute adrenal crisis should be suspected if they present in shock, especially when this is accompanied by anorexia, nausea, vomiting, weakness and abdominal pain with deep tenderness on palpation. Intravenous saline should be infused as required to normalise haemodynamic indices and care must be taken not to correct hyponatraemia too rapidly. Hypoglycaemia may be a rare presentation of acute adrenal insufficiency in adults.

Global issues

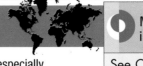

- As the incidence of HIV/AIDS increases, especially in developing countries, overt adrenal insufficiency may become more prevalent due to a necrotising adrenalitis secondary to cytomegalovirus infection or tuberculous involvement; Kaposi's sarcoma may also metastasise to the adrenal glands.
- Synacthen (ACTH$_{1-24}$) is not available in some developing countries.
- Assays for antibodies directed at the adrenal cortex are also not widely available in developing countries.
- Patients with chronic adrenal insufficiency must be advised to increase their salt intake during summer in countries with hot dry summers.

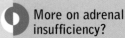

More on adrenal insufficiency?

See Chapter 20 of
Davidson's Principles and Practice of Medicine
(20th edn)

54

An elderly woman with recurrent spontaneous hypoglycaemia

M. W. J. STRACHAN

Presenting problem

A 78-year-old Caucasian woman is admitted to hospital in a coma (Glasgow Coma Score (GCS) 5). She was found collapsed at home by her husband, who reports that his wife has been experiencing increasingly frequent dizzy spells over the previous 4 months. These episodes typically occur first thing in the morning, before breakfast, or later in the day, particularly if she has been working in her large garden. These spells are often relieved by a cup of sweet tea and a biscuit. She is an otherwise fit woman and her only medication is low-dose aspirin and simvastatin.

On the patient's arrival in the Accident and Emergency department, the triage nurse performs a capillary blood glucose test, and a level of 1.3 mmol/l (23.4 mg/dl) is recorded on the meter. Venous blood samples are taken and the patient is given 50 ml of 50% dextrose intravenously. Within 5 minutes her GCS has risen to 15. The laboratory glucose is subsequently reported at 1.6 mmol/l (28.8 mg/dl).

What would your differential diagnosis include before examining the patient?

The differential diagnosis of acute hypoglycaemia is very extensive. In the first instance, of course, it is crucial to confirm that you are dealing with a hypoglycaemic disorder and, for that, all constituents of Whipple's triad should be met (Box 54.1). In addition, laboratory confirmation of the low blood glucose concentration is essential, because bedside meters are not sufficiently accurate in the hypoglycaemia range. Clearly, though, your patient should not have treatment deferred while awaiting the pronouncement from the laboratory, and intravenous dextrose (or intramuscular glucagon) should be administered when venous blood samples have been taken.

Often the cause of acute hypoglycaemia is obvious. The husband does not report that his wife has diabetes mellitus and he looks affronted when excess alcohol consumption is suggested! Pituitary and adrenocortical

> **BOX 54.1**
>
> **Whipple's triad**
>
> - The patient must have symptoms of hypoglycaemia
> - The patient must have biochemical evidence of hypoglycaemia
> - The symptoms must resolve when the hypoglycaemia is corrected.

insufficiency rarely cause acute hypoglycaemia in adults, but can in children. Disorders of carbohydrate metabolism would also have presented in early life and acute liver failure, sepsis and kidney failure are much less likely, given the prolonged history. This implies a more insidious process, such as endogenous insulin excess (insulinoma) or a non-islet cell tumour causing hypoglycaemia. Drug-related causes should always be considered in an individual with hypoglycaemia. Aspirin can cause hypoglycaemia, but only in very high doses. If the patient's husband has diabetes (or a close family member or friend), then the possibility of factitious or felonious hypoglycaemia should not be discounted.

Examination

The lady is apyrexial and cardiovascularly stable, with good peripheral perfusion. The skin is normal and she is well nourished, if indeed slightly overweight. A left-sided hemiparesis is noted on arrival in the department, but this quickly resolves on correction of the hypoglycaemia. No abnormal masses are noted on palpation of the abdomen.

Has examination narrowed down your differential diagnosis?

Transient neurological phenomena are not uncommon in elderly patients and it is important to exclude hypoglycaemia in anyone with acute neurological symptoms and/or signs. The cardiovascular stability and the rapid recovery with intravenous dextrose essentially exclude severe acute illness. Non-islet cell tumour-induced hypoglycaemia usually occurs in the context of large retroperitoneal sarcomas, which may already have been diagnosed and are often palpable on abdominal examination. Further narrowing down of the differential diagnosis requires further analysis of the blood samples.

Further investigations

Routine biochemistry and liver function tests are normal and salicylate concentrations are not elevated. Serum insulin and C-peptide concentrations are elevated at 70 pmol/l (9.76 mU/ml) and 4 µg/l (4 pg/ml) respectively.

Has the diagnosis been clinched?

Measurements of serum insulin and C-peptide concentrations during the episode of hypoglycaemia are essential in establishing the cause of hypoglycaemia when there is no obvious precipitant. If further information comes to light when the patient recovers from the acute episode, then the samples can be discarded before being assayed. However, unnecessary provocation tests (e.g. prolonged fasting) can be avoided if samples are taken during the acute episode.

The finding of elevated insulin and C-peptide concentrations, taken with the chronic history, points very strongly to this patient having an underlying insulinoma. Exogenous insulin would have caused elevation of only the serum insulin, and other causes of acute hypoglycaemia, e.g. sepsis, liver disease and non-islet cell tumour-induced hypoglycaemia, would have been associated with undetectable levels of both. The only other possibility is sulphonylurea poisoning, but this can be detected in the initial blood sample.

Definitive investigations

There is no detectable sulphonylurea activity in the blood sample. A computed tomography scan (CT) of the pancreas shows no abnormality, but an endoscopic ultrasound scan reveals a 1.5 cm rounded lesion in the tail of the

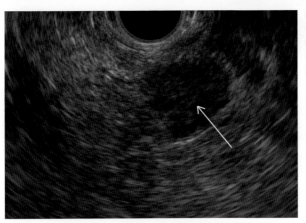

Fig. 54.1 Endoscopic ultrasound scan showing 10 mm lesion in the tail of the pancreas (arrow).

pancreas (Fig. 54.1). Biopsy confirms the presence of neuroendocrine cells, with heavy staining for insulin.

How will you treat this patient?

The definitive treatment is surgery. Insulinomas are usually benign and can often be 'shelled out' by an experienced surgeon. While surgery is awaited, or if the patient is not deemed to be fit for an operation, oral diazoxide will suppress insulin secretion and prevent recurrent hypoglycaemia. It is often helpful to teach the patient home blood glucose monitoring and to provide dietary advice on the treatment of hypoglycaemia and the need for regular meals and snacks, particularly prior to exercise.

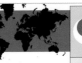

Global issues

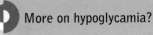 More on hypoglycamia?

- World-wide, insulin and sulphonylurea-treated diabetes are the most common causes of hypoglycaemia.

- In developed countries, alcohol excess is a common cause of hypoglycaemia in non-diabetic individuals.

- Patients with severe *falciparum* malaria should be monitored frequently for the development of hypoglycaemia.

- Toxic hypoglycaemia syndrome can result from the consumption of unripe ackee fruit, which grows in the Caribbean and in West Africa.

See Chapter 20 of
Davidson's Principles and Practice of Medicine (20th edn)

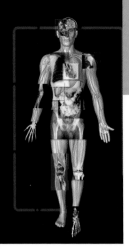

55

An obese middle-aged woman with recently discovered hyperglycaemia

S. BANERJEE

Presenting problem

An obese 46-year-old woman presents with recurrent attacks of pruritus vulvae and mild dysuria. She is an office assistant, of lower middle income group. She has no history of polyuria, polyphagia or polydipsia, and has not noticed any recent changes in body weight. She is a non-smoker and does not drink alcohol; she is not on any regular medication. She has two children and reports that high blood glucose levels were noted during her second pregnancy, though no intervention was required. Her mother and elder brother both developed diabetes in their early fifties and are managed with tablets. Her father died of coronary artery disease and hypertension.

A routine urine examination, performed by her general practitioner, shows the presence of glucose and a trace of albumin. No ketonuria is noted. Her fasting plasma glucose is 8 mmol/l (144 mg/dl); 2 hours after a 75 g glucose load, the plasma glucose is 15 mmol /l (270 mg/dl). A vaginal swab reveals the presence of *Candida albicans*.

What would your differential diagnosis include before examining the patient?

The GP has done the main work here, as the blood tests are certainly diagnostic of diabetes. This lady has a classic history for a new presentation of type 2 diabetes. She is overweight, has osmotic symptoms and has a strong family history. Moreover, she probably had gestational diabetes during her second pregnancy. The possibility of other aetiologies of diabetes should always be considered, though, because occasionally someone with a classic phenotype for type 2 diabetes turns out to have something completely different.

Type 1 diabetes would need to be considered if there were a history of recent unexplained weight loss, particularly in a thin person, and if ketonuria had been identified. Diabetes may also occur in people with pancreatic pathology, most commonly following acute or chronic pancreatitis. Haemochromatosis is a rare trap for the unwary and only causes 'bronze diabetes' in very advanced cases. Diabetes secondary to endocrinopathies, i.e. Cushing's syndrome, acromegaly and phaeochromocytoma, should be obvious clinically, but the overlap between Cushing's syndrome and simple central obesity means that distinguishing the two is not always straightforward. Steroid-induced diabetes should never pose diagnostic difficulty if a careful drug history is taken. Finally, there are rare

BOX 55.1

Further investigations

Urea	6.3 mmol/l (17.6 mg/dl)
Creatinine	94 µmol/l (1.06 mg/dl)
HbA$_{1C}$	10.4%
Total cholesterol	5.5 mmol/l (213 mg/dl)
LDL cholesterol	3.3 mmol/l (128 mg/dl)
HDL cholesterol	0.85 mmol/l (33 mg/dl)
Triglyceride	2.6 mmol/l (228 mg/dl)
Bilirubin	22 µmol/l (1.29 mg/dl)
ALT	68 U/l
GGT	30 U/l
Alkaline phosphatase	97 U/l
Urine albumin:creatinine	3.1 mg/mmol (normal range 0–3.5)

monogenic disorders that cause diabetes and these should be considered in patients whose presentation does not quite fit the bill: for example, a young person who is not overweight, has not lost any weight and does not have ketonuria.

Examination

On examination, the patient is 1.68 m tall and weighs 89.1 kg, giving a body mass index of 31. Her waist:hip ratio is 1.04. She looks well, has no features of Cushing's syndrome or acromegaly, and is not clinically dehydrated. She has normal pulses, which are equal in all the limbs. Her blood pressure is 160/90 mmHg supine and 150/86 mmHg erect. Ankle jerks on both sides are normal, but vibration sense and monofilament sensation test in the feet are diminished. The interdigital spaces and toenails are normal and there is no callus formation. Fundal examination shows no evidence of diabetic retinopathy. Abdominal examination is unremarkable.

Has examination narrowed down your differential diagnosis?

Examination has essentially excluded the coexistence of an endocrinopathy and confirms the impression of central obesity. Blood pressure is elevated in the majority of people with type 2 diabetes, and this remains the most likely diagnosis.

Further investigations

A full blood count is within normal limits. Further blood test results are shown in Box 55.1. A 12-lead electrocardiogram (ECG) is normal. An ultrasound scan of the abdomen reveals an echo-bright liver consistent with fatty infiltration.

Does this narrow down your differential diagnosis?

Type 2 diabetes is associated with central obesity and resistance to the peripheral actions of insulin (metabolic syndrome). This lady has a typical lipid profile for someone with the metabolic syndrome, i.e. borderline high total cholesterol, low HDL cholesterol and borderline high triglycerides. The elevated ALT and the ultrasound features are consistent with non-alcoholic fatty liver disease,

BOX 55.2	
Therapeutic targets in type 2 diabetes	
Fasting blood glucose	4–7 mmol/l (72–126 mg/dl)
2 hrs after food	4–10 mmol/l (72–180 mg/dl)
HbA$_{1C}$	< 7%
BP	< 130/80 mmHg
LDL cholesterol	< 2.60 mmol/l (100 mg/dl)
HDL cholesterol	> 1 mmol/l (40 mg/dl)
Triglyceride	< 1.5 mmol/l (150 mg/dl)
Ideal body weight	Body mass index 20–25

which is now increasingly recognised as being a component of the metabolic syndrome. The elevated glycated haemoglobin indicates that she has had elevated blood glucose concentrations for at least several months. She does not have microalbuminuria — this is good news, because in someone with type 2 diabetes this is an additional risk factor for cardiovascular disease.

How will you treat this patient?

Type 2 diabetes is strongly associated with premature cardiovascular disease and so reduction in cardiovascular risk is one of the main overall goals of modern diabetes therapy. Given her young age, she is also at risk of microvascular complications of diabetes, i.e. retinopathy, nephropathy and neuropathy. In fact, the neurological findings suggest that she may already have a degree of peripheral neuropathy.

Therapeutic targets are shown in Box 55.2. Lifestyle modification underpins all of the therapy that will be prescribed for this lady. She should see a dietitian and be advised to lose weight and take regular exercise. She does not smoke, but if she did she would need to be strongly advised to stop. Most guidelines say that in an individual like this, antidiabetic therapy should not be prescribed for 3–4 months to determine whether lifestyle measures result in improved metabolic parameters. It is highly likely, though, that this lady will require an oral hypoglycaemic agent and metformin would be the first-line choice. It has, at worst, a neutral effect on weight and on its own does not cause hypoglycaemia.

Blood pressure should be aggressively targeted, with an angiotensin-converting enzyme (ACE) inhibitor in the first instance. Most guidelines recommend statin treatment for all people with type 2 diabetes over the age of 40 years. Aspirin is indicated in people over the age of 50 years, provided there are no contraindications.

This lady will require long-term review by a multidisciplinary diabetes team. She should be screened annually for diabetic eye, kidney and foot disease and should receive regular lifestyle reminders. Given her peripheral neuropathy, she should receive detailed foot care advice, particularly about avoiding overtight shoes and high-risk activities, such as walking barefoot. The likelihood is that she will require multiple medications to control her blood pressure and, as time progresses (and her pancreatic β cell reserve falls), she will need increased medication, including insulin, to maintain good glycaemic control.

Global issues

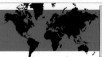

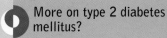

More on type 2 diabetes mellitus?

See Chapter 21 of
Davidson's Principles and Practice of Medicine
(20th edn)

- The incidence of diabetes mellitus, particularly type 2, is increasing globally.

- Increasing longevity and the global epidemic of obesity are to blame for the rising incidence of type 2 diabetes.

- Type 2 diabetes mellitus can be asymptomatic in its early stages and is often diagnosed late by routine screening or accidental detection.

- More than 20% of people with newly diagnosed type 2 diabetes mellitus have complications at the time of presentation.

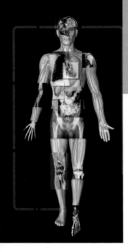

56

A woman with type 1 diabetes, a cough and breathlessness

B. M. FRIER

Presenting problem

A 33-year-old Caucasian woman with type 1 diabetes is admitted to hospital with a 2-week history of increasing shortness of breath and a cough, productive of green sputum. She has stopped taking her insulin for 2 days preceding admission because she has lost her appetite, has been feeling nauseated and has not been eating. She has had previous admissions to hospital with diabetes-related problems and seldom attends the diabetes outpatient clinic. In the Accident and Emergency department, a capillary blood sample registers high on the glucose meter, and venous blood samples are sent for urgent laboratory estimations. Urinalysis is also performed. The results are shown in Box 56.1.

What would your differential diagnosis include before examining the patient?

The elevated white cell count and C-reactive protein (CRP), in association with the history of increasing shortness of breath, cough and purulent sputum, suggest that she has a lower respiratory tract infection. The presence of a metabolic acidosis (HCO_3 6.1 mmol/l (meq/l)) and of ketonuria indicates severe metabolic decompensation. The International Diabetes Federation (IDF) criteria for significant diabetic ketoacidosis (DKA) comprise:

1. hyperglycaemia (plasma glucose > 11 mmol/l (198 mg/dl))
2. metabolic acidosis with an arterial bicarbonate (HCO_3) concentration of < 15 mmol/l (meq/l) or arterial H^+ of > 49 nmol/l (pH < 7.31) associated with ketonaemia (β-hydroxybutyrate > 0.27 mmol/l).

In addition to DKA, the differential diagnosis includes starvation and alcohol-induced ketoacidosis. However, in those circumstances it is rare for the blood glucose to exceed 14 mmol/l (252 mg/dl) and for the plasma HCO_3 to fall below 18 mmol/l (meq/l).

Examination

On examination, the patient is pyrexial (temperature 38.3°C), tachycardic (120 beats/min), and hypotensive (98/54 mmHg). She appears dehydrated with a dry tongue, and her breath has a 'fruity' odour. Heart

56

BOX 56.1

Initial investigations

Sodium	132 mmol/l (meq/l)
Potassium	5.5 mmol/l (meq/l)
Chloride	96 mmol/l (meq/l)
Bicarbonate	6.1 mmol/l (meq/l)
Urea	12.2 mmol/l (34.14 mg/dl)
Creatinine	150 µmol/l (1.69 mg/dl)
Glucose	39.2 mmol/l (706 mg/dl)
CRP	248 mg/l
Urinalysis	
Blood	+
Protein	+
Glucose	+++
Ketones	++++
WCC	25.1×10^9/l (10^3/mm^3)
Haemoglobin	149 g/l (14.9 g/dl)
Platelets	322×10^9/l (10^3/mm^3)
MCV	90.3 fl

auscultation and abdominal palpation are unremarkable. Her breathing is noted to be rapid and deep. Auscultation of her chest reveals upper right-sided coarse crepitations and bronchial breathing.

Has examination narrowed down your differential diagnosis?

In addition to the signs of a right upper lobe infection, a few characteristic signs of DKA are present. The relative insulin deficiency and excessive secretion of counter-regulatory hormones that occur in DKA allow uncontrolled lipolysis and result in high circulating levels of free fatty acids, which are metabolised in the liver where they are oxidised to ketone bodies. This produces the classical 'fruity' smell (said to resemble pear drops) on the patient's breath. In an attempt to compensate for the metabolic acidosis of DKA, a respiratory alkalosis is induced via rapid deep breathing (called Kussmaul respirations).

Further investigations

Arterial blood gases reveal H$^+$ 96.9 nmol/l (pH = 7.01), PO_2 9.89 kPa (74.2 mmHg), $PCO2$ 1.84 kPa (13.8 mmHg), HCO$_3$ 5.9 mmol/l (meq/l) and base excess −23.0 mmol/l (meq/l), confirming that she has a severe metabolic acidosis. A chest X-ray shows a right upper zone pneumonia (Fig. 56.1).

Has the diagnosis been clinched?

The clinical examination and investigations demonstrate the presence of a lobar pneumonia, and the severe bacterial infection has precipitated DKA in this patient. The patient stopping her insulin inappropriately has aggravated the metabolic decompensation. Common precipitating factors of DKA include new presentation of untreated type 1 diabetes, intercurrent infection, non-compliance with insulin therapy, psychological factors adversely affecting self-management

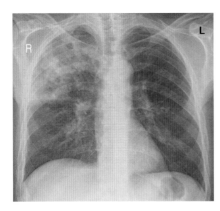

Fig. 56.1 Chest X-ray showing right upper zone pneumonia.

(especially in adolescents and young adults), myocardial infarction and drugs such as steroids.

How will you treat this patient?

There are several different issues that need to be considered for this patient.

1. *Fluid replacement.* The total body water deficit in DKA is usually between 5 and 8 litres. Between 1 and 2 litres of isotonic saline should be administered intravenously in the first hour. Thereafter, 250–500 ml/hr of 0.9% saline should be given and continued until the patient is volume-replete. When the blood glucose declines to ~15 mmol/l (270 mg/dl), intravenous 5% glucose should be added to allow sufficiently high concentrations of intravenous insulin to continue to be administered to switch off ketogenesis.
2. *Insulin therapy.* Add 50 U of soluble (short-acting) insulin to 50 ml 0.9% saline and administer intravenously by infusion pump, initially at 6 U/hour. Thereafter, give a continuous intravenous infusion of 1–3 U/hr, depending on hourly blood glucose measurements. Aim for a fall in blood glucose of 3–6 mmol/l (54–108 mg/dl) per hour; then maintain blood glucose between 10 and 12 mmol/l (180–216 mg/dl). Continue intravenous infusion for 12–24 hours after the ketosis has resolved and the patient is eating and drinking.
3. *Electrolyte replacement.* The initial serum potassium is elevated because of the insulin deficiency and acute renal failure, but patients with DKA usually have profound total body potassium deficits. This patient will need lots of potassium. Give potassium replacement by intravenous infusion, but not in the first litre of fluid.
4. *Other measures.* The pneumonia should be treated with a broad-spectrum antibiotic depending on the most likely local organisms and their common sensitivities. In the UK, amoxicillin is often used as the first-line drug, plus or minus a macrolide. In view of the severity of the illness, though, intravenous ceftriaxone 2 g daily might be a better option. The patient should be admitted to a high-dependency unit for close observation. Urine output, heart rate and blood pressure should be monitored, and if the patient were to remain anuric despite volume replacement, a urethral catheter should be inserted. A nasogastric tube would be required if the patient was semiconscious to reduce the risk of aspiration pneumonia. Sodium bicarbonate should not be administered, as it may worsen intracellular acidosis.

Most patients make a complete recovery from DKA and spend only a few days in hospital. Cerebral oedema is a rare but devastating complication that can occur in children and young adults.

Prior to discharge she should be seen by the diabetes team and reminded about the need to monitor blood glucose frequently during intercurrent illness, to increase (rather than decrease) insulin doses and to maintain a high intake of clear fluids. She should be encouraged to re-attend the diabetes clinic.

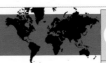

Global issues

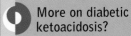

More on diabetic ketoacidosis?

- The mortality rate associated with DKA is around 5–10% in Western countries, and is reported to be up to 25% in developing countries where access to intensive clinical and laboratory facilities may not be available.

- While DKA is rare in type 2 diabetes, an increase in incidence has been reported in African-Americans and other ethnic groups with type 2 diabetes.

See Chapter 21 of
Davidson's Principles and Practice of Medicine
(20th edn)

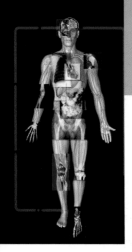

57

A middle-aged man with poorly controlled diabetes and a non-healing foot ulcer

A. RAMACHANDRAN

Presenting problem

A 55-year-old gentleman with type 2 diabetes mellitus of 15 years' duration is hospitalised for control of his diabetes and management of a non-healing ulcer on the right heel, which developed following a thorn prick 2 months earlier. The patient also complains of numbness in his feet and pain in both legs on walking distances of more than 100 m; the pain subsides after a few minutes' rest. He has been a heavy smoker for the last 30 years. His right first and second toes were amputated 2 years ago and he had laser therapy for diabetic retinopathy last year. He takes several medications, including metformin and glibenclamide for his diabetes, as well as aspirin and enalapril. Prior to referral his general practitioner had performed some investigations and the results are provided in Box 57.1.

What would your differential diagnosis include before examining the patient?

The foot is a frequent site for complications in patients with diabetes mellitus, and for this reason foot care is extremely important. Tissue necrosis in the foot is a common reason for hospital admission in diabetic patients. These admissions

BOX 57.1	
Initial investigations	
Haemoglobin	72 g/l (7.2 g/dl)
WCC	$15.8 \times 10^9/l$ ($10^3/mm^3$)
Fasting blood glucose	14.3 mmol/l (258 mg/dl)
Post-prandial blood glucose	25.4 mmol/l (458 mg/dl)
HbA_{1c}	13.5%
Urea	12 mmol/l (78 mg/dl)
Creatinine	168 µmol/l (1.9 mg/dl)
Urine examination	
Albumin	++
ECG	T wave inversions in V_1–V_4 suggestive of anteroseptal ischaemia; normal R–R interval

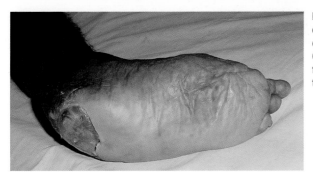

Fig. 57.1 Large ulcer on the heel following debridement. Note the Charcot deformity of the foot and the previous toe amputations.

tend to be prolonged and may end with amputation. A non-healing foot ulcer in a patient with diabetes mellitus requires differentiation from other types of neuropathic, ischaemic and neuro-ischaemic ulcers. Since this patient has diabetes, is a chronic smoker and has symptoms suggestive of both peripheral neuropathy and intermittent claudication, the diagnosis favours a neuro-ischaemic ulcer.

Examination

The patient is conscious, oriented, febrile and pale. The respiratory rate is 18/min. He is mildly dehydrated and has xanthelasma palpebrarum on the right side. Bilateral pitting oedema is present. His pulse rate is 100/min regular. Blood pressure readings supine and standing are 160/90 mmHg and 150/80 mmHg, respectively. The pulsations of both carotid and subclavian arteries are equal on both sides. The pulsations of the popliteal, posterior tibial and dorsalis pedis arteries are absent in both lower limbs. The first and second toes on the right side are amputated with well-healed scars. The nervous system examination reveals absent ankle jerks and decreased vibration sense and proprioception on both sides. The left foot is swollen and its skin is dry and hairless. There is a non-healing ulcer 3 × 3 cm on the right heel (Fig. 57.1), with foul-smelling pus discharge and erythema and swelling of the surrounding skin. There is flattening of the arch of the right foot with features of an early Charcot deformity. Non-proliferative diabetic retinopathy, with laser photocoagulation scars, is present in both eyes on fundus examination.

Have examination and initial investigations narrowed down your differential diagnosis?

This gentleman has a royal flush of diabetes complications. He has known retinopathy, while blood and urine tests strongly suggest the presence of diabetic nephropathy. He has electrocardiogram (ECG) evidence of coronary artery disease and clinical evidence of peripheral vascular disease and peripheral neuropathy.

Various mechanisms could have produced the initial foot ulceration, including somatic neuropathy (diminished proprioception), autonomic neuropathy (dry skin, fissures, Charcot neuropathy) and peripheral vascular disease (claudication and absent arterial pulsations in lower limbs). Secondary infection of the ulcer has caused surrounding cellulitis.

In addition to diabetes mellitus, other conditions can also produce persistent foot ulcers and these include Hansen's disease, thromboangiitis obliterans (Buerger's disease) and vasculitis; however, given the overwhelming evidence diabetes has to be the likely culprit here.

Further investigations

X-ray right foot	Early Charcot arthropathy
Doppler test of lower limb	
Right ankle brachial index	0.6
Left ankle brachial index	0.8
Biothesiometry	Severe neuropathy (sensation felt at 45 V of current by vibrating method)
Monofilament test	Protective sensation absent with 10 g monofilament in all arches of foot
Colour arterial Doppler	Monophasic pulsations present in posterior tibial artery, dorsalis pedis artery and popliteal artery in right lower limb, suggestive of peripheral vascular disease
Nerve conduction study	Severe sensory motor neuropathy in both lower limbs

Further investigations

Box 57.2 provides the results of further investigation of the right foot.

Does this narrow down your differential diagnosis?

The results confirm the clinical impression that this man has severe sensory motor neuropathy, as well as peripheral vascular disease. These abnormalities, as well as uncontrolled hyperglycaemia and anaemia, have produced a non-healing ulcer in the right foot. There is secondary infection of the ulcer, surrounding cellulitis and an early Charcot deformity of the foot.

How will you treat this patient?

Strict glycaemic control should be ensured with conversion of this gentleman's treatment to insulin therapy. Broad-spectrum antibiotics should be administered according to the culture and sensitivity of the organisms grown from a swab taken from the ulcer. Necrotic tissue should be debrided aggressively. Regular dressings and follow-up will be essential; pressure relief is essential — appropriate footwear should be provided, with insoles that redistribute pressure around the foot and away from the ulcerated area. Total contact casting and intravenous bisphosphonate therapy have been advocated for patients with an acute Charcot arthropathy, but the former would be ill advised here, given the presence of active ulceration. The patient should be initiated into a rehabilitation programme comprising education regarding footwear and footcare (e.g. avoiding barefoot walking, regular inspection of the feet for new abnormalities).

Consideration should also be given to the feasibility of vascular reconstruction. If available, magnetic resonance imaging (MRI) angiography should be performed to assess the patency of the large vessels in the leg. The gentleman should be given strong advice and help to stop smoking. He is already taking aspirin and an angiotensin-converting enzyme (ACE) inhibitor, but his blood pressure is poorly controlled. This needs to be aggressively targeted (to below 120/70 mmHg) with additional antihypertensive therapy, given his retinopathy and nephropathy. He would also derive prognostic benefit from being commenced on a statin, irrespective of his total cholesterol concentration.

Global issues

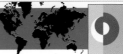

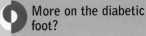
More on the diabetic foot?

See Chapter 21 of
Davidson's Principles and Practice of Medicine
(20th edn)

- Diabetic foot disease is one of the most frequent causes of hospitalisation and is one of the most expensive complications of diabetes.

- Diabetic foot ulceration is common among people who walk bare foot.

- Diabetic foot disease places a heavy burden on socioeconomic resources of families and countries, particularly developing countries.

- The magnitude of the problem in developing countries calls for epidemiological research to enable and encourage policymakers and health administrators to address the problems caused by this dreaded complication of diabetes mellitus.

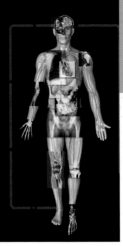

58

A middle-aged man with dysphagia

I. D. R. ARNOTT

Presenting problem

A 55-year-old man presents to his general practitioner with a 4-week history of progressive dysphagia. He is able to swallow all liquids, but the ingestion of solid food leads to regurgitation and vomiting. He also complains of some non-specific but occasionally severe retrosternal discomfort that is relieved by regurgitation or vomiting. There is no odynophagia or early satiety. Over the duration of his history he has lost 3 kg weight and has also noticed a decreased appetite. He has suffered from gastro-oesophageal reflux for many years, being woken approximately 3 times a week with symptoms of nocturnal reflux.

His past medical history is notable for a non-ST elevation myocardial infarction 4 years ago. A coronary artery stent was inserted and he has been asymptomatic since then. He is also known to have hypertension. His current medication includes aspirin, atenolol, simvastatin and lisinopril. He lives with his wife and is able to complete all activities of daily living. He gave up smoking following his heart attack, having smoked 15 cigarettes per day since the age of 27. He consumes approximately 32 units of alcohol per week.

What would your differential diagnosis include before examining the patient?

The most important diagnosis to confirm or exclude is oesophageal cancer. The progressive nature of his symptoms makes this most likely. It is of note that he is able to tolerate liquids but not solids. The differential diagnosis includes a benign oesophageal stricture. The history for benign disease is often longer but the same pattern for solids and liquids exists. The other main differential diagnosis is achalasia or other dysmotility syndromes. Again, a longer history would be expected and individuals often experience symptoms with liquids as well as solids. It is common to have some evidence of weight loss with all of the above, but this is much greater with malignant causes. General well-being and weight are often maintained in the early stages of oesophageal cancer and so the absence of these does not exclude the diagnosis. Odynophagia is more commonly caused by reflux oesophagitis and infections such as candidiasis, but can also occur in oesophageal cancer.

Examination and initial investigations

There is no evidence of lymphadenopathy or pallor. The patient's body mass index is 30. Pulse is 68/min and venous pressure is not raised. Heart sounds are normal and there is no peripheral oedema. The chest is clear. The abdomen is soft and non-tender, with no masses or organomegaly.

Initial investigations, comprising full blood count, serum biochemistry and liver function tests, are normal and a chest X-ray is also normal.

Have examination and initial investigations narrowed down your differential diagnosis?

No. The differential diagnosis remains the same. Although there are physical findings that do point to a particular diagnosis, it is more common for examination not to influence your decision-making at this stage. An upper gastrointestinal endoscopy is urgently required.

Further investigations

Anatomically, the cricopharyngeus is normally 20 cm from the incisors, and at endoscopy this marks the proximal extent of the evaluable oesophagus. The gastro-oesophageal junction lies 40 cm from the incisors.

The patient undergoes an upper gastrointestinal endoscopy 4 days following clinic review. There is evidence of columnar lined oesophagus from 32 cm, extending to the gastro-oesophageal junction. At 38 cm there is an exophytic, macroscopically malignant tumour arising from the oesophageal wall, which causes narrowing of the lumen; the endoscope will not pass through this (Fig. 58.1). Multiple biopsies are taken from the mass and from the columnar lined oesophagus above. Biopsies of the tumour mass reveal adenocarcinoma and those from above reveal specialised intestinal metaplasia, i.e. Barrett's oesophagus.

To stage the patient's oesophageal tumour a computed tomography (CT) scan of the chest and abdomen is performed. This confirms concentric thickening of the distal oesophagus and some peri-tumour lymph nodes. On the scan, these do not reach size criteria for tumour spread, but they do raise suspicion of lymph node involvement. The scan does not show any solid organ metastatic disease.

CT cannot adequately stage the tumour within the oesophagus and further imaging is therefore required: namely, endoscopic ultrasound (EUS). This confirms the presence of tumour at 38 cm within the oesophagus; although it involves the mucosa and submucosa, it has not breached the muscularis mucosae and is therefore staged as T2. The lymph nodes noted on CT are enlarged up to 1 cm but there are no enlarged coeliac axis nodes. In view of the relatively early tumour stage, these enlarged nodes have more significance. To classify them further, EUS-guided fine needle aspiration is undertaken. This reveals malignant cells in 2 out of 3 nodes sampled.

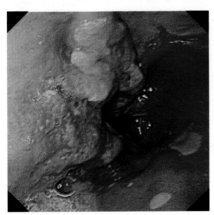

Fig. 58.1 An exophytic cancer seen in the distal oesophagus at upper gastrointestinal endoscopy.

Has the diagnosis been clinched?

These investigations have confirmed a distal oesophageal adenocarcinoma arising in an area of Barrett's oesophagus. Investigations have staged this tumour as T2N1M0. The Barrett's oesophagus has occurred as a consequence of long-term acid reflux. Risk factors for oesophageal cancer are shown in Box 58.1 and can be remembered using the mnemonic 'BELCH-SPAT'.

BOX 58.1

Risk factors for oesophageal cancer

- Barrett's oesophagus
- Ethanol abuse
- Lye stricture
- Coeliac disease
- Head and neck tumours
- Smoking
- Plummer–Vinson syndrome
- Achalasia
- Tylosis

How will you treat this patient?

The priority is to relieve the dysphagia and this is usually achieved by endoscopic balloon dilatation. At endoscopy, a controlled radial expansion balloon may be placed through the stricture under direct vision and then inflated to approximately 3 atmospheres pressure. This corresponds to a balloon diameter of 15 mm.

Tumours of this stage, specifically because of the lymph node spread, are not generally considered curable by surgery alone. This gentleman should, therefore, undergo two cycles of neoadjuvant chemotherapy with cisplatin and 5-fluorouracil. Current protocols suggest that further staging following this is needed before decisions about surgery can be made. If the restaging CT shows evidence of tumour shrinkage, then the patient should be a good candidate for cardio-oesophagectomy with curative intent. Recovery from such surgery is typically prolonged, and on discharge this man will need strict dietary and nutritional instructions to help him maintain his weight.

Survival rates, despite best treatment, remain low. For oesophageal carcinoma overall, the 1-year survival is 27% and the 5-year survival is approximately 9%. For this gentleman, given best treatment, 2-year survival is in the region of only 45%. A guarded prognosis, therefore, must be conveyed to the patient.

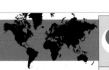

Global issues

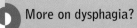

More on dysphagia?

- The incidence of oesophageal carcinoma varies world-wide. Squamous cell cancer occurs commonly in parts of China, Iran, Central Asia, Siberia, Mongolia, Afghanistan, parts of Africa, Iceland and Finland, whereas adenocarcinoma occurs in Western populations.

- Invasive oesophageal candidiasis can present with odynophagia, particularly in areas with a high prevalence of human immunodeficiency virus (HIV).

- In developing nations, tuberculosis should be included in the differential diagnosis of odynophagia. Tuberculosis can rarely involve the oesophagus; however, mediastinal lymphadenopathy and a cold abscess can produce similar symptoms.

See Chapter 22 of
Davidson's Principles and Practice of Medicine
(20th edn)

59

A middle-aged man with a recent haematemesis

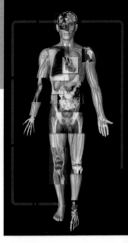

S. M. W. JAFRI

Presenting problem

A 42-year-old male patient presents to the Accident and Emergency department with a 1-day history of vomiting fresh blood. He also reports the passing of black-coloured stools for the last 3 days and feeling generally unwell for almost 6 weeks. His main complaint is of easy fatiguability and he is unable to carry on his work beyond 3 p.m. He is privately employed as a driver and does not drink alcohol. His past medical history is uneventful, with the exception that he has had three episodes of jaundice: the first when he was 20 years old, then 4–5 years after that and a further episode about 3 years ago. Each time he was seen by a herbal practitioner, who prescribed some herbs, and after a few days the patient felt better. He did not have any blood tests. His main reason for not seeking medical attention, other than the herbal practitioner, was financial constraints, as he thought that a doctor would order lots of tests that he could not afford.

What would your differential diagnosis include before examining the patient?

The key facts are that this 42-year-old male patient is presenting with haematemesis and melaena, with at least three previous episodes of jaundice. It is possible that he is suffering from chronic viral hepatitis B or C and has now developed cirrhosis, portal hypertension and bleeding from oesophageal varices, or else he may be suffering from a peptic ulcer which is bleeding. Other possibilities include oesophageal ulcers from chronic reflux oesophagitis, Mallory–Weiss tears and gastric carcinoma, but with this history these seem very unlikely.

Examination

Physical examination reveals an icteric and pale patient. His blood pressure is 110/70 mmHg and heart rate 90/min. Although oriented in place and person, he is somewhat confused and at times inattentive during examination. The liver is palpable about 2 cm below the costal margin and the spleen is palpable 4 cm below the costal margin. There is no shifting dullness or fluid thrill. On the chest and back there are a few spider angiomas.

Has examination narrowed down your differential diagnosis?

The mild confusion, hepatosplenomegaly, jaundice and spider angiomas suggest that this patient has portal hypertension secondary to cirrhosis. The haematemesis is most likely due to variceal hemorrhage. However, patients

BOX 59.1

Initial investigations

Haemoglobin	100 g/l (10 g/dl)
Platelets	54×10^9/l (10^3/mm^3)
WCC	2.3×10^9/l (10^3/mm^3)
Prothrombin time	18 sec
Urea	14.3 mmol/l (40.5 mg/dl)
Creatinine	65 µmol/l (0.73 mg/dl)
Bilirubin	74 µmol/l (4.33 mg/dl)
ALT	54 U/l
AST	46 U/l
Alkaline phosphatase	112 U/l
Albumin	28 g/l (2.8 g/dl)
α-fetoprotein	8 U/l (upper limit of normal 5.5 U/l)
Hepatitis B surface antigen and core antibody	Negative
Hepatitis C virus antibody	Positive

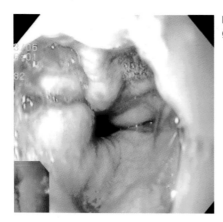

Fig. 59.1 Oesophageal varices at upper gastrointestinal endoscopy.

with cirrhosis do have a higher incidence of peptic ulceration, which at this stage cannot be ruled out.

Investigations

Blood test results are shown in Box 59.1. The patient has an emergency ultrasound carried out and this shows mild ascites, splenomegaly, altered echotexture of the liver, a dilated portal vein and varices around the splenic hilum. There is suspicion of a mass in the right lobe of the liver measuring 3.3 cm. As the α-fetoprotein is high in a patient who has a mass in a cirrhotic liver, further investigation with dynamic computed tomography (CT) is performed; this confirms the mass to be a hepatoma.

From the Accident and Emergency department, and following aggressive resuscitation with intravenous fluids, the patient is transferred to the endoscopy suite, where he has an upper gastrointestinal endoscopy. This reveals bleeding oesophageal varices (Fig. 59.1); the stomach contains about 200 ml of altered blood. There is no ulcer or erosions, but there is significant portal hypertensive gastropathy involving most of the stomach; there are no fundal varices.

Does this narrow down your differential diagnosis?

Yes; this patient has chronic hepatitis C with cirrhosis. He has two further complications: hepatic decompensation (ascites and mild hepatic encephalopathy) and a hepatoma. Hepatitis C is a chronic disease and, if not treated early, can result in cirrhosis in about 30% of patients after a delay of 25–30 years. After a further few years, hepatic decompensation and the development of hepatocellular cancer may occur. There are over 200 million patients with hepatitis C throughout the world and it has evolved as one of the major causes of chronic liver disease and reasons for liver transplantation as well.

How will you treat this patient?

Resuscitation with intravenous crystalloids and, if necessary, blood is essential prior to endoscopy. At endoscopy, the patient should be treated with band ligation of the oesophageal varices. This would require at least 2–3 endoscopic sessions to achieve complete eradication.

Once his condition has stabilised and the bleeding has been stopped, the patient should be commenced on propranolol at a dose that will lower his heart rate to around ≤ 60/min. This would reduce portal hypertension, which, in turn, should help his portal hypertensive gastropathy and further bleeding from varices. For mild ascites, he should be treated with a low-salt diet; if that is not enough, he should receive spironolactone at a small dose of 50 mg daily. Resection of the hepatoma is not feasible, as he already has hepatic decompensation. He should therefore receive either percutaneous ethanol injections (PEI), transcutaneous arterial chemo-embolisation (TACE) or radiofrequency ablation, depending on local expertise and facilities. All three modalities have shown comparative results. If he is being treated in a centre where transplant facilities are available, he should be evaluated for a liver transplant, as this would be his best chance for survival.

Global issues

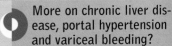

More on chronic liver disease, portal hypertension and variceal bleeding?

See Chapter 23 of
Davidson's Principles and Practice of Medicine
(20th edn)

- Chronic liver disease is extremely prevalent throughout the world but has different causes. Viral hepatitis B and C are behind most cases; the other important cause is alcohol.

- Patients with a history of jaundice should be properly evaluated with liver function tests and hepatitis B and C serology. They should be treated without delay if serology is positive.

- Effective treatment is available to control hepatitis B and to cure hepatitis C.

- Patients who have cirrhosis should be treated conservatively. If cirrhosis is complicated by ascites, encephalopathy, bleeding varices or a hepatoma, they should be treated in a specialised centre.

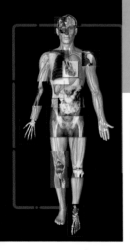

60

A boy with long-standing diarrhoea

G. K. MAKHARIA

Presenting problem

A 16-year-old boy presents to the outpatient department complaining of diarrhoea which he has had for 6 years. He passes 4–5 large-volume stools daily, which are frothy, greasy and foul-smelling, and contain undigested food material. The stools do not contain visible blood, mucus or pus. He has post-prandial bloating of the abdomen, generalised weakness and easy fatiguability. He has no abdominal pain, fever or joint pains. His parents mention that he is not growing well.

What would your differential diagnosis include before examining the patient?

The list of causes of chronic diarrhoea (diarrhoea lasting for more than 4 weeks) is extensive. It may be caused not only by diseases of the small and large intestine, but also by systemic diseases such as hyperthyroidism, diabetes mellitus, autonomic neuropathy and drugs (Box 60.1). We need to ask the following questions when approaching this patient:

1. Is the diarrhoea due to a functional disease (long-standing symptoms, no nocturnal diarrhoea) or an organic disease (weight loss, fever, short duration)?
2. Is the diarrhoea of small-bowel type (large volume, frothy, greasy, foul-smelling stool that contains undigested food material) or large-bowel type (more than six stools per day containing blood, mucus and/or pus, associated with tenesmus)?
3. Is the diarrhoea associated with features of malabsorption (bulky, frothy, greasy stool containing undigested food)?
4. Is there a systemic inflammatory response (such as fever, sweating or joint pains)?

From the history alone, it seems that the diarrhoea in this boy is chronic and of small-bowel type, and has features suggestive of malabsorption.

BOX 60.1

Causes of chronic diarrhoea and malabsorption

Small-bowel type
- Coeliac disease
- Tropical sprue
- Parasitic infections
- Immunodeficiency syndromes
- Crohn's disease
- Whipple's disease
- Abetalipoproteinaemia

Large-bowel type
- Irritable bowel syndrome
- Inflammatory bowel disease
- Microscopic colitis

Examination

The height, weight and body mass index of the patient are 150 cm, 32 kg and 14.2, respectively. He is pale and lacks secondary sexual characteristics. He has angular cheilitis and stomatitis.

Has examination narrowed down your clinical diagnosis?

The physical examination indicates that this patient has short stature (amounting to growth retardation), probable anaemia and nutritional deficiencies. These features support a diagnosis of malabsorption. Malabsorption in turn localises the site of disease to the small intestine. The causes of such chronic diarrhoea include coeliac disease, tropical sprue, parasitic infections (*Giardia lamblia*, *Cryptosporidium*, *Strongyloides*, *Microspora*, *Isospora*) and Crohn's disease (Box 60.1).

Investigations

The investigations in a patient with chronic diarrhoea with malabsorption include the following:

1. Haematological and biochemical tests to determine the type of anaemia and other effects of malabsorption (hypoproteinaemia, hypocalcaemia).
2. Tests to confirm the presence of malabsorption: d-xylose test, stool examination for fat globules, measurement of 72-hour stool fat excretion.
3. Endoscopic examination of the upper part of the intestine.
4. Intestinal mucosal biopsies. In the mucosal biopsies, a note is made on the crypt and villous architecture; these are most often graded using the Modified Marsh classification (grade 0 = normal crypt villous (CV) ratio = 1:3–4; grade 1= mild increase in intraepithelial lymphocytes (IEL), CV ratio 1:1; grade 2 = moderate villous atrophy, CV ratio < 1; grade 3 = flat mucosa with no recognisable villi).
5. Tests to determine the precise cause of the chronic diarrhoea and malabsorption, such as stool examination for ova and cysts of parasites, serological tests for coeliac disease (IgA-anti-endomysial antibody, IgA-anti-human tissue transglutaminase antibody, IgA or IgG antigliadin antibody), serum immunoglobulin profile (IgA, IgG and IgM levels), lipid profile and apolipoprotein levels, lactose hydrogen breath test (for lactose intolerance) and glucose hydrogen breath test (for bacterial overgrowth).

This patient's haemoglobin is 70 g/l (7.0 g/dl) and serum protein is 64 g/l (6.4 g/dl) (albumin 31 g/l (3.1 g/dl), globulin 33 g/l (3.3 g/dl)). After 5 g d-xylose ingestion, his 5-hour urinary d-xylose excretion is 0.5 g (normal > 1 g); his daily stool fat excretion is 8.0 g/day. Upper gastrointestinal endoscopy reveals attenuated and scalloped duodenal mucosal folds. The mucosal biopsy reveals a flat mucosa, an increase in intra-epithelial lymphocytes, and infiltration of the lamina propria with chronic inflammatory cells (Fig. 60.1); there are no parasites or abnormal macrophages. Serum IgA anti-human tissue transglutaminase antibody and IgA anti-endomysial antibody are positive. Serum levels of IgG, IgA and IgM are within normal limits. A glucose hydrogen breath tests and a lactose hydrogen breath test are normal. Stool examination reveals cysts of *Giardia lamblia*. The serological tests for human immunodeficiency virus (HIV) 1 and 2 are negative.

Have further investigations narrowed down your differential diagnosis?

Laboratory investigations show severe villous abnormality and a positive coeliac serological test. The diagnosis of coeliac disease is based on the Modified European Society of Paediatric Gastroenterology Hepatology and Nutrition (ESPGHAN) criteria, which include typical clinical manifestations, and suggestive histology (villous atrophy) and response to gluten-free diet. Therefore, based on clinical, histological and serological features, our patient has coeliac disease. In addition, he has *Giardia lamblia* infection, which might have contributed to his diarrhoea and malabsorption.

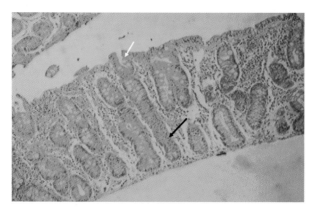

Fig. 60.1 Photomicrograph of an intestinal mucosal biopsy showing severe villous atrophy (flattening of villi, white arrow) and hyperplasia of crypts (black arrow) (H&E ×20).

How will you treat this patient?

Coeliac disease is a common autoimmune disorder, which occurs in genetically predisposed individuals and is induced by ingestion of a protein called gluten. Gluten is present in cereals such as wheat, barley and rye. The hypersensitivity to gluten in patients with coeliac disease is permanent: 'Once a coeliac, always a coeliac.' Therefore, the treatment of coeliac disease is withdrawal of gluten from the diet, which should continue on a life-long basis. These patients usually have deficiency of several nutrients and therefore a complete nutritional assessment is essential. This man should also be treated with a nitroimidazole for *Giardia lamblia* infection.

Although patients start feeling well 2–4 weeks after the institution of a gluten-free diet, normalisation of the histological picture may take a few months. During the initial days of treatment, vitamins and haematinics should be supplemented. The most important cause of failure to respond to treatment is poor or incomplete dietary compliance. The treatment should be continued under the supervision of a dietitian.

Global issues

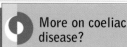

More on coeliac disease?

See Chapter 22 of
Davidson's Principles and Practice of Medicine (20th edn)

- Coeliac disease affects about 1% of the general population the world over.

- The wide belief that coeliac disease is a disease of childhood is not true. Adult patients with coeliac disease may present with either typical (chronic diarrhoea) or atypical (short stature, refractory anaemia, metabolic bone disease and infertility) manifestations.

- Coeliac disease shows an iceberg phenomenon; for every symptomatic patient, 3–10 patients remain undetected, i.e. are minimally symptomatic or asymptomatic. Such people may be picked up in screening programmes of 'at-risk individuals', such as those with type 1 diabetes and other autoimmune disorders.

- Abnormalities in coeliac disease may not be limited to the intestine; patients may also have involvement of other organs, such as skin, liver and brain.

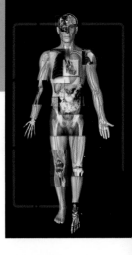

61

A young woman with constipation

I. D. PENMAN

Presenting problem

A 28-year-old woman is referred with a 2-year history of constipation, passing hard stools with difficulty only once per week. She has to strain, complains of a sensation of incomplete emptying, discomfort around her perianal area on defaecation, and also diffuse lower abdominal discomfort and bloating. In the last few months she has noticed mucus per rectum and small amounts of bright red blood, mainly on the toilet paper when she wipes herself. On systematic enquiry she reports a lack of energy and fatigue but no fever, sweats, diarrhoea or upper abdominal symptoms. She denies any urinary or gynaecological symptoms.

Past history includes investigations for headaches, but no serious cause was found. She takes codeine intermittently for these headaches and has had a brief period of time off work for anxiety and stress. The patient says her diet is reasonable, but does not contain much fruit. She works in a large office building as an operator in a call centre.

Prior to referral, her general practitioner checked some routine blood tests including urea, electrolytes, glucose, full blood count and erythrocyte sedimentation rate; these were all normal.

What would your differential diagnosis include before examining the patient?

In the majority of young adults with constipation the problem is one of 'simple' constipation without any underlying structural, inflammatory or other colonic disorder. In the developed world, diet and lifestyle factors are common causes of constipation and many young adults have a diet lacking in sufficient fibre, fruit, vegetable and fluid intake. Medications are a common cause of constipation (Box 61.1); the patient is taking codeine and this could well be contributing. Systemic disease (e.g. endocrine or neurological) can sometimes be associated with constipation and this should be sought. In this lady's case there may be many explanations for small amounts of blood and mucus per rectum, but it does raise the possibility of colorectal disease such

as proctitis (which can sometimes be associated with proximal constipation) or with neoplasia. All of these must be considered, but the diagnosis can usually be reached by a careful history, abdominal and rectal examination, and a few relatively simple investigations.

Examination

The patient looks generally well with no signs to suggest a systemic disorder, but is a little overweight. Abdominal examination is normal, rectal examination is tender but otherwise normal, and the rectum is empty. There is no obvious evidence of neurological abnormality.

Has examination narrowed down your differential diagnosis?

As is often the case, clinical examination has ruled out some obvious and serious conditions, but has not significantly narrowed down the differential diagnosis. Colorectal polyps and cancer are rare in people of this age and the patient appears well with no history or examination findings to suggest intestinal obstruction. Proctitis, rectal cancer and other rectal disorders, however, have not been completely excluded. Had proctoscopy or rigid sigmoidoscopy been performed in the clinic, this might have helped. Positive findings are useful (e.g. proctitis, ulcerative colitis, rectal cancer), but in practice the views are often limited and a negative rigid sigmoidoscopy does not adequately exclude problems more proximally in the rectosigmoid or left colon. The bleeding and mucus cannot be ignored and some further investigations are necessary.

Further investigations

A repeat full blood count, along with C-reactive protein (CRP), thyroid function tests and serum calcium, is normal, excluding hypercalcaemia and hypothyroidism; these are unusual but well-known causes of constipation. The patient undergoes a flexible sigmoidoscopy with examination of the colon up to the splenic flexure. Total colonoscopy is not performed, as bright red blood per rectum almost always originates in the distal colon or rectum and colon cancer is very rare at this age and with this presentation. There is considerable stool present despite bowel preparation, something that is often found in patients with chronic constipation. On the anterior wall of the distal rectum is an area of oedematous, friable, inflamed mucosa with ulceration, and this is biopsied. Histology shows non-specific inflammation, excess collagen and muscle thickening, features consistent with solitary rectal ulcer syndrome (SRUS).

Subsequently, an intestinal transit marker study is performed. The patient swallows capsules containing different-shaped pellets on each of 3 consecutive days and an abdominal X-ray is taken on day 5. While most or all of the pellets should be excreted by day 5, in this patient a large number of pellets are still retained in a uniform distribution throughout the colon (Fig. 61.1). These features are typical of 'slow-transit' constipation and the solitary rectal ulcer has probably resulted from repeated trauma of the rectal mucosa, a consequence of prolapse and ischaemia during straining at defaecation.

Does this narrow down your differential diagnosis?

The clinical picture, normal blood tests and findings from the flexible sigmoidoscopy and intestinal marker study confirm the diagnosis and further investigation is unnecessary.

How will you treat this patient?

By the time patients are referred to specialist clinics with constipation most of the simple measures have already been tried: stopping any constipating medications, increasing fluid intake to at least 2 litres daily, increasing dietary fibre, fruit and

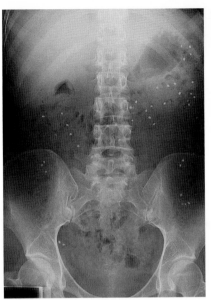

Fig. 61.1 Abdominal X-ray (day 5) after the patient ingests capsules containing different-shaped pellets on days 1, 2 and 3. Over 40 of the 60 pellets are still present, diffusely distributed throughout the colon.

vegetable intake, and regular exercise. Setting aside a regular, unhurried time for defaecation and availability of adequate toilet facilities and privacy are also important. None of these measures has proved effective in this patient; nor has therapy with a bulking agent (ispaghula), which worsened the bloating. Laxatives, including senna, lactulose and bisacodyl, are also of limited benefit.

In very difficult cases of chronic constipation several newer methods are sometimes effective. A combination approach may be necessary using agents such as a solution of inert polyethylene glycol salts (e.g. Movicol), which acts as an osmotic agent, glycerol suppositories (which can improve rectal emptying), and prokinetics such as metoclopramide or 5-HT$_4$ agonists. Other approaches that may be successful include biofeedback, in which a trainer helps the patient to retrain the coordination of rectal sensation and muscular control of defaecation over a number of sessions. It is labour-intensive and not widely available, but good results have been reported. In a minority of severely affected individuals, colectomy with ileorectal anastomosis is necessary, but this is a last resort and requires further careful evaluation and discussion.

Global issues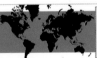

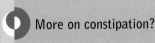 More on constipation?

- While more common in the developed world, chronic constipation is a world-wide problem, especially in hot climates.

- In the developing world, tuberculosis and chronic amoebiasis can present with constipation alternating with diarrhoea.

- Complex investigations are rarely necessary and most patients can be managed without resort to expensive medications.

See Chapter 22 of
Davidson's Principles and Practice of Medicine (20th edn)

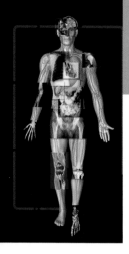

62

A woman with chronic abdominal pain

S. M. W. JAFRI

Presenting problem

A 35-year-old lady from Karachi in Pakistan presents to an outpatient clinic with a history of abdominal pain for the last 5 years. The pain generally starts around the umbilicus and radiates to almost the whole of the abdomen. It is colicky in nature and lasts from a few minutes to an hour on most of the occasions it occurs. She has had 3 or 4 attacks per year, but in the last 6 months she has had several episodes and now seeks medical advice. On previous occasions, she just attended the Accident and Emergency department of her local hospital; an injection to lessen the pain was given but few investigations were performed. She belongs to a low socioeconomic class and is the mother of five children; her husband earns a modest salary as a domestic servant. At the age of 14 she was ill for almost 6 months and remembers that she lost a lot of weight and at that time also had a persistent cough with haemoptysis. She was treated by a general practitioner for 18 months and was told that she possibly had tuberculosis. She is mostly constipated and moves her bowels 2 or 3 times a week. Her stools are otherwise normal with no mucus or blood. Recently, she has also noticed that she has lost some weight. On further questioning, she admits to having a mild fever but this has not been recorded.

What would your differential diagnosis include before examining the patient?

This lady belongs to a low socioeconomic class and, almost certainly, had tuberculosis at the age of 14, which was treated by her GP. Putting this important historical fact into perspective, her current abdominal pain could be due to abdominal tuberculosis. Mild fever and weight loss, although not documented, would also favour tuberculosis. Other than this diagnosis, she could be suffering from a peptic ulcer, renal or biliary colic, pancreatitis or an intra-abdominal lymphoma. Multiple worm infestation is also a possibility.

Examination

On examination it is apparent that the patient has lost some weight. She is pale. There is no icterus and a few insignificant small lymph nodes are palpable in the cervical region. Chest examination is normal but on abdominal examination there is a palpable mass in the right iliac fossa. The rest of the examination is normal, as is digital examination of the rectum.

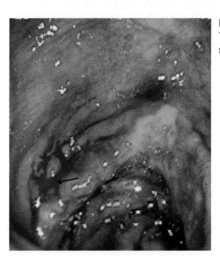

Fig. 62.1 Findings at colonoscopy. There is ulceration (arrow) with a surrounding cobblestone appearance.

Has examination narrowed down your differential diagnosis?

The mass in her right iliac fossa would fit well with the initial probable diagnosis of tuberculosis; however, this needs further evaluation before it is confirmed. There is nothing on examination that points to renal or gallbladder pathology. Lymphoma and chronic pancreatitis have still to be excluded.

Further investigations

The patient's haemoglobin is 100 g/l (10 g/dl). White blood cell and platelet counts are normal. The erythrocyte sedimentation rate (ESR) is 66 mm/hr. A Mantoux test is positive using 5 tuberculin units. Enzyme-linked immunosorbent assay (ELISA) for *Entamoeba histolytica* is negative. Chest X-ray and stool examinations are normal, as is ultrasound of the abdomen. A barium follow-through examination shows evidence of narrowing in the terminal ileum and caecum. Upper gastrointestinal endoscopy is also normal and duodenal biopsies do not show any villous atrophy. Colonoscopy reveals several ulcers in the ascending colon (Fig. 62.1), as well as in the terminal ileum, and biopsies reveal granulomatous inflammation (Fig. 62.2). Stains for acid-fast bacilli and fungi are negative and *Entamoeba histolytica* is not seen. Cultures of the biopsies are negative for acid-fast bacilli.

Does this narrow down your differential diagnosis?

A normal stool examination and the negative ELISA for *E. histolytica* rule out parasitic infestation. The colonic examination and the biopsy reports confirm granulomatous colitis and ileitis; hence the differential diagnosis narrows down to intestinal tuberculosis and Crohn's disease. In South-east Asia, tuberculosis is far more common than Crohn's disease; however, Crohn's disease does exist and should be considered. Unfortunately, it is very difficult to obtain positive cultures for acid-fast bacilli from intestinal biopsies, as abdominal tuberculosis is a pauci-bacillary disease. If available, polymerase chain reaction (PCR) for mycobacterial DNA can be performed on tissue biopsies, and this has a higher sensitivity than culture. If in doubt regarding the final diagnosis between tuberculosis and Crohn's disease, then antituberculous treatment should be given before starting steroids for Crohn's disease.

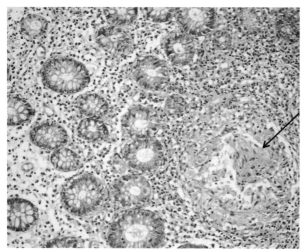

Fig. 62.2 Colonic mucosal biopsy. There is a non-caseating granuloma (arrow) suggesting tuberculosis or Crohn's disease.

How will you treat this patient?

Given her past history, this patient should be treated with isoniazid, rifampicin, pyrazinamide, ethambutol and streptomycin for a period of 2 months followed by the first four drugs for another month and, thereafter, rifampicin, isoniazid and ethambutol should be continued for a further 5 months (category 11 WHO regimen). The duration of treatment for extrapulmonary tuberculosis is the same as for pulmonary tuberculosis; however, the duration may be extended in individual cases on the basis of clinical evaluation and the results of repeat imaging tests at the end of 8 months. Before starting anti-tuberculosis treatment, liver function tests should be checked and thereafter monitored periodically. Eye examination should be carried out at the start and during treatment with ethambutol. Possible adverse effects of antituberculosis treatment should be thoroughly discussed with the patient before starting treatment. Crohn's disease should be actively considered if her symptoms do not respond to antituberculosis therapy, but even in this situation the final diagnosis may still be tuberculosis!

Global issues

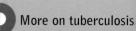 More on tuberculosis

- Both pulmonary and extrapulmonary tuberculosis are found world-wide.

- With the emergence of human immunodeficiency virus (HIV) infection, tuberculosis has again become one of the world's major health problems.

- In the developing world, tuberculosis still causes major morbidity and significant mortality. The emergence of multidrug resistance makes it important for patients to be investigated properly, not only to confirm the diagnosis but also to assess drug sensitivities.

- In the developing world, amoebomas (localised inflammatory masses due to *E. histolytica*) can be confused with caecal or colonic masses due to tuberculosis. The disease should be treated with anti-amoebic drugs after appropriate investigations.

See Chapters 19 and 22
Davidson's Principles and Practice of Medicine (20th edn)

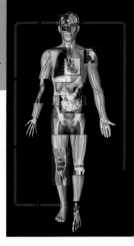

63

A young woman with fever and jaundice during pregnancy

A. L. KAKRANI

Presenting problem

A 20-year-old female working as a farm labourer is admitted to a teaching hospital in India with a low-grade, intermittent fever, which she has had for 3 days. The onset of fever was followed by yellowish discoloration of her eyes with nausea, vomiting and a decrease in appetite. She is 32 weeks pregnant. This is her second pregnancy; her first was uneventful.

What would your differential diagnosis include before examining the patient?

Several diseases can produce these symptoms during pregnancy. In tropical countries, an acute febrile illness with jaundice should raise the suspicion of acute viral hepatitis (e.g. due to hepatitis viruses A, B, C and E), *falciparum* malaria and leptospirosis. The clinical presentation of hepatitis E is similar to hepatitis A. Both viruses are spread via the faecal–oral route, whereas B and C are transmitted per-cutaneously. Acute symptoms in hepatitis C virus infection are usually trivial and there is no clue to suggest acute hepatitis B virus infection in this patient. The pro-dromal symptoms of acute viral hepatitis are systemic and variable. Constitutional symptoms include anorexia, nausea, vomiting, fatigue, malaise, myalgia, headache, photophobia, cough and coryza-like symptoms. These usually precede the onset of jaundice by 1–2 weeks. Fever is usually low-grade. The gastrointestinal symp-toms are frequently associated with changes in taste and olfaction. Dark-coloured urine and clay-coloured stools may occur about 1–5 days prior to the onset of clinical jaundice. In *falciparum* malaria jaundice is common due to haemolysis and hepatic dysfunction, and anaemia develops rapidly. Hypoglycaemia can occur in malaria. Leptospirosis presents with fever, haemorrhages, jaundice, and hepatic and renal dysfunction; conjunctival hyperaemia frequently occurs.

Pregnancy-associated liver diseases should also be considered. Intrahepatic cholestasis of pregnancy usually occurs in the third trimester of pregnancy. The condition is characterised by itching and liver function tests (LFTs) suggesting cholestasis; however, the bilirubin may be normal and the liver biochemistry may be hepatitic. Acute fatty liver of pregnancy is more common in twin and first pregnancies. Clinical manifestations occur between 31 and 38 weeks of pregnancy, with vomiting and abdominal pain followed by jaundice. Lactic acidosis, coagulopathy, encephalopathy and renal failure may occur in severe cases. These patients have a high serum uric acid and no haemolysis. The HELP (haemolysis, elevated liver enzymes and low platelets) syndrome is a variant of pre-eclampsia. The liver disease is associated with hypertension, proteinuria and fluid retention; hepatic infarction and rupture can occur. Gallstone disease with common bile duct (CBD) obstruction also requires consideration, as gallstones are more common during pregnancy and a stone might move into the common bile duct causing biliary colic and cholestatic jaundice.

Examination

On examination, the patient is conscious and alert. She is febrile and has moderate icterus and mild pallor. Her blood pressure is 120/84 mmHg. The uterus is palpable and fetal movements are normal. The liver and spleen are not palpable. No scratch marks are seen on the skin. The patient does not have conjunctival hyperaemia or haemorrhages.

Has examination narrowed down your differential diagnosis?

Acute viral hepatitis and pregnancy-associated liver disease still remain in the differential diagnosis. Infectious causes such as *falciparum* malaria and leptospirosis seem less likely.

BOX 63.1

Initial investigations

Haemoglobin	90 g/l (9 g/dl)
WCC	10.5 × 10⁹/l
	(10³/mm³)
Differential count	
Neutrophils	70%
Lymphocytes	28%
Eosinophils	2%
Bilirubin	
Total	136 µmol/l
	(8 mg/dl)
Direct	88.4 µmol/l
	(5.2 mg/dl)
ALT	2400 U/l
AST	2000 U/l
Alkaline phosphatase	200 U/l
Uric acid	256 mmol/l
	(4.3 mg/dl)
HbsAg	Negative
Anti-HBc	Negative
IgM-HAV	Negative
IgM-HEV	Positive
Anti-HCV	Negative
Serum HEV RNA	Positive

Investigations

The results of initial investigations are provided in Box 63.1.

Has the diagnosis been clinched?

A hepatitic pattern of LFTs suggests acute viral hepatitis. It is now certain that the hepatitis is due to hepatitis E virus (HEV).

About 24 hours after admission, the patient becomes irritable and drowsy. The jaundice deepens and the area of hepatic dullness becomes grossly reduced (less than two percussion spaces). She develops a flapping tremor. Abdominal ultrasound examination performed at this time shows a reduction in hepatic size and increased echogenicity. A computed tomogram (CT) of the brain suggests the presence of cerebral oedema.

HEV normally causes a self-limiting acute hepatitis like hepatitis A and does not lead to chronic disease. However, it differs from hepatitis A because infection during pregnancy can lead to acute liver failure; a mortality of up to 20% is recorded in various studies. In view of the rapid deterioration in the patient's condition, with diminishing consciousness and reduction in liver size, it is clear that she has developed fulminant hepatic failure.

How will you treat this patient?

She is given a bowel washout. A nasogastric tube is inserted and she is given lactulose, 60 ml as a starting dose and later 30 ml 6-hourly, along with vancomycin 250 ml 6-hourly (preferred to neomycin and metronidazole) due to her pregnancy. She is transferred to the intensive care unit and requires intubation,

63

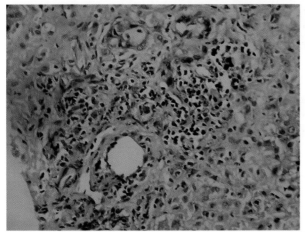

Fig. 63.1 Liver necropsy in acute viral hepatitis due to HEV, showing the portal triad with heavy neutrophilic infiltrate and ballooning of hepatocytes in places.

ventilation and inotropic support. Nutrition is provided by a low-protein formulation via the nasogastric tube. Liver transplantation, though ideal in this setting, is not possible in the treating hospital. She continues to pursue a downhill course and dies on the sixth day of hospitalisation. Liver necropsy is performed and the histopathology is seen in Figure 63.1.

Global issues

- HEV infection spreads by the faecal–oral route and is commonly seen in regions with over-crowding and poor sanitation.

- The disease occurs primarily in India, Asia, Africa and Central America. In Europe and USA infection is usually seen in travellers to an endemic area.

- In developing countries a febrile illness with jaundice should raise the suspicion of acute viral hepatitis due to A and E viruses, *falciparum* malaria and leptospirosis.

- Yellow fever should also be considered in the differential diagnosis in sub-Saharan Africa.

- Large epidemics of hepatitis E can occur after contamination of water supplies from monsoon flooding or contamination of drinking water supply lines with sewage. The disease usually occurs in young adults who are immune to hepatitis A virus (HAV).

- For reasons largely unknown, HEV infection in pregnant females is associated with a poorer outcome, and the risk of developing fulminant hepatic failure is high.

- Presently, there is no commercially available vaccine for the disease.

> More on viral hepatitis and pregnancy-associated liver disease?
>
> See Chapter 23 of **Davidson's Principles and Practice of Medicine** (20th edn)

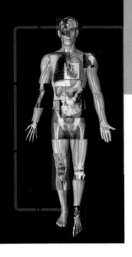

64

A man with worsening jaundice and confusion

C. L. LAI

Presenting problem

A 55-year-old Caucasian businessman is admitted with increasing mental dullness over the past 2 days. He has had severe anorexia and nausea, mild diarrhoea, and a low-grade fever associated with right upper abdominal discomfort for 2 weeks. For the last 10 days, he has been aware of a gradual darkening of his urine. His wife has noticed progressive yellow discoloration of his skin and sclera. He is a social drinker. He went to Shanghai for a trade conference 6 weeks ago. There is no history of drug-taking.

BOX 64.1

Common causes of acute hepatitis associated with acute hepatic failure

- Viral hepatitis A–E* (the most common cause globally)
- Drugs (paracetamol overdose being the most common cause in Western countries)
- Fulminant Wilson's disease
- Autoimmune hepatitis
- Pregnancy (including hepatitis E infection)
- Other viruses (mostly in immunocompromised patients): cytomegalovirus, herpes simplex, Epstein–Barr virus
- Other rare causes: extensive malignancy of the liver

*Acute hepatitis C is the least likely to give rise to acute hepatic failure.

What would your differential diagnosis include before examining the patient?

The severe prodromal symptoms, followed by jaundice, are typical of acute hepatitis irrespective of aetiology. The development of mental dullness 2 weeks after the onset of the symptoms of acute hepatitis should alert the physician to the possible complication of acute hepatic failure. The classification of acute liver failure is based on the interval between the development of jaundice and hepatic encephalopathy; less than 7 days is defined as 'hyperacute', between 8 and 28 days as 'acute', and between 29 days and 12 weeks as 'subacute'. Our patient falls into the 'acute' category.

The causes of acute hepatitis associated with acute hepatic failure are listed in Box 64.1.

The travel history to Shanghai would indicate a definite risk for acute hepatitis A, Asian countries being endemic for this virus. The other diagnoses are easily excluded. Sexual exposure to hepatitis B is possible, but the short incubation period of 4 weeks makes it highly unlikely. A negative drug history rules out drug-induced hepatitis. Wilson's disease presenting with fulminant hepatitis usually occurs in childhood or adolescence. Autoimmune hepatitis is much more common in women. The patient is not immunocompromised.

Examination

The patient is deeply jaundiced, drowsy and apathetic, though arousable. He has fetor hepaticus and a flapping tremor. His liver is normal in size. A spleen tip is palpable.

Has examination narrowed down your differential diagnosis?

Fetor hepaticus and a flapping tremor are indicative of hepatic encephalopathy, confirming the development of acute hepatic failure as a complication of acute hepatitis. The clinical grading for his encephalopathy is grade 2 out of 4. However, as expected, physical examination does not help in identifying the cause of the acute hepatitis. Analysis of blood samples is required for this. The mild splenomegaly is a common finding in acute hepatitis.

Investigations

The patient's liver function tests are as follows: bilirubin 330 μmol/l (19 mg/dl); alanine aminotransferase (ALT) 5500 U/l; aspartate aminotransferase (AST) 4700 U/l; albumin 37 g/l (3.7 g/dl). Alkaline phosphatase and γ-glutamyl transferase (GGT) are normal. Prothrombin time is prolonged to 70 seconds. Arterial ammonia is raised to five times above the normal range. His renal function tests and blood glucose level are normal.

IgM anti-hepatitis A virus (anti-HAV) is positive. He is negative for other viral hepatitis markers and antinuclear antibody. He has a normal serum copper and caeruloplasmin.

Has the diagnosis been clinched?

The patient is suffering from acute fulminant viral hepatitis A complicated by acute hepatic failure. This complication is uncommon, occurring in 0.1% of patients, but the incidence becomes higher with increasing age of infection. ALT and AST levels are of little prognostic value for acute hepatitis, whereas the plasma bilirubin and the prothrombin time reflect the severity of the liver damage. The prothrombin time is dependent on factors V and VII, both of which have short half-lives of less than 24 hours. The prothrombin time is therefore a very reliable prognostic index of the course of the acute hepatic failure, and should be monitored on a daily or twice-daily basis. Arterial ammonia is less sensitive than the prothrombin time as an index of liver failure, but can also be used to monitor the course of the disease.

How will you treat this patient?

The patient should be monitored in the intensive care unit for the development of further complications. If there is any evidence of progressive mental deterioration, intracranial pressure monitoring should be instituted, since cerebral oedema is a known and dreaded complication of acute hepatic failure. Hypoglycaemia is also a common complication. The blood glucose level should be monitored

---

BOX 64.2

Poor prognostic criteria in acute hepatic failure

Non-paracetamol causes

- Prothrombin time
  >100 seconds

or

- Three of the following five criteria:
  Age < 10 or > 40 years
  Time from jaundice to
  encephalopathy > 7 days
  Bilirubin > 300 μmol/l
  (17.6 mg/dl)
  Prothrombin time > 50 sec
  Non-viral hepatitis causes

or

- Factor V level < 15%
  and grade 3 or
  4 encephalopathy: less
  commonly used criteria

Paracetamol overdose

- pH < 7.3 24 hrs after the
  ingestion of paracetamol

or

- Serum creatinine
  >300 μmol/l (3.38 mg/dl)
  and prothrombin time
  >100 sec *and* grade
  3 or 4 encephalopathy

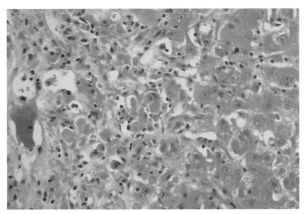

Fig. 64.1 The hepatitic changes are predominantly periportal, with inflammatory infiltrate consisting of plasma cells and lymphocytes. Periportal parenchymal necrosis is striking (H&E X40). (Histology section courtesy of Dr Philip P. C. Ip, Department of Pathology and Clinical Biochemistry, Queen Mary Hospital, Hong Kong.)

at 2-hourly intervals. Interestingly, cerebral oedema and hypoglycaemia, though common in acute liver failure, are much less likely to develop with liver failure in chronic liver disease such as cirrhosis of the liver.

Renal function and urine output should also be closely monitored for the development of the hepatorenal syndrome. If facilities are available, the surgeons should be alerted early for the consideration of liver transplantation. Patients with poor prognostic criteria (Box 64.2) have $\geq 90\%$ mortality and should receive liver transplantation at the earliest opportunity, since further clinical deterioration may cause irreversible cerebral oedema as well as increasing the risk of transplantation. This patient has four of the five poor prognostic criteria listed in Box 61.2. Liver transplantation is definitely indicated. The histology of the explanted liver is shown in Figure 64.1.

Global issues

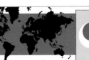

- The prevalence of hepatitis A is high in Africa, Russia and Central America, intermediate in Asia, and low in North America, Western Europe and Australia.

- Travellers from countries of low endemicity to those of high or intermediate endemicity are at risk of infection and should receive hepatitis A vaccination as prophylaxis.

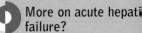

More on acute hepatic failure?

See Chapter 23 of
Davidson's Principles and Practice of Medicine
(20th edn)

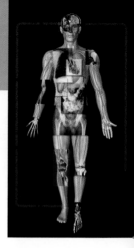

65

A confused man with jaundice and abdominal distension

J. COLLIER

Presenting problem

A 50-year-old man is referred to the medical admissions unit with a 4-week history of increasing abdominal distension and anorexia, followed by 2 weeks of jaundice. There has been no change in bowel habit or vomiting and he denies any weight loss. His wife has noticed him to be confused over the last 24 hours. He takes no regular medication. He has drunk 8 pints of beer a day for about 10 years, but stopped 10 days ago when he started to feel unwell. The general practitioner has checked some blood tests, which are shown in Box 65.1.

What would your differential diagnosis include before examining the patient?

Abdominal distension in the absence of symptoms of bowel obstruction suggests either an abdominal mass or ascites, of which the most common causes in a previously fit man are cirrhosis and malignancy. Cirrhosis is usually asymptomatic until portal hypertension develops and synthetic liver function worsens; then symptoms of chronic liver failure, such as ascites, appear quite quickly.

BOX 65.1	
Initial investigations	
Sodium	130 mmol/l (meq/l)
Potassium	3.8 mmol/l (meq/l)
Urea	0.9 mmol/l (2.56 mg/dl)
Creatinine	89 μmol/l (1.39 mg/dl)
Albumin	25 g/l (2.5 g/dl)
Bilirubin	90 μmol/l (5.29 mg/dl)
Alkaline phosphatase	400 U/l
ALT	150 U/l
AST	180 U/l
Haemoglobin	110 g/d (11 g/dl)
WCC	8×10^9/l (10^3/mm^3)
Platelets	70×10^9/l (10^3/mm^3)
Prothrombin time	20 sec

The presence of jaundice indicates either liver disease, which may be acute or chronic, or obstruction to the biliary tree, which is usually due to malignancy.

Acute liver disease can be excluded, as this is not associated with ascites. However, the presence of jaundice with ascites does not differentiate carcinoma of the head of the pancreas with peritoneal metastases from chronic liver failure.

Investigations in this case do narrow down the differential diagnosis, as the presence of pancytopenia suggests chronic liver disease. Platelets are often disproportionately lower than the rest of the blood count in cirrhosis due to a combination of splenomegaly and reduced hepatic thrombopoietic production. The prolonged prothrombin time and low albumin can be seen in both chronic liver failure and biliary obstruction, but in the latter the prolonged clotting is reversible with vitamin K.

It is common for individuals to stop drinking about 2 weeks before jaundice develops in alcoholic liver disease because they feel so unwell; alcohol detoxification will not, therefore, be needed in this man.

Examination
The patient has 5–6 spider naevi on his upper chest wall. He has a 6 cm firm, non-tender palpable liver. Ascites is confirmed on abdominal examination. Asterixis (flapping tremor) is demonstrated.

Does this narrow down your differential diagnosis?
The finding of stigmata of chronic liver disease makes the diagnosis of cirrhosis most likely. However, it is important to remember that not everyone with decompensated chronic liver disease will have these cutaneous stigmata. A large liver is also frequently seen in individuals with cirrhosis due to alcohol.

Alcohol excess increases the risk of progression to cirrhosis in chronic liver disease due to other causes such as chronic viral infection, hepatitis B and C, and haemochromatosis. These conditions must also be excluded before concluding that the liver disease is due to alcohol alone.

Jaundice in an alcoholic with cirrhosis may either reflect end-stage liver disease or be due to a superimposed alcoholic hepatitis. The latter can only be confirmed histologically, but in practice it is usually assumed that alcoholic hepatitis is present if there is jaundice.

The patient's confusion in the presence of a hepatic flap is likely to be due to hepatic encephalopathy. Other causes of confusion in an alcoholic that need to be excluded are subdural haematomas, occurring after a head injury, when there may be focal neurological signs present. Wernicke's encephalopathy can be difficult to exclude, but frequently coexists with nystagmus and is often treated empirically.

BOX 65.2

Ascitic tap

Albumin	4 g/l (0.4 g/dl)
WCC	600 × 10⁹/l (10³/mm³)
Neutrophils	90%

Further investigations
Ultrasound shows that the liver is enlarged and has a coarse texture; the spleen is also enlarged but there is no bile duct dilatation. No focal lesions are seen within the liver and the main portal vein is patent. The results of the ascitic tap are shown in Box 65.2 and in Figure 65.1.

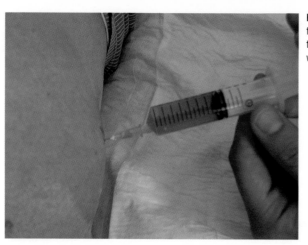

Fig. 65.1 Clear ascitic fluid being aspirated at the time of an ascitic tap with a 10 ml syringe.

The chronic liver disease screen tests indicate that the patient is hepatitis C antibody-positive. It is only on more detailed questioning that he is found to have used intravenous drugs once when he was aged 20.

Does this narrow down your differential diagnosis?

Ultrasound is very good at excluding an obstructive cause for jaundice. A classically irregular cirrhotic liver is not always seen on ultrasound but the liver texture is usually abnormal, as in this case. Splenomegaly suggests portal hypertension and would not be expected with the other causes of ascites. A transudative ascites is also consistent with cirrhosis. This has been complicated by spontaneous bacterial peritonitis, as shown by the elevated ascitic white cell count.

How will you treat this patient?

Spontaneous bacterial peritonitis carries a high mortality. Either intravenous cephalosporins or oral quinolones are effective and should be given while awaiting bacterial culture results. Secondary prophylaxis is then needed to reduce the risk of further infections. Spironolactone, which blocks an activated renin–angiotensin system, should also be started. However, this should be stopped if any evidence of intravascular dehydration occurs, indicated by a rising urea or creatinine or by the serum sodium falling to less than 125 mmol/l, as this can exacerbate encephalopathy.

The mild hepatic encephalopathy will probably improve with treatment of the infection, but lactulose should also be given orally. Constipation is a common precipitant of hepatic encephalopathy, and if lactulose cannot be given orally because of reduced conscious level, then phosphate enemas are an alternative.

An upper gastrointestinal endoscopy will be needed to look for varices, even though there is no history of bleeding, as β-blocker prophylaxis will reduce the risk of bleeding from asymptomatic large varices.

Long-term abstinence from alcohol is crucial; it will prevent progression of liver disease in most cases and may lead to improvement in liver function over the next 6 months. Treatment of the patient's hepatitis C will need to be considered when his liver function has improved.

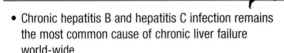
More on chronic hepatic failure?

See Chapter 23 of
Davidson's Principles and Practice of Medicine (20th edn)

- Chronic hepatitis B and hepatitis C infection remains the most common cause of chronic liver failure world-wide.

- Non-cirrhotic portal hypertension is common in Africa and in other areas where schistosomiasis is prevalent. It usually presents with variceal bleeding. Liver function is preserved and ascites does not occur.

- Tuberculosis is a common cause of ascites in endemic areas.

- Patients with chronic Budd–Chiari syndrome (thrombosis of the large hepatic veins and sometimes the inferior vena cava) may present with features of chronic liver disease and portal hypertension.

- Veno-occlusive disease (occlusion of central hepatic veins) has similar clinical features to Budd–Chiari syndrome. It may result from exposure to pyrrolizidine alkaloids in *Senecio* and *Heliotropium* plants, which are used to make teas, and following administration of cytotoxic drugs and hepatic irradiation.

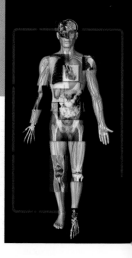

66

A middle-aged man in sub-Saharan Africa with vomiting, anorexia, weight loss and abdominal pain

J. A. KER

Presenting problem

A 45-year-old male patient, married with two children, complains of loss of appetite with subsequent weight loss, nausea and vomiting for 3 weeks. A few days after the nausea and vomiting started, he developed a constant abdominal pain, localised to the right hypochondrium. He is currently unemployed and has not travelled outside his home city of Pretoria, South Africa.

He has never been ill before and does not suffer from any chronic medical problems. He takes alcohol sparingly and only on special occasions. He is a non-smoker. On specific enquiry he has no other symptoms. A family history is negative for any major illnesses.

What would your differential diagnosis include before examining the patient?

The interpretation of nausea, vomiting and abdominal pain remains a challenging exercise. Great judgement is required, but a meticulously executed history and physical examination will go a long way in assisting the correct approach to such a complaint. An acute surgical abdomen must be excluded. The constant right hypochondrial pain must put pathology of the liver or gallbladder high on the list of causes of this man's symptoms.

Examination

The patient is fully alert, but generally looks ill with signs of weight loss. Oral temperature is 37.5°C. No jaundice, cyanosis or significant pallor is noted and he has no lymphadenopathy. His pulse is 80/min and blood pressure is 160/90 mmHg.

His abdomen is generally tender but there is no obvious rebound tenderness. The liver is tender on palpation and the left lobe is palpable 2 cm below the xiphisternum. The liver span is 15 cm. There is no splenomegaly and no fluid thrill. Bowel sounds and digital rectal examination are normal. No abnormalities are noted in the remainder of the physical examination. Routine urine dipstick testing is normal, with no bilirubin detected.

Has examination narrowed down your differential diagnosis?

The patient does not have an acute surgical abdomen. The examination points to liver pathology and further investigations should focus on this organ. The tender rather than painful abdomen and the absence of fever make cholecystitis unlikely. Further basic investigations, particularly liver function tests, are needed. The results are listed in Box 66.1.

Initial investigations	
Haemoglobin	89 g/l (8.9 g/dl)
MCV	88.1 fl
Platelets	$553 \times 10^9/l$ ($10^3/mm^3$)
WCC	$11.1 \times 10^9/l$ ($10^3/mm^3$)
Neutrophils	90%
Blood smear	Anisocytosis, microcytes, ovalocytes, rouleaux formation and auto-agglutination of the red cells
U&E	Normal
Bilirubin	14 μmol/l (0.82 mg/dl)
ALT	34 U/l
Alkaline phosphatase	115 U/L
GGT	103 U/L
Albumin	31 g/l (3.1 g/dl)
Total protein	103 g/l (10.3 g/dl)
Protein electrophoresis	Polyclonal elevation of IgG and IgA

Has the diagnosis been clinched?

Not yet. This 48-year-old male has been sick for 3 weeks with nausea, vomiting and abdominal pain, and he has an enlarged tender liver. Blood tests reveal an anaemia of chronic disease and a polyclonal gammopathy. The liver function pattern could fit in with a space-occupying lesion and the most appropriate test at this stage would be an ultrasound scan of the liver. A human immunodeficiency virus (HIV) test should also be carried out to exclude this common cause of polyclonal gammopathy in sub-Saharan Africa.

Further investigations

Liver ultrasonography reveals a large mass (8 cm diameter) in the right lobe of the liver due to either a tumour or an abscess (Fig. 66.1). The HIV test is non-reactive. The most likely diagnosis is a liver abscess (short history, anaemia of chronic disease, elevated white cell count and increased absolute neutrophil count) and in sub-Saharan Africa this is most likely to be due to an amoebic infection.

How will you treat this patient?

Although the diagnosis has not yet been confirmed, time is of the essence and the patient should be started straight away on metronidazole 800 mg per mouth 8-hourly for 10 days. A luminal agent, such as diloxanide furoate 500 mg per mouth 8-hourly for 10 days, should be given to eliminate intestinal colonisation to all patients following completion of metronidazole therapy. Meanwhile, an α-fetoprotein level is checked and found to be in the normal range, making a hepatocellular carcinoma unlikely. Amoebic serology is performed: amoeba haemagglutination test 2.5 (N < 1.0) with amoeba fluorescent antibody IgG and IgM positive. This confirms recent amoebic infection.

The patient responds to treatment in a dramatic way (he starts eating and his nausea, pain and fever settle), and it is decided that aspiration of the liver

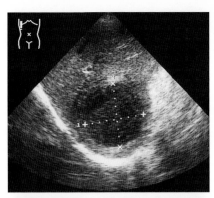

Fig. 66.1 Ultrasound of the right lobe of the liver showing an echogenic mass measuring 8 × 8 cm.

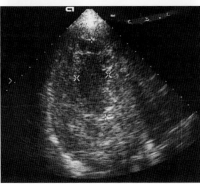

Fig. 66.2 Repeat ultrasound examination 16 days later, following therapy with metronidazole. The mass has decreased in size and now measures 3 × 7 cm.

abscess is not necessary. The anaemia slowly resolves, as does the polyclonal gammopathy. A repeat ultrasound examination of the mass 16 days later shows significant reduction in the dimensions of the abscess (Fig. 66.2). It is important to note that diarrhoea is often absent in amoebic liver abscess and that the diagnosis can be difficult.

Global issues

More on amoebic liver abscess?

- Amoebiasis is an important public health problem and is the second leading cause of death from parasitic diseases world-wide.

- Travellers to endemic areas are at high risk of developing this disease, which can present months to years after travel. Therefore, a careful travel history is essential.

See Chapter 13 of **Davidson's Principles and Practice of Medicine** (20th edn)

- Amoebic liver abscess is the most common extra-intestinal manifestation of disease. Amoebic liver abscess most commonly affects males between the ages of 18 and 50.

- Amoebic liver abscess usually presents with acute symptoms (< 10 days) but a chronic presentation, as with the present case, can occur.

- In some Mexican populations, susceptibility to amoebic liver abscess is associated with HLA-DR3 and complotype SC01.

- At present no vaccine is available for humans.

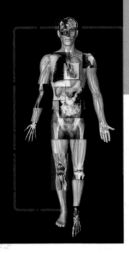

67

A 65-year-old woman with anaemia and macrocytosis

J. I. O. CRAIG

Presenting problem

A 65-year-old woman is referred to the haematology clinic with a 6-month history of general malaise, tiredness and a 2-month history of shortness of breath on moderate exertion. She has been on thyroxine replacement for 5 years. She has not had any operations. On direct questioning she admits to a sore tongue and pins and needles in her feet, but has no other complaints. She is on no other medication and has no history of excessive alcohol intake. Her diet is good. She remembers a maternal aunt who required injections for anaemia. The general practitioner has performed a full blood count, which shows a macrocytic anaemia, mild leucopenia and thrombocytopenia (Box 67.1).

<table>
<tr><td colspan="2">**BOX 67.1**</td></tr>
<tr><td colspan="2">**Initial investigations**</td></tr>
<tr><td>Haemoglobin</td><td>72 g/l
(7.2 g/dl)</td></tr>
<tr><td>MCV</td><td>123 fl</td></tr>
<tr><td>WCC</td><td>3.5 × 10⁹/l
(10³/mm³)</td></tr>
<tr><td>Platelets</td><td>110 × 10⁹/l
(10³/mm³)</td></tr>
</table>

What would your differential diagnosis include before examining the patient?

The major cause of a marked macrocytosis with these blood results is megaloblastic anaemia due to vitamin B_{12} or folate deficiency. These occur in quite different clinical circumstances, which can usually be gleaned from the history. The patient's relatively long history of breathlessness on exertion is likely to be due to the slow development of anaemia. Both vitamin B_{12} and folate are required for the synthesis of DNA and will cause systemic symptoms, such as malaise and a sore tongue, in addition to anaemia, leucopenia and thrombocytopenia. Only vitamin B_{12} deficiency, however, is associated with neurological problems. The most common cause of vitamin B_{12} deficiency is pernicious anaemia, an autoimmune disorder causing lack of intrinsic factor and hence vitamin B_{12} malabsorption. It is often associated with other autoimmune disorders in the patient or family. This woman had hypothyroidism and an aunt has probable vitamin B_{12} deficiency ('anaemia requiring injections' — vitamin B_{12} is given by intramuscular injection). Her diet is good — she is not a vegan, eats meat and vegetables, and has no symptoms to suggest malabsorption. The stores of folate in the body are short, lasting only a few months, and deficiency is associated with an inadequate diet — in particular, lack of green vegetables. Folate deficiency can be a manifestation of coeliac disease, although she has no overt symptoms of this.

Examination

On examination this lady appears pale, with a hint of jaundice. Her tongue is beefy-red. She is not tachypnoeic, but has an elevated regular pulse of 90/min with a flow murmur on auscultation of her heart. There are no overt signs of cardiac failure. The spleen tip is just palpable on deep inspiration. She has bilateral reduction in pin-prick sensation in her feet to the level of the ankles.

Investigations

The initial full blood count (FBC) results are shown in Box 67.1. Blood film reveals big oval red cells and hypersegmented neutrophils (Fig. 67.1). The bilirubin is elevated at 50 μmol/l (2.93 mg/dl) and is predominantly unconjugated. Other liver function tests and thyroid function tests are normal. Urinalysis shows an increased urobilinogen only. Bone marrow aspirate shows a megaloblastic marrow. Serum B_{12} is low at 50 pg/ml, with normal levels of folate and ferritin.

Have examination and initial investigations narrowed down your differential diagnosis?

The history and the FBC have been the most helpful here in suggesting the diagnosis. Examination confirms a moderate anaemia with pallor, tachycardia and a flow murmur. There are signs of sensory peripheral neuropathy, which would be consistent with vitamin B_{12} deficiency. The mildly enlarged spleen is consistent with haemolysis of the abnormal red cells, confirmed by the findings of increased urinary urobilinogen and unconjugated serum bilirubin.

Further investigations

To determine the cause of B_{12} deficiency, a Schilling test is performed. This test assesses the absorption of radio-labelled vitamin B_{12} (indirectly determined by measuring the amount of radio-labelled vitamin B_{12} in a 24-hour urine collection) before and after administration of intrinsic factor. Normal recovery is 7.5–12%. The following results are obtained: part 1 (without intrinsic factor), < 1% recovery of radio-labelled B_{12}; part 2 (with intrinsic factor),

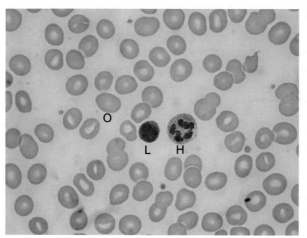

Fig. 67.1 Blood film in megaloblastic anaemia. A blood film showing large oval red cells (oval macrocyte, O) and a neutrophil with many lobes in the nucleus (hypersegmented neutrophil, H). This is typical of megaloblastic anaemia. Usually the red cells are the same size as the nucleus of a lymphocyte (L) and there is a maximum of five lobes in the nucleus of a neutrophil.

10% recovery of radio-labelled B_{12}. Gastric parietal cell antibodies and intrinsic factor antibodies are positive.

Does this narrow down your differential diagnosis?

The results confirm no absorption of B_{12} until intrinsic factor is given. This confirms that the terminal ileum can absorb B_{12} as long as intrinsic factor is provided. Autoantibodies to gastric parietal cells and to intrinsic factor are positive, confirming the diagnosis of pernicious anaemia.

How will you treat this patient?

She will require life-long supplementation with parenteral vitamin B_{12} (hydroxy-cobalamin). This is given intramuscularly, initially at a dose of 1 mg, 3 times a week for 2 weeks, then life-long every 2–3 months. Response can be confirmed by finding a high reticulocyte count about a week after starting treatment.

Global issues

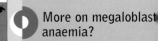

More on megaloblast
anaemia?

- Nutritional deficiency of vitamin B_{12} is the most common cause of megaloblastic anaemia in Hindu vegetarians and is a significant problem in Mexico, South and Central America, and some areas of Africa.

- There is little racial variation in the incidence of pernicious anaemia.

See Chapter 24 of
**Davidson's
Principles and
Practice of
Medicine**
(20th edn)

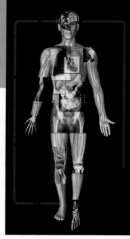

68

A middle-aged man with an elevated haemoglobin concentration

T. DAS

Presenting problem

A 45-year-old man attends the medical outpatient department with a 6-week history of fronto-parietal headache, insomnia, loss of concentration and a generalised itch that is worse after a hot bath. He also complains of a dragging discomfort in the left upper abdomen and early satiety accompanied by weight loss for 1 month. He was treated for pulmonary tuberculosis 4 years ago, but has no other past history of note. He is a fishmonger and does not smoke or drink. Family history is unremarkable.

What would your differential diagnosis include before examining the patient?

Headache, insomnia and loss of concentration are non-specific symptoms. The weight loss and early satiety are of concern and raise the possibility of gastric pathology. Itch after a hot bath is not uncommon, but is a feature of polycythaemia rubra vera (PRV).

Examination

On examination, the patient has stigmata of recent weight loss, but there is no dehydration, cyanosis, jaundice or oedema. His face has a plethoric look and bilateral conjunctival suffusion is present. His pulse is 80/min regular and blood pressure is 130/80 mmHg. Abdominal examination reveals that the spleen is palpable 5 cm below the left costal margin; it is non-tender. The liver is palpable 2 cm below the right costal margin; it is firm and non-tender.

Has examination narrowed down your differential diagnosis?

Examination has been extremely helpful and confirms that this man has a significant systemic disorder. The differential diagnosis at this stage will include causes of hepatosplenomegaly. Chronic liver disease with portal hypertension would be high up the list of potential diagnoses, but there are no peripheral stigmata of liver disease; he is not jaundiced and there are no features of portal hypertension such as ascites and abdominal wall vein distension. Chronic malaria and kala-azar are ruled out because of the absence of fever, and chronic schistosomiasis is excluded because features of portal hypertension are absent.

Haematological causes of hepatosplenomegaly seem more likely. Chronic haemolytic anaemias, such as sickle cell anaemia and the thalassaemia syndromes, are generally associated with jaundice and often there is a history of repeated blood transfusions in the past; there is frequently a positive family history too. Lymphoma may be characterised by pruritus, but generalised lymphadenopathy is likely to be present. Chronic myeloid leukaemia and myelofibrosis are possibilities, but this man is relatively young and there is no anaemia. Polycythaemia rubra vera is characterised by itch after bathing, plethoric facies and splenomegaly, with or without hepatomegaly, and seems the most likely diagnosis in the present case. Blood tests are clearly required.

Investigations

The blood test results are shown in Box 68.1. The haemoglobin is markedly increased. The red blood cell (RBC) indices are normal. A peripheral blood film (Fig. 68.1) shows numerous RBCs which are normochromic and normocytic. The red cell mass is increased. No abnormal or immature cells of the erythroid series are seen. The urine examination

BOX 68.1	
Initial investigations	
Haemoglobin	227 g/l (22.7 g/dl)
Haematocrit	0.69
RBC	$7.86 \times 10^{12}/l$ ($10^6/mm^3$)
WCC	$14.3 \times 10^9/l$ ($10^3/mm^3$)
Differential count	
Neutrophils	87%
Lymphocytes	9%
Monocytes	3%
Eosinophils	1%
Platelets	$490 \times 10^9/l$ ($10^3/mm^3$)
ESR	5 mm/1st hr

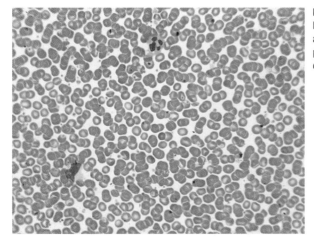

Fig. 68.1 Peripheral blood film from a patient with polycythaemia, showing elevated red cell count.

is normal. The chest X-ray and electrocardiogram (ECG) are normal. Biochemical parameters show normal blood glucose, urea, serum creatinine and liver function tests. Serum uric acid is 348 µmol/l (5.8 mg/dl). Serum ferritin is 22.9 µg/l (ng/ml). The serum erythropoietin level is at the lower end of the normal range. The oxygen saturation is 95% while breathing ambient air. An ultrasound scan of the abdomen shows mild hepatomegaly and moderate splenomegaly.

Does this narrow down your differential diagnosis?

The striking laboratory finding is the presence of a high haemoglobin, which is defined as haemoglobin values > 165 g/l (16.5 g/dl) in females and > 180 g/l (18.0 g/dl) in males. The common causes of a high haemoglobin are given in Box 68.2. High haemoglobin may be due to an increase in the number of red blood cells (true polycythaemia) or a reduction in the plasma volume (relative polycythaemia). In this patient there is no evidence of dehydration, diuretic therapy or alcohol consumption, so haemoconcentration giving rise to relative polycythaemia is ruled out.

True polycythaemia is caused either by increased erythropoiesis in the bone marrow due to increased erythropoietin production (secondary polycythaemia), or by primary increase in marrow activity (primary proliferative polycythaemia). Chronic hypoxaemia can give rise to secondary polycythaemia, but the arterial oxygen saturation is normal in this patient. There is neither a history of living at high altitude nor any evidence of lung or cyanotic heart disease. There are no features of renal disease or other tumours. The serum erythropoietin level is also normal.

The presence of a raised red cell mass and splenomegaly and the absence of any cause of secondary polycythaemia confirms the diagnosis of primary proliferative polycythaemia or PRV. In addition, the raised neutrophil and platelet count are also minor criteria for PRV.

BOX 68.2
Causes of high haemoglobin
Relative polycythaemia
• Haemoconcentration (plasma volume is decreased)
Secondary polycythaemia
• High altitude
• Chronic lung disease
• Cyanotic heart disease
• Renal disease — hydronephrosis, cysts, carcinoma
• Other tumours — hepatomas, bronchogenic carcinoma, uterine fibroids, phaeochromocytoma, cerebellar haemangioblastoma
Primary polycythaemia
• Polycythaemia rubra vera

How will you treat this patient?

Periodic phlebotomy (venesection) serves to maintain the red cell mass within normal limits and prevents thrombosis. The target haemoglobin level is 140 g/l (14 g/dl) or less in men and 120 g/l (12 g/dl) or less in women. Between 400 and 500 ml of blood are removed and venesection is initially repeated every 5–7 days until the haematocrit is reduced to below 45%. Thereafter, venesections may be performed at 3-month intervals. Aspirin is indicated to reduce thrombotic risks, unless there is a contraindication to its use. Cytotoxic agents like hydroxyurea or interferon (IFN)-α may be used to treat symptomatic splenomegaly and myeloproliferation, e.g. raised platelets. Intravenous radioactive phosphorus (5 mCi of ^{32}P) may be considered in older patients, but its use is associated with a significant increase in risk of transformation to acute leukaemia. Rarely, massive splenomegaly may require splenectomy. Allogeneic bone marrow transplantation can be curative in the occasional young patient, but there is significant mortality associated with the procedure.

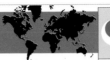

- PRV, a Philadelphia (Ph)-negative myeloproliferative disorder, is a clonal disorder involving multipotent haematopoietic progenitor cells.

- A single mutation, *V617F* in the *JAK2* gene, has been found in > 90% of patients with PRV. Thus, if an individual is positive for this mutation, it obviates the need for red cell mass/bone marrow studies.

- The prevalence is 1–3 cases per 100 000 population.

- There is frequent concomitant iron deficiency. Therefore, these patients may present with a normal haemoglobin, but iron-deficient indices and a raised red cell count.

- PRV appears to be more common in Jews of European origin than in non-Jews. Recently, a higher incidence has been reported from Sweden.

- In many patients with PRV, the leucocyte alkaline phosphatase level is increased and an elevated serum vitamin B_{12} or B_{12}-binding capacity may be present. Bone marrow aspirate and biopsy may reveal an abnormal karyotype and myelofibrosis.

See Chapter 24 of
**Davidson's
Principles and
Practice of
Medicine**
(20th edn)

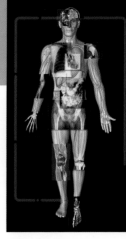

69

A 35-year-old woman with leucopenia

J. I. O. CRAIG

Presenting problem

A 35-year-old woman presents with a 1-week history of a sore throat and a 2-day history of fever. She had coryzal symptoms 2 weeks previously, which settled after 3 days. Her past medical history is unremarkable and there is no family history of note. She had taken paracetamol for the sore throat, but is on no other prescribed medicines; nor has she used any other drugs. A full blood count (FBC) and blood film show a leucopenia with a marked neutropenia and a borderline thrombocytopenia (Box 69.1).

What would your differential diagnosis include before examining the patient?

The main abnormality is a leucopenia, which is as a result of a neutropenia. The patient's sore throat could be either a manifestation of the cause of the neutropenia or a result of neutropenia itself (e.g. a secondary infection with thrush). Isolated neutropenia is commonly associated with viral infections and drugs. During viral infections it is transient, resolving after a few days. Drugs can cause neutropenia in expected or idiosyncratic ways. Neutropenia is an expected side-effect of chemotherapy and immunosuppressants such as azathioprine. It is known to occur occasionally in patients receiving antithyroid drugs such as carbimazole. Idiosyncratic reactions should be considered with any drug. This woman does not have a significant drug history. Less commonly, neutropenia can be due to lack of production of cells from the bone marrow, which is often associated with abnormalities in the other blood parameters such as haemoglobin and platelets. The patient does have a mildly reduced platelet count in addition to a marked neutropenia; therefore a primary bone marrow cause is a possibility and a bone marrow examination is indicated.

BOX 69.1	
Initial investigations	
Haemoglobin	115 g/l (11.5 g/dl)
WCC	1.6×10^9/l (10^3/mm^3)
Neutrophils	0.1×10^9/l (10^3/mm^3)
Lymphocytes	1.5×10^9/l (10^3/mm^3)
Platelets	140×10^9/l (10^3/mm^3)

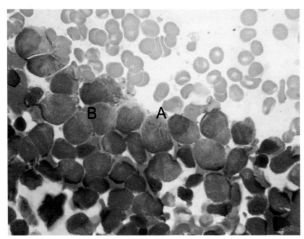

Fig. 69.1 Bone marrow aspirate. This bone marrow aspirate shows many granulated blasts (B), some of which contain a number of Auer rods (A). This is typical of acute promyelocytic leukaemia.

Examination

On examination this woman appears unwell and has a temperature of 38.5°C. She has white plaques over her soft palate, suggestive of oral candidiasis. There is no cervical lymphadenopathy. She has a tachycardia of 100/min, but her blood pressure is normal. Her chest is clear and other examination normal. There are no signs of skin or mucosal bleeding and funduscopy was normal.

Have examination and initial investigations narrowed down your differential diagnosis?

The examination reveals that this woman is unwell, with fever in the presence of marked neutropenia. She has a normal blood pressure but neutropenic sepsis can be life-threatening. She needs to be admitted to hospital urgently for intravenous broad-spectrum antibiotics and further investigation of the cause of neutropenia, including a bone marrow examination. It seems unlikely in this case that the patient's neutropenia is due to the more common causes such as viral infection or drugs.

Further investigations

A throat swab grows *Candida albicans*. Renal and liver function tests are normal. A bone marrow aspirate shows the marrow to be infiltrated with immature blasts consistent with acute leukaemia. There are many Auer rods in the blasts, which is consistent with acute myeloid leukaemia (AML, Fig. 69.1). The cytogenetics of the leukaemia show a translocation between chromosomes 15 and 17, which is found in acute promyelocytic leukaemia, a subtype of AML with a good prognosis.

Does this narrow down your differential diagnosis?

This establishes the diagnosis of neutropenia as a consequence of acute promyelocytic leukaemia.

How will you treat this patient?

Initially, she requires immediate skilled supportive care, including broad-spectrum antibiotics and oral antifungal treatment, e.g. fluconazole. Neutropenic sepsis is an emergency and empirical broad-spectrum antibiotics should be started immediately; they can be modified once microbiology results are available.

To treat the AML specifically, this woman requires chemotherapy and ATRA (all-*trans* retinoic acid) treatment. This differentiating agent has reduced the risks of life-threatening bleeding from the abnormal coagulation associated with this type of leukaemia. The prognosis is good, with an overall survival of around 75% at 5 years.

Global issues

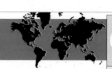

- The normal neutrophil count varies with age and race, and appropriate reference ranges must be used.

- Africans, black Americans and Afro-Caribbeans have a lower neutrophil count than Caucasians.

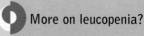 More on leucopenia?

See Chapter 24 of
Davidson's Principles and Practice of Medicine
(20th edn)

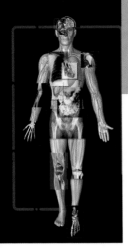

70

A young woman with a lump in her neck

J. M. DAVIES

Presenting problem

A 28-year-old woman is referred urgently to the haematology clinic by her general practitioner. She has noticed an enlarging lump on the left-hand side of her neck and is extremely anxious about what might be wrong. There is no previous history of note and she takes no regular medication.

She denies any antecedent upper respiratory tract infection and has no oropharyngeal symptoms of note. She does, however, admit to 4 weeks of exertional breathlessness and has noticed unintentional weight loss of approximately 10 kg over the last 6 months. She has not, however, noticed any night sweats and has not, as far as she has been aware, been febrile. There is no family history of note and her parents, brothers and sister have all been well. She is not aware of contact with any infectious disease and has not travelled outside the UK for 2 years. She has been in a stable relationship for 5 years and has never used drugs recreationally. She is a non-smoker and takes alcohol only very occasionally.

What would your differential diagnosis include before examining the patient?

The differential diagnosis here is wide, but the most common cause of a persistent neck lump presenting in this context would be cervical lymphadenopathy. Clearly, there are other neck masses which should be considered, including branchial cysts. Of importance here is the fact that the patient is unwell, reporting systemic symptoms in association with the neck mass. Both the GP and the patient herself are concerned about haematological malignancy, and the referral has been made essentially to confirm or exclude this diagnosis. The investigations performed by the GP (Box 70.1) confirm the systemic nature of the disorder, with an anaemia with normal indices, an elevated platelet count, an elevated white count due to a neutrophilia, but an associated lymphopenia. The erythrocyte sedimentation rate (ESR) is also elevated, which is a non-specific finding but does point to the presence of underlying systemic upset. Overall, the blood picture would be compatible with that seen in anaemia of chronic disease.

Examination

The patient looks pale and there is evidence of recent weight loss. Examination of the scalp, ears and oropharynx is normal. There is a 1.5×2 cm left supraclavicular fossa lymph node, which is firm and non-tender. There is

BOX 70.1	
Initial investigations	
Haemoglobin	98 g/l (9.8 g/dl)
MCV	82 fl
WCC	$14.6 \times 10^9/l$ ($10^3/mm^3$)
Neutrophils	$13.8 \times 10^9/l$ ($10^3/mm^3$)
Lymphocytes	$0.6 \times 10^9/l$ ($10^3/mm^3$)
Platelets	$524 \times 10^9/l$ ($10^3/mm^3$)
ESR	56 mm/hr

no convincing lymphadenopathy in either axilla. Examination of the abdomen reveals no enlargement of the liver or spleen, and the inguinal lymph nodes are not palpable. The patient is breathless on minimal exertion, and examination of the chest shows signs compatible with a right pleural effusion. There is no evidence of facial or upper limb oedema and the jugular venous pressure is not raised.

Has examination narrowed down your differential diagnosis?

Examining this patient provides two important clues as to what might be going on. Firstly, the left neck mass is an enlarged lymph node. Secondly, the examination confirms that the patient is unwell and has, in addition to the lymphadenopathy, further pathology involving the chest. Although the differential diagnosis is still wide, the chief possibilities are now lymphoma or some other disseminated malignancy: for example, metastatic carcinoma. Not excluded but less likely would be an infective process: for example, tuberculosis. What is clear, however, is that urgent further investigation is mandatory.

Further investigations

At the initial clinic visit the anaemia is confirmed. Renal function and liver function are normal. The serum urate is elevated, which may be indicative of increased cell turnover, and there is a polyclonal rise in immunoglobulins. The lactate dehydrogenase is normal, and although commonly elevated in lymphoproliferative disorders, a normal level does not exclude this as a potential diagnosis. The serum albumin is low and corrected calcium and phosphate are normal. A chest X-ray shows significant mediastinal widening and a right pleural effusion. A computed tomography scan (CT) of chest, abdomen and pelvis reveals massive mediastinal lymphadenopathy but no abnormality below the diaphragm (Fig. 70.1).

Echocardiography shows a pericardial effusion but with normal left ventricular function. The pleural fluid is an exudate but contains no malignant cells. An excision biopsy of the left supraclavicular lymph node confirms a diagnosis of nodular sclerosing Hodgkin's disease.

Does this narrow down your differential diagnosis?

The diagnosis here was clinched by obtaining tissue for histopathological analysis and this was done by excision biopsy. Where the differential diagnosis is wide or uncertain, then biopsy is essential for a formal diagnosis.

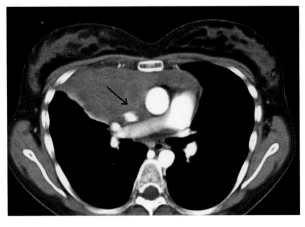

Fig. 70.1 CT of the chest showing mediastinal lymphadenopathy (arrow).

How will you treat this patient?

There are two key components to the management of this woman. Firstly, appropriate psychological support and open and honest communication are necessary from the start. In terms of the lymphoma, the patient is staged and any appropriate prognostic scoring performed. In a patient presenting in this way with Hodgkin's disease, the primary treatment is multi-agent chemotherapy. The prognosis in Hodgkin's disease is generally good to excellent, with predicted 5-year survival in younger patients in excess of 80%. Response may be monitored clinically and by cross-sectional imaging. Positron emission tomography (PET) has an important role to play in the evaluation of any residual mediastinal masses and radiotherapy may be used additionally to consolidate chemotherapy responses, particularly in the mediastinum.

Global issues

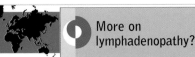

More on lymphadenopathy?

- Lymphadenopathy is common. Likely causes may, however, vary by geographical location, with infectious diseases such as tuberculosis and human immunodeficiency virus/acquired immunodeficiency syndrome (HIV/AIDS) being more common in certain populations than others.

See Chapter 24 of **Davidson's Principles and Practice of Medicine** (20th edn)

- Where the lymphadenopathy is due to metastatic malignant disease, there would again be variations as to the histopathology within populations, depending on risk exposure.

71

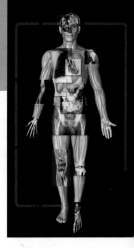

A young garment worker from Bangladesh with fever and massive splenomegaly

T. AHMED

Presenting problem

A 30-year-old garment worker from Bangladesh is admitted to hospital because of recurrent episodes of fever during the last 18 months and massive splenomegaly. Each episode of fever persists for an average duration of 2–3 weeks and recurs at intervals of about 2–3 weeks. The fever is associated with chills and rigors and usually occurs in the evening, with slight remission in the morning. The patient has taken three courses of chloroquine, without evidence of malarial parasites in the blood film, and several courses of ciprofloxacin on the basis of a positive Widal test. He has anorexia during the febrile episodes, but otherwise has a good appetite and feels well during afebrile periods. He has lost about 9 kg weight during the period of his illness. He has an occasional mild cough. The patient is married and has two healthy children. He has no history of headache, seizures, haematemesis or melaena. The patient has not received any blood transfusions and has no history of extramarital sexual exposure. Recently, he has gone to a traditional healer for the treatment of jaundice. His bowel and bladder habits are normal.

What would your differential diagnosis include before examining the patient?

When a patient from a tropical country presents with recurrent bouts of fever and massive splenomegaly, chronic malaria and visceral leishmaniasis (kala-azar) are at the top of the list in the differential diagnosis. Pancytopenia, with its consequent clinical manifestations, is a common feature in kala-azar. A diagnosis of tropical splenomegaly syndrome might also be entertained, depending on the patient's country of origin. In this syndrome, an exaggerated immune response to malaria, especially in malarious areas, produces splenomegaly. Tuberculosis involvement of liver and spleen should also be considered, as should other chronic infections, such as systemic fungal infections and chronic brucellosis.

In untreated patients, the fever of brucellosis shows an undulating pattern; the pyrexia persists for weeks before there is a period of apyrexia that may be followed by relapse. This patient is a garment worker and does not give a history of domestic exposure to infected animals or their products. In the absence of an occupational history, therefore, chronic brucellosis seems unlikely.

Fungal disease, especially histoplasmosis, can present with fever and hepato-splenomegaly. Fungal infections, although reported in immunocompetent individuals, are much more common in immunocompromised hosts. This patient's history does not provide any clue to immunosuppression. Moreover, chronic fungal infections left untreated for 18 months are often fatal. Therefore, fungal disease is unlikely in this patient.

Cirrhosis with portal hypertension should be considered in a patient with hepatosplenomegaly, but massive splenomegaly occurs rarely, except in extrahepatic portal hypertension. Hepatosplenomegaly is also a feature of lymphoproliferative or myeloproliferative diseases like lymphoma, chronic myeloid leukemia, chronic lymphatic leukemia, myelofibrosis, polycythaemia rubra vera and rarely Waldenström's macroglobulinaemia. Fever is an important symptom in patients with lymphoma; however, in other conditions it is not a presenting feature but can occur as a result of opportunistic infections. Patients with myelofibrosis and chronic myeloid leukaemia may develop massive splenomegaly.

Examination

Examination reveals that the patient is mildly anaemic and icteric, but otherwise appears well. His temperature is 40.3°C and pulse rate is 140/min. Peripheral lymph nodes are not palpable. The spleen is palpable 10 cm from the left anterior axillary line along its long axis. The liver margin is palpable 1.5 cm below the right costal margin. There is no ascites or stigmata of chronic liver disease. Examination of other systems reveals no abnormality.

Has examination narrowed down your differential diagnosis?

The presence of mild jaundice and hepatosplenomegaly, but the absence of recurrent fever, favour primary liver diseases. Jaundice may also occur in kala-azar (though rarely), chronic lymphocytic leukaemia and Hodgkin's disease. Absence of features of hyperviscosity excludes the likelihood of Waldenström's macroglobulinaemia. Absence of peripheral lymphadenopathy makes the diagnosis of chronic lymphocytic leukaemia and lymphoma unlikely but not impossible. Further narrowing down of the differential diagnosis requires a step-wise diagnostic approach starting with simple blood tests.

Investigations

Results of peripheral blood investigations are provided in Box 71.1.

The urine is yellow and on dipstick examination is positive for urobilinogen. Abdominal ultrasonography confirms splenomegaly without evidence of focal abnormalities, but not hepatomegaly. There is no free fluid and no apparent abdominal lymphadenopathy. A formal gel (aldehyde) test shows egg-white opacity within 20 minutes of adding formalin to the patient's serum (strongly positive). This is a non-specific test which suggests that there are high circulating immunoglobulin levels (Fig. 71.1).

An immunochromatographic test for kala-azar using rK39 antigen is positive. Bone marrow aspiration with examination for amastigotes (Leishman–Donovan (LD) bodies) on Giemsa stain yields a definitive diagnosis in approximately 80% of cases and is carried out here. The sensitivity approaches 100% in splenic aspirates. Despite the safety of splenic aspiration when aspiration is performed very rapidly with a small-bore needle, it is rarely done outside areas where kala-azar is endemic. Alternative but less sensitive diagnostic methods include liver biopsy and lymph node aspiration when lymphadenopathy is present. Culture is a time-consuming and expensive process and is rarely used for clinical purposes.

BOX 71.1

Initial investigations

Haemoglobin	96 g/l (9.6 g/dl)
WCC	5.5×10^9/l (10^3/mm³)
Differential count	
Neutrophils	65%
Lymphocytes	28%
Monocytes	05%
Eosinophils	02%
Platelets	250×10^9/l (10^3/mm³)
ESR	120 mm/1st hr
Peripheral blood smear	Anisochromia, anisocytosis
Thick and thin blood smears	Negative for malarial parasites
Bilirubin (total)	35.7 µmol/l (2.1 mg/dl)
Protein (total)	85 g/l (8.5 g/dl)
Albumin	35 g/l (3.5 g/dl)
ALT	32 U/l

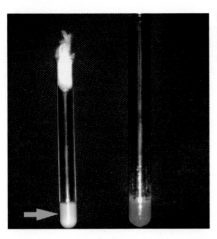

Fig. 71.1 Strongly positive formal gel (aldehyde) test (arrow). The tube on the right is a control tube showing no change when aldehyde is added to the patient's serum.

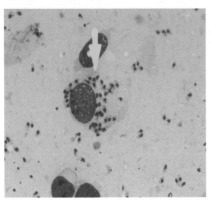

Fig. 71.2 Bone marrow aspirate showing intracellular and extracellular Leishman–Donovan (LD) bodies (arrow).

Has the diagnosis been clinched?

The presence of LD bodies in bone marrow confirms the diagnosis of kala-azar (Fig. 71.2). However, in a country where malaria, typhoid and tuberculosis are common, the diagnosis of one does not exclude the other.

How will you treat this patient?

The standard treatment of kala-azar is with one of the pentavalent antimonial compounds, e.g. sodium stibogluconate (100 mg/ml) or meglumine antimoniate (85 mg/ml). The daily dose is 20 mg/kg body weight, given either intravenously or intramuscularly for 28–30 days. The incidence of cardiotoxicity with pentavalent antimonial compounds is significant. Increasing the dose of stibogluconate, or the use of amphotericin B, pentamidine, paromomycin or oral miltefosine may be required for resistant cases or as the first-line drug where stibogluconate resistance is high.

Global issues

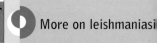 More on leishmaniasi

- Among chronic infectious diseases, chronic kala-azar and malaria are the most common causes of massive splenomegaly in the tropics.

- Travel history and endemicity of the disease are important for the diagnosis of splenomegaly.

- In countries where human immunodeficiency virus (HIV) infection is common, kala-azar is an important opportunistic infection and therefore should be considered in the differential diagnosis of all cases of splenomegaly.

- A few patients develop post-kala-azar dermal leishmaniasis (PKDL), manifested by skin lesions that are most prominent on the face. These lesions develop either during treatment or months to years after treatment.

- Chronic schistosomiasis due to *Schistosoma mansoni* may produce massive splenomegaly with portal hypertension in the tropics. Endemic areas include Africa, the Middle East, the Caribbean, Brazil and Venezuela.

See Chapter 13 of
**Davidson's
Principles and
Practice of
Medicine**
(20th edn)

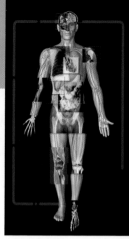

72

A 30-year-old woman with menorrhagia

C. A. LUDLAM

Presenting problem

A 30-year-old woman with a long history of menorrhagia is being considered for a hysterectomy and is referred for pre-operative assessment to establish whether she has a bleeding disorder. She already has a family consisting of two daughters and a son. As a child she underwent tonsillectomy and required a blood transfusion because of post-operative bleeding. Two wisdom teeth were extracted 7 years previously and bleeding started from one of the sockets 5 hours after surgery, and lasted 36 hours. A coagulation screen (consisting of an activated partial thromboplastin time (APTT), prothrombin time and fibrinogen) is normal (Box 72.1).

What would your differential diagnosis include before examining the patient?

Judging from the long history of haemorrhagic incidents, a congenital disorder is more likely than an acquired bleeding condition, e.g. secondary to liver or renal failure. This lady probably has a 'mild' bleeding disorder because excess bleeding has only occurred after surgery. A coagulation disorder, due to a reduction in one of the clotting factors, is more likely than a disorder of primary haemostasis (von Willebrand disease or a platelet disorder) because the bleeding started a few hours after, rather than at the time of surgery.

Statistically, von Willebrand disease would be the most likely diagnosis because it is relatively common, although in this condition bleeding usually starts immediately after trauma. This is because the von Willebrand factor facilitates the arrest of initial haemorrhage by promoting the adhesion of platelets to the damaged vessel wall. In thrombocytopenia or a platelet functional disorder (relatively uncommon) too, bleeding is usually immediate, again because of the poor development of platelet aggregates at the site of trauma. Bleeding which starts a few hours after surgery is more characteristic of a coagulation factor deficiency, e.g. factor VIII, IX or XI; in this situation the initial platelet haemostatic plug is poorly reinforced by fibrin strands formed by the coagulation system and it therefore disintegrates a few hours after formation.

Examination

On examination, no bruises or purpura are seen. Joints are normal and there is no evidence of limitation of range of movement or arthritis. No stigmata of chronic liver disease are present and no clinical hepatosplenomegaly is identified.

Has examination narrowed down your differential diagnosis?

Chronic liver disease or thrombocytopenia secondary to hypersplenism is unlikely. Neither is a severe coagulation disorder probable because there is no evidence of joint damage secondary to recurrent haemarthroses.

Further investigations

The platelet count and morphology on a blood film are normal. Heritable platelet functional disorders are uncommon (although that due to aspirin is common). Although the APTT and prothrombin time (PT) are normal, this does not exclude a mild bleeding disorder, as these global coagulation tests are insensitive to mild clotting factor deficiencies and levels have to be below about 25% of normal before the screening tests are prolonged. In this patient, assay of coagulation factors reveals a reduced factor VIII of 0.30 U/ml, but normal factor IX and XI levels.

Von Willebrand factor level is normal (Box 72.1), as is the binding of factor VIII to von Willebrand factor. Genetic analysis of the factor VIII gene on the X chromosome reveals that the patient is heterozygous for the intron 22 inversion. This is the most common genetic mutation that causes severe haemophilia A.

Does this narrow down your differential diagnosis?

A low factor VIII level is found in von Willebrand disease (and its Normandy variant), carriers of haemophilia A, acquired haemophilia (unlikely in this case because of the life-long history) and female haemophilia (very rare). Factor IX is measured because it may be reduced in carriers of haemophilia B (factor IX deficiency), which has a prevalence of about one-fifth that of haemophilia A; factor XI deficiency (haemophilia C) is the next most common congenital coagulation factor deficiency.

Von Willebrand factor has the dual function of being both the carrier protein for factor VIII (which it stabilises in the circulation) and the 'adhesive' that sticks platelets to damaged vessel walls. With a deficiency of von Willebrand factor there is a reduction in the factor VIII level (as factor VIII has a shorter half-life in the absence of its carrier protein), and primary platelet plug formation at the site of trauma is defective, resulting in immediate haemorrhage. The von Willebrand factor results exclude von Willebrand disease and its Normandy variant, in which levels of von Willebrand factor are normal but there is reduced binding of factor VIII.

BOX 72.1	
Initial investigations	
Platelets	$250 \times 10^9/l$ ($10^3/mm^3$)
Prothrombin time	14 sec
APTT	35 sec
Fibrinogen	2.1 g/l (0.21 g/dl)
Von Willebrand factor (by ristocetin assay)	0.7 U/ml (normal 0.5–1.5)
Factor VIII	0.30 U/ml (normal 0.5–1.5)
Factor IX	0.85 U/ml (normal 0.5–1.5)
Factor XI	0.90 U/ml (normal 0.5–1.5)

This woman, therefore, is a carrier of severe haemophilia A and has a mild bleeding disorder because of the reduced factor VIII level (secondary to random inactivation of X chromosomes, or lyonisation in early embryogenesis).

How will you treat this patient?

This woman's mild bleeding disorder, due to reduced factor VIII concentrations, may be predisposing her to menorrhagia. Desmopressin (DDAVP) would raise the level to over 0.50 U/ml for up to 12 hours. This vasopressin analogue probably releases factor VIII from endothelial cells (along with von Willebrand factor). It can be given either as a nasal spray, or as a subcutaneous or intravenous injection. The nasal spray at the time of menstruation, along with the fibrinolytic inhibitor, tranexamic acid, might lessen the menorrhagia and avoid the need for a hysterectomy.

If this does not reduce the menorrhagia and there is no other correctable gynaecological cause for the excess bleeding, desmopressin could be used preoperatively and the injections continued twice daily to maintain the factor VIII level above 0.50 U/ml after surgery. Tachyphylaxis may develop and it is often not useful to give more than about four injections. As factor VIII is an acute phase reactant, the stress of the surgery will also elevate the factor VIII level and therefore after 1 or 2 days further desmopressin is not likely to be necessary. Desmopressin has potent antidiuretic activity, which lasts about 24 hours and may complicate management of fluid balance in the immediate post-operative period. Instead of desmopressin, factor VIII concentrate could be used; infusions would need to be given 12-hourly initially, as its half-life is approximately 12 hours.

The patient should be informed that she is a carrier of severe haemophilia and counselled about the consequences. As a carrier, each of her daughters will have a 1 in 2 chance of being a carrier and a similar chance that each son will have severe haemophilia A.

If she wishes to add to her family, antenatal diagnosis could be offered. Fetal sex could be determined by detecting Y chromosomal DNA in a maternal blood sample after 6 weeks, or by chorion villus biopsy at 11 weeks' gestation. In a male fetus, using the same chorion villus sample, the intron 22 inversion mutation could be sought and, if present, would indicate that the fetus has severe haemophilia.

This woman's existing son should have his factor VIII level measured (even though he has not had any haemorrhagic symptoms), as he has a 50% chance of having severe haemophilia. The daughters should also have their factor VIII measured because each has a 50% of being a carrier of severe haemophilia and, like their mother, of having a mild bleeding disorder. A normal factor VIII in a daughter does not exclude carrier status. Genetic testing (to seek the intron 22 inversion and to give a definitive assignment of carrier status) should only be undertaken when the girl is able to understand the implications of the genetic issues and is able to give true informed consent, usually in her early teenage years.

If the woman has sisters and brothers, consideration should be given to offering to measure their factor VIII levels and undertake genetic studies (in the females who might be carriers and in the males if haemophilia is diagnosed).

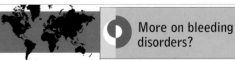

Global issues

More on bleeding disorders?

See Chapter 24 of
Davidson's Principles and Practice of Medicine
(20th edn)

- The incidence of haemophilia is the same throughout the world.

- If desmopressin is contraindicated or it does not raise the factor VIII level sufficiently, factor VIII concentrate could be used. Both recombinant and plasma-derived factor VIII concentrates are available (with the former being preferred). It is usual to offer immunity to hepatitis A and B by vaccination prior to concentrate therapy. If possible, concentrate should be avoided as there is a small risk of an inhibitory antibody developing to factor VIII, it is more expensive than desmopressin, and a plasma-derived concentrate exposes the recipient to the possibility of transfusion-transmitted infection. Plasma-derived factor VIII concentrates undergo at least one viral inactivation step in manufacture and hence they are exceedingly safe from hepatitis viruses and human immunodeficiency virus (HIV).

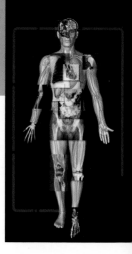

73

A woman with thrombocytopenia after hip surgery

C. A. LUDLAM

Presenting problem

A 40-year-old woman, para 4+0, is involved in a road traffic accident in which her left femur is fractured. The fracture is plated at surgery, during which she receives a transfusion of 3 units of red cell concentrate. For prophylaxis against venous thromboembolism she is given daily subcutaneous injections of a low molecular weight heparin. The post-operative period is complicated by a moderately severe wound infection, which necessitates her staying in hospital. A routine full blood count 8 days after surgery reveals her platelet count to be $60 \times 10^9/l$ ($10^3/mm^3$), with a haemoglobin of 109 g/l (10.9 g/dl) and a mildly elevated total white count of $12.1 \times 10^9/l$ ($10^3/mm^3$) (due to a mild neutrophilia). By the following day, the platelet count has dropped to $50 \times 10^9/l$ ($10^3/mm^3$). Her pre-operative platelet count was $160 \times 10^9/l$ ($10^3/mm^3$) and the haemoglobin and white count were normal.

What would your differential diagnosis include before examining the patient?

The two most likely diagnoses are disseminated intravascular coagulation (DIC) and heparin-induced thrombocytopenia (HIT). The patient has not been pre-scribed any drugs that might have suppressed her marrow platelet production. Other candidates in the differential diagnosis include thrombocytopenia due to occult liver disease or splenomegaly and two uncommon possibilities, thrombotic thrombocytopenic purpura (TTP) and post-transfusional purpura (PTP). The last two are important to consider because treatment is very specific, and without it, both have a high mortality. Causes of thrombocytopenia are listed in Box 73.1.

In TTP, platelet aggregates cause microvascular thrombosis and intravascular red cell haemolysis. The clinical consequences of microvascular occlusion are often renal failure or neurological impairment. PTP is a rare condition which occurs predominantly in multiparous women and presents with severe thrombocytopenia and sudden onset of extensive purpura and ecchymoses 10 days after a blood transfusion. It is usually due to the presence of an antibody against one of the platelet-specific antigens, PLA1, in a woman who is PLA1-negative but previously carried a PLA1-positive fetus. The anti-PLA1 antibody combines with the PLA1 antigen in the blood being transfused and the complex attaches to the patient's platelets by the Fc receptor on the platelet surface (as an innocent bystander);

hence the mother's platelets are cleared rapidly from the circulation by the reticulo-endothelial system. This is a life-threatening condition and should be treated immediately with intravenous immunoglobulin.

BOX 73.1

Causes of thrombocytopenia

Marrow disorders

- Hypoplasia
  Idiopathic
  Drug-induced: cytotoxics, antimetabolites, thiazides
- Infiltration
  Leukaemia
  Myeloma
  Carcinoma
  Myelofibrosis
  Osteopetrosis
- Vitamin B_{12}/folate deficiency

Increased consumption of platelets

- Disseminated intravascular coagulation (DIC)
- Idiopathic thrombocytopenic purpura (ITP)
- Viral infections, e.g. Epstein–Barr virus, human immunodeficiency virus (HIV)
- Bacterial infections, e.g. Gram-negative septicaemia
- Hypersplenism
- Thrombotic thrombocytopenic purpura
- Liver disease
- Connective tissue disease, e.g. systemic lupus erythematosus (SLE)

Examination and initial investigations

The patient looks generally well on examination; her temperature is 37.3°C and her pulse and blood pressure are normal. The orthopaedic wound is erythematous and a small abscess appears to be developing. There is no purpura, bruising or bleeding. No stigmata of liver disease are apparent and neither the liver nor the spleen is palpable.

Examination of the blood film confirms the thrombocytopenia and reveals normal red cell morphology. The activated partial thromboplastin time (APTT), prothrombin time and fibrinogen are all normal.

Have examination and initial investigations narrowed down your differential diagnosis?

Despite the infected wound, this woman's clinical state is good and so DIC and TTP seem unlikely. Red cell fragments are typically seen in TTP and these were not identified on the blood film. DIC is excluded by the normal coagulation screen. PTP is unlikely because the platelet count is much higher than would be customary for this condition.

In the absence of an alternative probable clinical diagnosis, HIT is the most likely. For this to be considered, the platelet count needs to have been observed to fall below the normal range after starting heparin, or to have decreased by more than 50% from the pre-heparin level. The characteristic feature of HIT is progressively worsening thrombocytopenia between 5 and 10 days after starting heparin (or earlier if the patient has received heparin within the previous 100 days). If the patient also has a new thrombosis at the time when the diagnosis is being considered, this increases the likelihood of a diagnosis of HIT.

Further investigations

It is important to make an expeditious diagnosis of HIT because to delay exposes the patient to the substantial risk of developing a thrombosis during the following 30 days. HIT is diagnosed in a patient in whom it is a likely diagnosis clinically and is confirmed by detecting antibody to heparin-platelet factor 4 (PF4) complex on the platelet surface. PF4 is a platelet alpha-granule constituent which is liberated during the platelet release reaction when the cells are activated. The antibody which attaches to the heparin-PF4 complex subsequently binds by its Fc portion to the platelet membrane Fc receptor, and in so doing, activates and cross-links platelets into aggregates. The anti-heparin-PF4 antibodies are usually detected using an enzyme-linked immunoassay (ELISA) solid phase binding assay. This technique has a high sensitivity but a relatively low specificity, i.e. it readily gives false positive results. There is also an assay for the antibody, which depends upon its ability to stimulate the release of serotonin from platelet-dense granules; this 'functional' test has a high sensitivity and specificity but is only available in specialist reference laboratories.

The finding of a strongly positive result in the heparin-PF4 antibody test, which is inhibited by excess heparin, makes the diagnosis of HIT in this clinical setting where it is considered a likely diagnosis. Interestingly, HIT has a higher incidence after orthopaedic and cardiac surgery than in medical settings.

How will you treat this patient?

HIT is associated with a high incidence of venous and, to a lesser extent, arterial thrombosis. By the time the diagnosis of HIT is made, about one-third of patients already have a clinical thrombosis, and even those in whom the heparin is discontinued have up to a 50% chance of subsequently developing a thrombus. The mortality of this complication of heparin therapy is high, at about 20–30% from thrombotic disease. Management is, therefore, to stop heparin immediately and to start an alternative non-vitamin K antagonist anticoagulant. The one most commonly used is recombinant hirudin (lepirudin, leach anticoagulant protein), which is a direct thrombin inhibitor. As this anticoagulant is excreted via the kidney, it is important to assess the creatinine prior to its use; in the presence of renal failure, a reduced dose should be given or bolus injections considered. The patient should receive a loading dose of hirudin, followed by a continuous infusion, as it has a short half-life. The dose should be monitored with the APTT to give a patient:control ratio of 1.5–2.5. An alternative anticoagulant is to use the heparinoid, danaparoid, at full anticoagulant dose. When the platelet count has returned to normal, an oral anticoagulant, e.g. warfarin, should be started; once the international normalised ratio (INR) is over 2.0 on 2 successive days, the hirudin can be discontinued. The warfarin should be continued for 4–6 weeks (even in the absence of an objectively confirmed thrombotic event).

Global issues

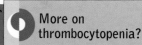

More on thrombocytopenia?

- A careful drug history is necessary to exclude other causes of drug-induced thrombocytopenia. Antibiotics, especially cephalosporins, penicillins, sulphonamides and thiazides, are all associated with thrombocytopenia.

- HIT is much more common with unfractionated heparin (UFH) than with low molecular weight heparin (LMWH). Moreover, bovine UFH is more likely to cause HIT than porcine UFH.

- Absolute confirmation of a diagnosis of HIT may not be possible in resource-limited nations because of a lack of availability of laboratory tests.

See Chapter 24 of
Davidson's Principles and Practice of Medicine
(20th edn)

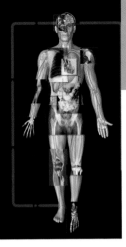

74

A woman with thrombocytosis noted after elective surgery

P. SHEPHERD

Presenting problem

A 75-year-old lady is admitted for an elective total knee joint replacement. Post-operatively she requires monitoring for a short period in the high-dependency unit and on discharge is noted to have a haemoglobin of 75 g/l (7.5 g/dl), white cell count of 20.3×10^9/l (10^3/mm^3) and platelets of 690×10^9/l (10^3/mm^3). Two months later she is referred to the local haematology clinic. Her blood count now shows: haemoglobin 135 g/l (13.5 g/dl), WCC 11.4×10^9/l (10^3/mm^3) and platelets 1346×10^9/l (10^3/mm^3). She is well and has had no previous problems with strokes, transient ischaemic attacks (TIAs), or cardiac or peripheral vascular disease.

BOX 74.1

Causes of thrombocytosis

Reactive disorders

- Infection, acute or chronic
- Bleeding, acute or chronic
- Neoplasia
- Inflammation, e.g. rheumatoid arthritis, connective tissue disease
- Post-splenectomy

Myeloproliferative disorders

- Primary thrombocythaemia
- Primary polycythaemia
- Chronic myeloid leukaemia
- Myelofibrosis
- Myelodysplasia with raised platelets

What would your differential diagnosis include before examining the patient?

Thrombocytosis may be reactive or due to an underlying myeloproliferative disorder. The initial results after her knee joint replacement could well be reactive in nature due to either bleeding or inflammation/infection. Other markers of inflammation may be present, such as an increase in the C-reactive protein (CRP) or the erythrocyte sedimentation rate (ESR). Most cases of thrombocytosis, particularly in the acute setting, are reactive in nature. However, if the thrombocytosis persists for a period of months in the absence of an ongoing inflammatory/infectious or neoplastic cause, then a myeloproliferative disorder should be suspected. There are no specific diagnostic features to separate a reactive thrombocytosis from a myeloproliferative disorder. In fact, the diagnosis of a myeloproliferative disorder is one of exclusion of reactive causes. The major causes of reactive thrombocytosis and of myeloproliferative disorders associated with increased platelets are shown in Box 74.1. The most common myeloproliferative disorder is primary thrombocythaemia, but other disorders should be excluded.

Examination and initial investigations

Examination shows a woman who looks well with no obvious problems. Her weight is steady and cardiorespiratory examination is normal. There is no hepatosplenomegaly. There is no obvious problem with her knee replacement and there are no features of inflammatory arthritis. Peripheral pulses are present and there is good capillary circulation in the feet.

The blood count is repeated and is similar to that above. The mean cell volume (MCV) is at the lower end of the normal range (79 fl). The blood film shows a normal white cell differential and no abnormal red or white cells. ESR is 14 mm/hour and CRP is 3 mg/l. Urea and electrolytes are normal, apart from a slightly elevated potassium of 5.6 mmol/l. Lactate dehydrogenase (LDH) is high at 840 U/l and urate is normal. The chest X-ray is normal.

Have examination and initial investigations narrowed down your differential diagnosis?

There are no positive findings on examination that support or refute the differential diagnosis. However, the duration of the thrombocytosis and the absence of any systemic symptoms or an underlying obvious inflammatory/infective/neoplastic lesion would support an underlying myeloproliferative disorder. If splenomegaly were present, this would be a strong pointer to a myeloproliferative disorder. However, with the ready availability of blood counts and possibly earlier diagnosis, this is frequently not present in many myeloproliferative disorders. In addition, the normal ESR, normal CRP and elevated LDH and potassium would point towards a myeloproliferative disorder. The particular type of myeloproliferative disorder is probably primary thrombocythaemia. There are no features on the blood film to suggest myelodysplasia or myelofibrosis. The normal haemoglobin generally excludes primary polycythaemia, provided there is no associated iron deficiency.

Further investigations

Bone marrow examination shows a hypercellular marrow with increased megakaryocytes, many of which are large and clustered in the marrow spaces (Fig. 74.1). Erythropoiesis and myelopoiesis appear to be maturing normally. Fine reticulin fibres are present throughout (grade 2). Iron stores are absent. Cytogenetic examination shows a normal female karyotype, and molecular studies using probes for BCR and ABL exclude a BCR-ABL fusion gene. JAK2 V617F mutation screening is negative.

Does this narrow down your differential diagnosis?

The blood and bone marrow findings exclude chronic myeloid leukaemia, myelofibrosis and myelodysplasia as a cause of the increased platelets. Iron-deficient primary polycythaemia can present with normal or low haemoglobin. In many of these cases the red cell count will be increased and the cells may be hypochromic and microcytic. If indicated, a short trial of iron therapy may suggest the true diagnosis of primary polycythaemia and the haemoglobin will exceed the normal range. In this case the likely diagnosis is primary thrombocythaemia. A single mutation in the JAK2 gene (V617F) on chromosome 9 is frequently found in myeloproliferative disorders, being present in over 90% of cases of primary polycythaemia and 50% of cases of primary thrombocythaemia and myelofibrosis. If positive, the test is helpful in diagnosing myeloproliferative disorders; if negative, it does not refute the diagnosis.

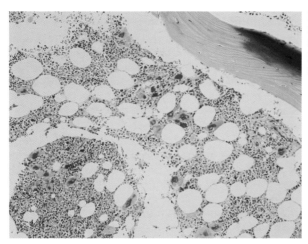

Fig. 74.1 Bone marrow biopsy Giemsa stain × 100 showing large clustered megakaryocytes.

How will you treat this patient?

The major risk with primary thrombocythaemia is that of occlusive arterial events such as a stroke, TIAs or digital ischaemia. Venous thrombosis can also occur. The risk of thrombosis does not correlate with the level of the platelet count. Some patients, particularly those with platelet counts over $1500 \times 10^9/l$ ($10^3/mm^3$), may have bleeding problems due to abnormal platelet function. Such patients may present with retroperitoneal haemorrhage or excessive tissue bleeding, e.g. after trephine biopsy of the bone marrow. For most patients aspirin 75 mg daily is indicated to inhibit platelet activation. This often relieves digital pain or erythromelalgia (red, hot and painful extremities on exposure to heat) due to platelet aggregation in the capillary circulation. Aspirin should in general not be used until the platelet count is less than $1500 \times 10^9/l$ ($10^3/mm^3$). Other contributing factors to arterial occlusion should be looked for and treated appropriately, e.g. hypertension, hypercholesterolaemia, smoking history, diabetes and so on. The risk of occlusive events is related to age, particularly over the age of 60, and the presence of other contributing factors.

If a thrombotic history is present or the patient is over 60 years, cytoreductive therapy should be offered with hydroxycarbamide (hydroxyurea), an RNA inhibitor, which aims to reduce the platelet count to below $400 \times 10^9/l$ ($10^3/mm^3$). Monitoring of the blood count at regular intervals is required to determine the optimum dose and efficacy. This agent, given orally, is usually very well tolerated. Since this is a clonal stem cell disorder, there is a low risk ($< 5\%$) that further abnormalities in the stem cell compartment can occur and lead to transformation to acute leukaemia over the years. The use of chemotherapy can increase this risk, particularly with alkylating agents such as busulfan, and the use of radioactive phosphorus (^{32}P). The risk of this occurring with hydroxycarbamide alone is significantly lower, but may be slightly above the baseline risk. Reducing the platelet count does, however, reduce the risk of occlusive events significantly and is recommended for this high-risk group. For those under 60 years old who have had no occlusive events and have a platelet count less than $1500 \times 10^9/l$ ($10^3/mm^3$), the use of chemotherapy to reduce the count is unproven, although trials are in progress. For young people under 40 years and with platelets less than $1500 \times 10^9/l$ ($10^3/mm^3$), aspirin alone is recommended.

Other agents can be used, particularly if treatment is indicated for younger people or those who are intolerant of hydroxycarbamide. These include anagrelide, a vasodilator that reduces platelet production from megakaryocytes, and interferon-α, neither of which is leukaemogenic. However, a randomised study comparing anagrelide with hydroxycarbamide showed a higher rate of occlusive events and a higher rate of myelofibrotic transformation in those treated with anagrelide. Thus, hydroxycarbamide is currently used as first-line treatment in the UK (and is markedly cheaper than anagrelide or interferon). Interferon-α has to be given by injection and has many side-effects. It is particularly useful when patients need treatment when other drugs are contraindicated: for example, in pregnancy.

Global issues

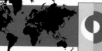

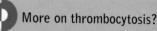
More on thrombocytosis?

- Reactive causes of thrombocytosis are more common than myeloproliferative disorders, particularly where chronic infections such as tuberculosis are present.

- *JAK2* mutation screening is not necessary for diagnosis.

See Chapter 24 of
Davidson's Principles and Practice of Medicine (20th edn)

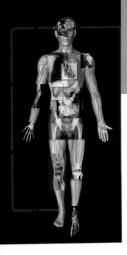

75

A woman with a reaction to a blood transfusion

M. L. TURNER

Presenting problem

A 69-year-old woman with myelodysplastic syndrome receives a transfusion of 2–3 units of red cell concentrate every 4 weeks to maintain her haemoglobin. During the current admission she receives her first unit of red cell concentrate (Fig. 75.1) without incident, but halfway through her second unit she complains of feeling unwell; in particular, she feels cold and slightly sick, and complains of back pain. The nurse temporarily stops the transfusion and asks you to review the patient urgently.

What would your differential diagnosis include before examining the patient?

A wide variety of different reactions can occur during red cell transfusion. A modest rise in temperature (less than 1.5°C) with no other clinical signs would suggest a febrile non-haemolytic transfusion reaction, whilst an urticarial rash would suggest a mild allergic reaction. More serious possibilities include ABO incompatibility or a haemolytic reaction to other red cell alloantibodies, a severe allergic reaction, or bacterial contamination of the red cell unit. Finally, there is the possibility of fluid overload or transfusion-related acute lung injury (TRALI).

Examination

The patient has a temperature of 39°C and looks flushed. General examination reveals no evidence of urticaria or other generalised rash. Her cardiovascular examination reveals a modest tachycardia at a 100/min and a drop in her blood pressure to 100/60 mmHg, but is otherwise normal. Respiratory examination is normal; in particular, there is no evidence of dyspnoea or wheeze. Her abdomen is soft and non-tender.

Has examination narrowed down your differential diagnosis?

It is clear that this cannot be dismissed as a mild allergic or febrile non-haemolytic transfusion reaction, and there is no evidence of fluid overload. There is no evidence of acute respiratory distress and therefore TRALI can also be dismissed. A severe allergic reaction would be expected to demonstrate relevant signs such as bronchospasm, angioedema or urticaria, along with hypotension. ABO incompatibility, other red cell alloantibody incompatibility and bacterial contamination all remain high on the list of differential diagnoses.

Fig. 75.1 A unit of red cell concentrate.

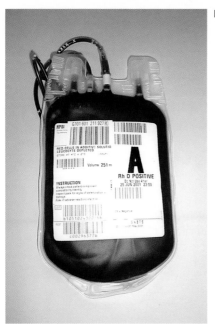

Further investigations

Close inspection of the red cell pack and prescription sheet show a discrepancy in the date of birth and hospital number with the patient's wristband. A patient of with a similar name is also regularly transfused within the same ward.

Does this narrow down your differential diagnosis?

It seems most likely that the blood sample from this patient has been inadvertently mixed up with that of another patient with a similar name. Major ABO incompatibility can cause these symptoms and signs as a result of acute haemolysis. A reaction to other red cell alloantibodies and bacterial contamination cannot be formally excluded at present.

How would you treat this patient?

The unit of blood should be taken down and returned intact to the hospital blood bank, along with a fresh blood sample from the patient correctly labelled for repeat ABO grouping, red cell alloantibody screen, direct antiglobulin test and cross-match. Intravenous saline infusion should be commenced and the urine output carefully monitored by catheterisation, if necessary. It is important to maintain urine output at > 100 ml/hr and diuretics should be used if necessary. The full blood count and coagulation screen should be monitored for evidence of disseminated intravascular coagulation, and the renal function and biochemistry for any evidence of renal failure. Blood cultures should be taken. The hospital blood bank should be alerted immediately. Steps clearly need to be taken to prevent a recurrence of this incident and the precise measures to be implemented would be determined by local policy. In the UK, the transfusion should be reported through the Hospital and Blood Service's incident reporting systems to both the Serious Hazards of Transfusion (SHOT) and the Medicines and Healthcare Products Regulatory Agency (MHRA). Audit of hospital practice and educational intervention/retraining might be necessary.

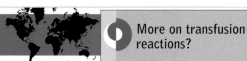
- ABO-incompatible blood transfusion remains the most common serious hazard of transfusion, with an overall incidence of around 1 per 100 000 transfusions.

- Most are due to errors in identification of the patient at the time of labelling the sample tube for pre-transfusion testing and/or in identifying the patient correctly against the blood pack at the time of transfusion.

- If the diagnosis is missed during the early stage of the transfusion and it continues, then the risk of severe morbidity or mortality is high.

See Chapter 24 of
Davidson's Principle and Practice of Medicine
(20th edn)

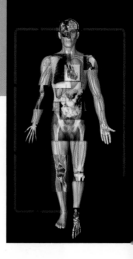

76

An elderly woman with an acute-onset monoarthritis

R. GUPTA

Presenting problem

A 70-year-old lady with known diabetes mellitus presents to the Accident and Emergency department with pain and swelling of the right knee joint for the preceding 24 hours. Yesterday morning she got out of bed without difficulty, but by the afternoon noticed a mild pain and swelling in the right knee joint which rapidly became unbearable and made her virtually immobile. She now feels unwell and has developed a fever. She denies any history of trauma. Five years ago the lady was diagnosed with osteoarthritis of the knees and was prescribed anti-inflammatory drugs by her general practitioner; she has been taking these from time to time. She has had type 2 diabetes for the last 10 years and takes oral hypoglycaemic drugs on a daily basis. Her recent records show good glycaemic control.

What would your differential diagnosis include before examining the patient?

The two most important causes of monoarthritis in someone of this age are septic arthritis and a crystal-associated arthritis (gout and pseudogout). Other causes of monoarthritis include monoarticular presentation of oligo-articular or poly-articular arthritis (e.g. reactive, psoriatic or other seronegative spondarthritides and rheumatoid arthritis), but these usually present at a younger age. Trauma or haemarthrosis associated with clotting abnormalities will also cause an acute monoarthritis, but there is no history to make either of these likely possibilities.

Examination

The patient looks slightly pale. She is febrile (38.3°C), with a pulse rate of 92/min and blood pressure of 140/80 mmHg. Her right knee joint is warm, swollen and tender with a moderate effusion. She has severe limitation of movements of the right knee joint and is unable to flex the joint because of pain. Other joints are normal, except for the presence of Heberden's nodes in the second, third and fifth fingers of both hands. Systematic examination is otherwise unremarkable.

Has the examination narrowed down your differential diagnosis?

Not really! The prime possibilities of septic arthritis and crystal arthropathy still remain. Fever can occur with either cause and the examination may not be discriminatory. It is crucial that septic arthritis is actively considered, as this

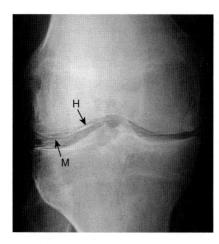

Fig. 76.1 X-ray of the right knee showing calcification of the fibrocartilaginous menisci (M) and articular hyaline cartilage (H).

H

M

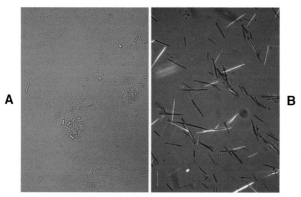

A

B

Fig. 76.2 Compensated polarised light microscopy of synovial fluid.
A. Calcium pyrophosphate crystals showing weak birefringence.
B. Compare with monosodium urate crystals, which show bright birefringence and needle-shaped morphology.

condition can be easily treated with antibiotics, but is potentially devastating if untreated. Gout seldom involves the knee joint in a first attack and is unlikely in patients over the age of 65 without a prior history of primary gout or chronic diuretic therapy. Pseudogout is the most common cause of acute monoarthritis in the elderly and the knee joint is the most commonly affected site. Synovial fluid analysis is the pivotal investigation in patients suspected of having septic arthritis or crystal-associated arthritis, and should be performed in all patients with acute monoarthritis, especially if there is overlying erythema.

Investigations

An X-ray of the right knee joint shows features of osteoarthritis with calcification of the cartilage (Fig. 76.1). The right knee is aspirated under aseptic conditions. Examination of the synovial fluid, using compensated polarised light microscopy, shows a weakly positive birefringence for calcium pyrophosphate dihydrate (CPPD) crystals (Fig. 76.2). Moreover, an urgent Gram stain of the synovial fluid is negative and culture of the synovial fluid after 48 hours is sterile.

Results of other less discriminating laboratory tests show: haemoglobin 112 g/l (11.2 g/dl), white cell count 11.6×10^9/l (10^3/mm³) with

80% polymorphs, and an erythrocyte sedimentation rate (ESR) of 70 mm/hr. A blood culture is sterile. Rheumatoid factor and antinuclear antibodies (ANA) are negative.

Has the diagnosis been clinched?

Yes. The presence of characteristic crystals and the absence of organisms in the synovial fluid suggest a diagnosis of pseudogout, which results from the deposition of CPPD crystals. It is important to wait for the synovial fluid culture report, as the presence of PPD crystals and calcification of the cartilage may be coincidental in someone of this age. It is also important to remember that a high neutrophil count in synovial fluid does not necessarily indicate infection.

How will you treat this patient?

The patient should be treated with non-steroidal anti-inflammatory drugs (NSAIDs), such as indometacin or diclofenac. If the symptoms are not controlled with NSAIDs alone, then the patient may be given an intra-articular injection of corticosteroids, provided infection has been confidently excluded. Pseudogout is associated with a wide array of underlying causes (Box 76.1). It is important that these are considered and investigated; in particular, serum calcium should be measured to exclude primary hyperparathyroidism.

BOX 76.1

Conditions associated with CPPD crystal arthritis

- Ageing
- Osteoarthritis
- Metabolic disease
  Haemochromatosis
  Hyperparathyroidism
  Hypophosphatasia
  Hypomagnesaemia
  Wilson's disease
- Familial predisposition

BOX 76.2

Causes of chronic monoarthritis

- Infections (tuberculosis and fungi)
- Chronic sarcoidosis
- Monoarticular presentation of:
  Rheumatoid arthritis
  Seronegative spondarthritis
  Enteropathic arthritis
  (e.g. Crohn's disease)
  Juvenile idiopathic arthritis
- Pigmented villonodular synovitis
- Foreign body (e.g. plant thorn)
- Synovial chondromatosis

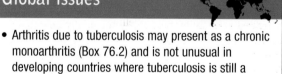

Global issues

 More on monoarthritis?

- Arthritis due to tuberculosis may present as a chronic monoarthritis (Box 76.2) and is not unusual in developing countries where tuberculosis is still a common problem. This may be more important in countries where human immunodeficiency virus (HIV) is a major public health problem. Tuberculosis commonly involves the spine, hip and knee joints.

See Chapter 25 of

Davidson's Principles and Practice of Medicine (20th edn)

- The incidence of pseudogout is highest in the elderly (> 65 years) and increases with advancing age.

- Osteoarthritis is the most common joint disease world-wide and the knee joint is the most common site of involvement. CPPD crystal deposition is favoured in a joint with osteoarthritis.

- Pseudogout (CPPD deposition disease) is very rare at a young age; if it is diagnosed, the associated conditions mentioned in Box 76.1 should be sought.

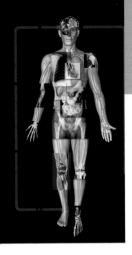

77

A 30-year-old woman with pain in multiple joints

E.R. McRORIE

Presenting problem

A 30-year-old woman presents with a 3-month history of joint pain and swelling affecting her hands, feet and right knee. She is stiff in the morning for around 1 hour and also tends to stiffen up in the evening. Due to the severity of her symptoms she has been experiencing increasing difficulty with fine hand function and mobility, and has been off work (she is a primary school teacher) for the past 4 weeks. Medication is ibuprofen 400 mg 12-hourly and occasional paracetamol. Past medical history is unremarkable, save for the diagnosis of a duodenal ulcer at endoscopy 5 years previously. Her mother had an unspecified form of arthritis that resulted in a right hip replacement. There is no family history of psoriasis. On direct questioning, she reports recent grittiness of the eyes and has noticed that her fingers turn pale in cold weather. There is no history of rashes, photosensitivity, orogenital ulceration, alopecia or recurrent miscarriages. She smokes 10 cigarettes per day.

What would your differential diagnosis include before examining the patient?

The character of her symptoms — joint pain and stiffness, the latter with a diurnal variation, and the reported definite joint swelling — is suggestive of an inflammatory arthropathy. Rheumatoid arthritis (RA) with associated Raynaud's phenomenon and keratoconjunctivitis sicca is the most likely diagnosis, given the distribution and relative symmetry of her symptoms. A connective tissue disease (CTD), such as systemic lupus erythematosus (SLE), is another possibility, as is psoriatic arthritis; although typically asymmetrical, this can occur in a symmetrical form. Parvovirus arthropathy is also part of the differential diagnosis, particularly as this woman's employment puts her at increased risk of parvovirus exposure. The persistence of her symptoms, however, makes this diagnosis less likely. The duration of the symptoms also effectively excludes septic arthritis, which is typically an acute monoarticular illness. The absence of preceding infective symptoms such as diarrhoea or urethritis, as well as the pattern of joint involvement, makes a reactive arthritis unlikely. A crystal arthropathy is very unlikely, given her age and gender.

Examination

On examination the patient is found to be apyrexial. There is tenderness and slight swelling of the proximal interphalangeal joints and the metacarpophalangeal joints, and a tense effusion in the right knee, where

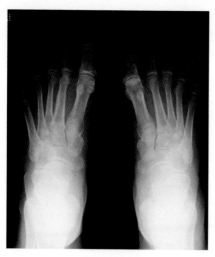

Fig. 77.1 X-ray of the feet showing periarticular erosions. No periarticular osteoporosis is evident on these films, but it is often observed in people with rheumatoid arthritis.

flexion is restricted to 120°. The metatarsal squeeze test is positive. There is no psoriasis, subcutaneous nodules, cutaneous vasculitis, sclerodactyly or nailfold capillary dilatation. Cardiorespiratory and abdominal examination is normal and there are no neurological signs. Urinalysis is clear. Schirmer tear testing reveals 3 mm of moisture after 5 minutes.

Initial investigations

X-rays of the hands, wrists and feet reveal periarticular osteoporosis and periarticular erosions (Fig. 77.1). Blood test results are shown in Box 77.1.

Have examination and initial investigations narrowed down your differential diagnosis?

The diagnosis of an inflammatory arthritis that is likely to be persistent has been established by the duration of the patient's symptoms and the presence of erosions. The negative family history and absence of psoriasis on examination exclude psoriatic arthritis. The absence of prominent extra-articular features, along with the raised C-reactive protein and the findings on autoimmune serology and X-rays, makes RA a more likely diagnosis than a CTD such as SLE or systemic sclerosis.

BOX 77.1	
Initial investigations	
Haemoglobin	108 g/l (10.8 g/dl)
MCV	88 fl
WCC	11.1 × 10⁹/l (10³/mm³)
Neutrophils	90%
Platelets	289 × 10⁹/l (10³/mm³)
ESR	50 mm/1st hr (Westergren)
CRP	24 mg/l
U&E, serum creatinine and LFTs	Normal
RF	Positive, 110 U/ml (0–20)
ANF	Positive, 1:80

Further investigations

If available, a positive test for anticyclic citrullinated peptide antibodies offers increased specificity, compared with rheumatoid factor (RF) testing in RA. Other autoimmune serology, such as antibodies to double-stranded DNA or extractable nuclear antigens, is likely to be negative, given the clinical picture and the presence of erosions.

How will you treat this patient?

Treatment with second-line (disease-modifying antirheumatic drug, DMARD) therapy should be commenced. This is likely not only to lead to a significant improvement in symptoms, but also to retard radiological progression and thus improve the long-term outcome. Opinion varies as to whether this should be sequential DMARD monotherapy, combination DMARD therapy, or step-up combination DMARD therapy based on disease activity. Examples of DMARDs include methotrexate, sulfasalazine and leflunomide. Treatment using therapy directed against tumour-necrosis factor-α (TNF-α) is increasingly used in early disease if local resources permit, particularly if initial DMARD treatment is ineffective or not tolerated. The early development of radiological erosions is a poor prognostic sign and emphasises the need for rapid disease control. As a temporising measure, the right knee should be aspirated and injected with a long-acting steroid. Treatment with plain analgesics will afford some additional pain relief but non-steroidal anti-inflammatory drugs (NSAIDs) should be avoided, if at all possible, as the past history of duodenal ulcer increases the risk of NSAID-induced peptic ulcer disease. As Schirmer tear testing has revealed inadequate tear production, treatment with artificial tears is likely to be of benefit. Disease education is also an important part of the management. The patient should be referred to occupational therapy for advice on joint protection and physiotherapy for instruction in quadriceps exercises. Stopping smoking is important not only as a general health measure, but also because it is likely to improve the symptoms of Raynaud's phenomenon. In addition, modification of vascular risk factors is an important part of the long-term management of individuals with RA.

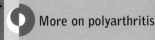

Global issues

More on polyarthritis

- Many of the DMARDs used to treat inflammatory arthritis carry a risk of acquiring opportunistic infection, or reactivating previous latent infection.

- Autoimmune serology could be considered a luxury! Remember that the diagnosis of a CTD is primarily clinical and supported by the results of autoimmune serology, not the other way round. If in doubt, treat with a DMARD but keep your diagnostic eyes open. Most of the extra-articular manifestations of inflammatory arthritis, other than renal involvement, cause symptoms, so continue to monitor urinalysis and blood pressure if the possibility of a CTD remains.

- Treatment with anti-TNF-α biological agents is highly effective; however, access to these agents in resource-poor nations may be limited due to their high cost.

- Patients being considered for anti-TNF-α therapy should be carefully selected and should not have active tuberculosis. Patients with latent tuberculosis infection (LTBI) should ideally be screened with interferon-γ release assays (IGRAs), but in developing nations the tuberculin skin test (TST) may be more cost-effective.

See Chapter 25 of **Davidson's Principles and Practice of Medicine** (20th edn)

78

An elderly woman with back pain

S. H. RALSTON

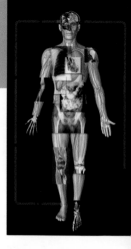

Presenting problem

A 76-year-old Caucasian woman is referred to the outpatient clinic with gradual onset of back pain of several months' duration. She has angina and hypertension, which are well controlled with atenolol, bendroflumethiazide and simvastatin. She has a past history of breast cancer, which has been in clinical remission for 15 years following surgery, radiotherapy and tamoxifen, which she took for 5 years but which has now been stopped. She suffered a wrist fracture about 10 years previously, which occurred when she tripped and fell whilst out shopping with her daughter. She does not smoke or drink alcohol, has a normal diet, and her menopause occurred at the age of 42 years. Prior to referral, her general practitioner checked some routine blood tests (Box 78.1).

BOX 78.1	
Initial investigations	
Haemoglobin	125 g/l (12.5 g/dl)
ESR	15 mm/hr
Creatinine	110 µmol/l (1.24 mg/dl)
Sodium	140 mmol/l (meq/l)
Potassium	3.6 mmol/l (meq/l)
Calcium	2.45 mmol/l (9.46 mg/dl)
Albumin	45 g/l (4.5 g/dl)

What would your differential diagnosis include before examining the patient?

Back pain is a common complaint and could be due to a variety of conditions, including osteoarthritis of the lumbar spine, soft tissue rheumatism, ankylosing spondylitis and osteoporotic vertebral fracture. Bone metastases from breast cancer would also be possible, although the history of early menopause increases the likelihood of osteoporosis as a cause for the patient's symptoms. Aortic aneurysm would also enter into the differential diagnosis in view of the history of hypertension, but the chronic nature of the pain would make this less likely.

Examination

The patient is apyrexial and looks well. Her height is 1.53 m and weight is 52 kg. When informed of these measurements, the patient reports that her weight is steady but she thinks that her height has fallen by about 6 cm from when she was younger. There is an obvious kyphosis mainly affecting the upper thoracic spine, but physical examination is otherwise unremarkable.

Has the examination narrowed down your differential diagnosis?

The height loss and kyphosis point strongly towards vertebral osteoporosis as the cause of this lady's symptoms. Bone metastases from breast cancer would be possible but are less likely in view of the fact that the patient looks well and has not lost weight. Ankylosing spondylitis can be associated with height loss, due to fixed flexion deformity of the spine, but it would be very unusual for ankylosing spondylitis to present at this age. Soft tissue rheumatism and osteoarthritis remain possible diagnoses and could be contributing to the back pain, but neither condition would explain the height loss and kyphosis.

Further investigations

Dual energy X-ray absorptiometry (DEXA) reveals that bone mineral density (BMD) values are reduced to within the osteoporotic range at the lumbar spine (T-score −3.7), and the femoral neck (T-score −2.6). The lateral imaging DEXA shows evidence of vertebral compression fractures (Fig. 78.1). X-rays of the thoracic and lumbar spine reveal evidence of osteoporosis with several wedge compression fractures in the thoracic and lumbar spine. Degenerative changes are also noted in the lumbar spine and at the thoracolumbar junction. An isotope bone scan reveals linear areas of increased tracer uptake in the thoracic spine consistent with benign vertebral collapse. Further biochemistry is performed to exclude secondary causes of osteoporosis, including thyroid function tests, calcium, phosphate and immunoglobulins, but these are normal.

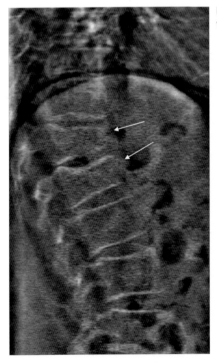

Fig. 78.1 Lateral DEXA scan image showing vertebral wedge fractures (arrows).

Does this narrow down your differential diagnosis?

These investigations would be consistent with a diagnosis of osteoporosis and vertebral fractures as the cause of this patient's back pain and height loss. Osteoarthritis of the spine could be contributing to the back pain but could not explain such dramatic height loss or the kyphosis, and the isotope bone scan appearances make metastatic disease unlikely. The normal biochemistry and haematology are consistent with post-menopausal osteoporosis and are helpful in excluding secondary causes of osteoporosis, such as thyrotoxicosis, myeloma and primary hyperparathyroidism.

How will you treat this patient?

This lady has established osteoporosis of the spine and hip, and fragility fractures affecting the spine and wrist. She is at increased risk of future fractures and the aims of therapy are to reduce this risk. The first choice would be one of the bisphosphonates: either alendronate 70 mg once weekly or risedronate 35 mg once weekly in combination with calcium and vitamin D supplements. Alternative treatments would include strontium ranelate (2 g daily) or parathyroid hormone (20 µg daily for 18 months), which have both been shown to reduce the risk of vertebral and non-vertebral fractures. Hormone replacement therapy would be contraindicated in view of the history of breast cancer. Raloxifene or calcitonin might be an option if the patient were intolerant of other medications, but neither of these agents has been shown to reduce the risk of non-vertebral fractures, which are a concern in a patient of this age.

Global issues

 More on osteoporosis?

- Post-menopausal osteoporosis is a common problem world-wide, although the disease is less common in some ethnic groups such as African-Americans, probably because of genetic factors.

- DEXA may not be available in low-resource settings. Although it has confirmed the diagnosis of osteoporosis in this case, the presence of vertebral fractures and radiological osteopenia in this patient would have been sufficient to clinch the diagnosis, even without a DEXA examination.

See Chapter 25 of **Davidson's Principles and Practice of Medicine** (20th edn)

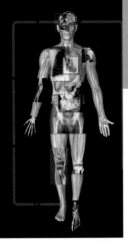

79

Repeated abortions and a stroke in a young woman

R. GUPTA

Presenting problem

A 28-year-old woman presents to the Accident and Emergency department with a 5-hour history of throbbing headache and sudden onset of weakness of the right upper and lower limbs. She stumbles while walking and also has difficulty in talking. There is no previous history of any significant medical illness. She has been married for 4 years and has no children. Although she has been pregnant three times, all ended in abortions. She sought the first abortion at the age of 18 years, as she was unmarried at that time and was not ready to start a family. She had two more spontaneous abortions at the age of 25 and 28 years. The last miscarriage occurred about 3 months ago and was attributed to a state of mental stress and trivial trauma. She has never been subjected to detailed investigation.

BOX 79.1

Causes of stroke in the young

- Subarachnoid haemorrhage
- Primary intracerebral haemorrhage
- Cardiac source of embolism
- Premature atherosclerosis
- Systemic lupus erythematosus
- Vasculitis
- Antiphospholipid antibody syndrome
- Thrombophilia
- Homocystinuria

What would your differential diagnosis include before examining the patient?

The differential diagnosis of stroke in a young person is extensive (Box 79.1). The most likely cause of a stroke in this woman is a subarachnoid or intracerebral haemorrhage, cerebral thrombosis or embolism. When embolism is suspected, a source of emboli from cardiac disease (e.g. valvular heart disease) or vascular disease should be sought. Other causes of stroke to be considered are systemic vasculitis or thrombosis because of thrombophilia. The absence of other clinical features makes systemic vasculitis in this young lady most unlikely, but this needs to be investigated further. The antiphospholipid antibody syndrome should be considered as a possibility in view of her poor obstetric history.

Examination and initial investigations

The patient is apyrexial and looks comfortable and well oriented; her pulse is 96/min and blood pressure is 130/76 mmHg. There are no skin lesions, oral ulcers or alopecia. Cardiovascular examination reveals normal peripheral pulses and no obvious abnormality of the heart. Neurological examination reveals a hemiparesis on the right side. Some urgent investigations are necessary.

A 12-lead electrocardiogram (ECG) and chest X-ray are normal, while an emergency non-contrast computed tomography scan (CT) of the brain reveals an acute infarct in the territory of the left middle cerebral artery, with no evidence of haemorrhage (Fig. 79.1A). Initial blood investigations show haemoglobin 135 g/l (13.5 g/dl); white cell count 7.8×10^9/l (10^3/mm^3); platelet count 98×10^9/l (10^3/mm^3); and erythrocyte sedimentation rate (ESR) 24 mm/hr. Renal and liver function tests are normal, as is a dipstick examination of urine.

Have the examination and initial investigations narrowed down your differential diagnosis?

Yes. This young woman has unfortunately had an acute ischaemic stroke, but the underlying cause has still to be determined. Examination has not revealed any abnormality of the heart or any other potential source of embolism, but there could yet be structural carotid artery or cardiac lesions, and a thrombophilic disorder still has to be excluded. As discussed earlier, systemic vasculitis or a connective tissue disease seems unlikely in view of the unremarkable history, examination and results of initial investigations. The antiphospholipid antibody syndrome is beginning to seem much more likely, but more blood tests and imaging are required.

Further investigations

A repeat full blood count confirms a mild thrombocytopenia. A transthoracic echocardiogram and Doppler studies of the carotid arteries are normal. A magnetic resonance imaging scan (MRI) of the brain confirms an infarct in the territory of the left middle cerebral artery (MCA) (Fig. 79.1B). Further tests show antinuclear antibodies (ANA) — negative, antinuclear cytoplasmic antibodies (ANCA) — negative, anticardiolipin antibodies (aCL) IgG — 52 GPL U/ml (normal < 12 GPL U/ml), aCL IgM — 26 MPL U/ml (normal < 12 MPL U/ml) and anti-β2 glycoprotein I antibodies (IgG) — 22 U/ml (normal < 8 U/ml). Lupus anticoagulant is positive, but proteins C and S, and antithrombin III concentrations are normal.

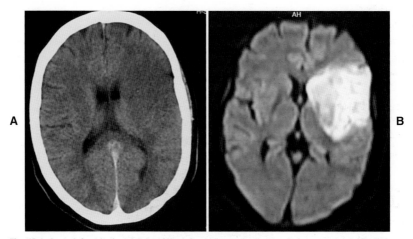

A   B

Fig. 79.1 Acute infarct in the territory of the left middle cerebral artery. A. A non-contrast CT of the head shows an acute infarct in the territory of the left middle cerebral artery. B. A corresponding image seen on the MRI diffusion weighted image suggests acute infarct in the same place.

Has the diagnosis been clinched?

Yes; the presence of strongly positive antiphospholipid antibodies in this young lady with recurrent abortions and a stroke has confirmed the diagnosis of antiphospholipid antibody syndrome. This syndrome may be primary or secondary. The secondary antiphospholipid antibody syndrome is common in patients with connective tissue diseases such as systemic lupus erythematosus (SLE). In the primary antiphospholipid syndrome, no such cause is usually seen. This woman has a primary antiphospholipid syndrome, as no underlying connective tissue disease has been found.

There are several types of antiphospholipid antibody. Those most commonly detected in clinical practice are anticardiolipin antibodies (IgG and IgM) and the lupus anticoagulant. Recently, antibodies against cofactor $\beta 2$ glycoprotein I have been used in the diagnosis of this syndrome. It is important to remember that these antibodies may be present transiently in low titres in many other conditions, such as infections, and following the use of drugs, such as sodium valproate and chlorpromazine. It is therefore recommended that repeat tests for antiphospholipid antibodies are performed after 6 weeks.

How will you treat this patient?

This lady has presented too late for thrombolytic therapy to be considered. She should be commenced on aspirin therapy and will require intensive input from a multidisciplinary stroke team to optimise her functional recovery. As well as arterial thromboembolic disease, the antiphospholipid syndrome is associated with venous thromboembolic disease. She will, therefore, require long-term anticoagulation. There is a risk of haemorrhage into the infarct if warfarin is commenced too soon after the acute event, and so this is best delayed for some days.

The patient will need to be counselled about future pregnancies. As well as miscarriage, there is a real risk of fetal intra-uterine growth retardation. At the time of pregnancy, warfarin should be replaced by subcutaneous injections of low molecular weight heparin.

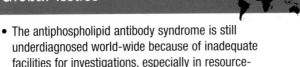

Global issues

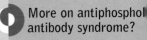

More on antiphospholipid antibody syndrome?

See Chapter 24 of
Davidson's Principles and Practice of Medicine (20th edn)

- The antiphospholipid antibody syndrome is still underdiagnosed world-wide because of inadequate facilities for investigations, especially in resource-limited settings.

- None of the currently available tests is sensitive enough to diagnose the condition in all patients. In the future, the availability of more sensitive tests, such as antibodies against $\beta 2$ glycoprotein I, will enable the diagnosis to be made in many more cases.

- MRI is not as widely available as CT. Diffusion weighted imaging can detect ischaemia earlier than CT, and other MRI sequences can be used to demonstrate abnormal perfusion. MRI is more sensitive at detecting strokes affecting the brain stem and cerebellum.

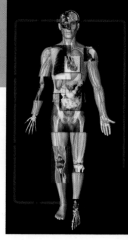

80

A 65-year-old man with a sudden headache

R. J. DAVENPORT

Presenting problem

A 65-year-old man develops a sudden-onset headache (i.e. of maximal intensity immediately) whilst masturbating, at the point of orgasm. There are no other symptoms other than nausea. He is otherwise well, apart from treated hypertension, and his only medication is bendroflumethiazide and aspirin. Embarrassment prevents him from seeking immediate medical attention, but 48 hours later he is seen in the Accident and Emergency department, where the examination is normal; he is discharged with simple analgesia. Ten days later the headache and nausea persist, and he reattends.

What would your differential diagnosis include before examining the patient?

The concern here is that this is a secondary rather than primary headache syndrome, and the most obvious worry is subarachnoid haemorrhage (SAH). SAH is no more likely to occur during physical activity (including sex) than other benign primary headache syndromes, and this may turn out to be either thunderclap headache or headache associated with sexual activity (previously called benign sex headache or coital cephalgia). The problem is that the history is insufficient to distinguish benign from potentially sinister headaches, and thus all sudden-onset headaches (maximal immediately or within minutes) must be assumed to be sinister until proved otherwise and require investigation. SAH may present with headache alone in between 10 and 20% of cases. Cigarette smoking, hypertension, a family history (first-degree) and alcohol intake of more than 2 units per day are all independent risk factors for SAH. SAH is not the only potential serious cause, however, and other diagnoses, including cerebral venous thrombosis, arterial dissection, infectious meningoencephalitis, subdural haematoma and pituitary apoplexy, should all be included in the differential diagnosis. Temporal arteritis is a potentially treatable cause of headache in older patients (usually over 60 years), but an abrupt onset such as this would be very unusual.

Examination

The patient is orientated and his Glasgow Coma Score is 15. He looks tired and fed up but not unwell. His blood pressure is 190/100 mmHg, his pulse is 85/min, and there are no physical signs. His neurological examination is normal and there is no neck stiffness. The results of initial investigations are shown in Box 80.1.

BOX 80.1

Initial investigations

Full blood count	Normal
ESR	30 mm/1st hour
U&E, glucose	Normal
12-lead ECG	Voltage criteria for left ventricular hypertrophy; otherwise normal
CT brain scan (unenhanced)	Normal

BOX 80.2

Further investigations

Opening pressure	28 cm CSF
Cell count	312 red blood cells, 1 white cell/mm³
Protein	700 mg/l (0.07 g/dl)
CSF appearance	Yellow compared against white background to naked eye
Spectrophotometric analysis	Positive for oxyhaemoglobin and bilirubin

Have examination and initial investigations narrowed down your differential diagnosis?

No. Blood tests are rarely helpful in identifying serious intracranial disease in this scenario, although hyponatraemia (due to cerebral salt wasting rather than inappropriate antidiuretic hormone secretion) is common in SAH. The electrocardiogram (ECG) is consistent with the history of hypertension, although it is not an accurate guide to left ventricular hypertrophy; never assume that headache is due to hypertension outside of hypertensive encephalopathy (which is clearly not the case here, as the patient is not encephalopathic). ECG changes of ischaemia may be seen in SAH, but this is very non-specific. The normal computed tomography (CT) brain scan would have been much more reassuring if it had been performed within 48 hours of the initial onset, but after that the sensitivity of CT for subarachnoid blood falls rapidly and a normal scan never excludes SAH.

Given the delayed presentation and the suspicion of SAH from the history, this man requires a lumbar puncture to exclude SAH.

Further investigations

A lumbar puncture is performed by an experienced operator and is successful at first pass. The sample is hand-delivered to laboratory without delay. The results are shown in Box 80.2.

Does this narrow down your differential diagnosis?

The lumbar puncture has confirmed a diagnosis of SAH. At this late stage of presentation (10 days after the initial onset) and with a normal brain CT, the cell count is unlikely to be relevant and we are more concerned with the pigment analysis. As the red blood cells lyse, they lend a yellowish tinge to the cerebrospinal fluid (xanthochromia); this can be seen with the naked eye, although samples should also be sent to the laboratory (by hand, as soon as possible, and protected from light if there is any delay). Oxyhaemoglobin alone can be seen after traumatic taps, as it may form in vitro, but the presence of bilirubin is much

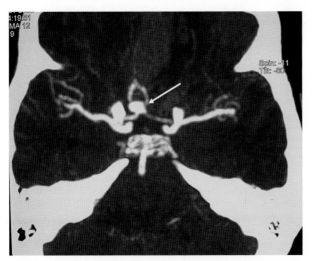

Fig. 80.1 CT angiogram showing an anterior communicating artery aneurysm (arrow).

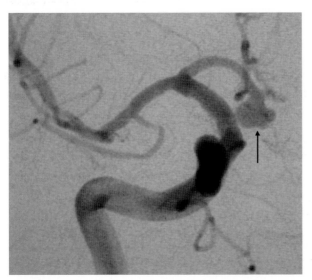

Fig. 80.2 Conventional catheter angiogram of the aneurysm before treatment (arrow).

more persuasive because this only occurs in vivo (provided the sample has not been left to degrade in light, when deoxyhaemoglobin can be broken down into bilirubin).

The next step is to identify the underlying cause, with intracranial aneurysms found in at least 85% of SAH; the remainder are due to perimesencephalic bleeds (good prognosis), and rarer vascular malformations such as arterio-venous malformations. Although conventional catheter angiography has been the preferred test in the past, many centres now undertake CT angiography as the initial test. In this case, it confirms an anterior communicating artery aneurysm (Fig. 80.1).

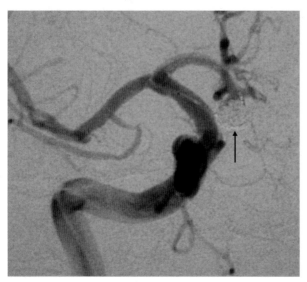

Fig. 80.3 Catheter angiogram after endovascular coiling is completed, showing total occlusion of the aneurysm (arrow).

How will you treat this patient?

He should be transferred immediately to a neuroscience centre, unless already there. Analgesia and stool softeners should be prescribed, along with antiemetics if required. He should rest in bed and a careful fluid balance chart should be recorded, with regular monitoring of his electrolytes. He should receive 3 litres of normal saline/24 hrs and be prescribed nimodipine 60 mg 4-hourly. His aneurysm should be secured as soon as practicable, either by endovascular coiling or surgical clipping (Figs 80.2 and 80.3).

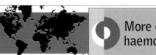

Global issues

- The overall incidence of SAH is 6–8 per 100 000 per annum.

- The risk of SAH is about twice as high for black people compared with white.

- Studies from Finland and Japan have produced much higher incidences of SAH: over 20/100 000 per annum.

More on subarachnoid haemorrhage?

See Chapter 26 of
Davidson's Principles and Practice of Medicine
(20th edn)

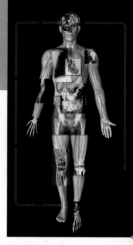

81

A 47-year-old woman with chronic headache

R. AL-SHAHI SALMAN

Presenting problem

You are asked to see a 47-year-old counsellor who has been referred by her general practitioner because she has headaches on most days of the month. When you assess her, the headaches are occurring on alternate days; she finds them worst early in the morning when they wake her from sleep. She is feeling depressed.

Since her thirties she has tended to have a day-long headache around the time of every wedding anniversary; these headaches are severe and unilateral, are preceded by visual fortification spectra lasting for an hour, and are accompanied by photophobia and vomiting, all of which compel her to lie down in a darkened room. Over the year prior to your assessment, she has suffered hot flushes and her periods have become infrequent. Her annual headaches have now become much more frequent, but oral sumatriptan has not been particularly effective in relieving them. She has resorted to over-the-counter (OTC) combination analgesics, obtained from her daughter who suffers from frequent migraine.

What would your differential diagnosis include before examining the patient?

This woman has chronic daily headache (CDH), defined by the International Headache Society as headache occurring on 15 or more days each month. CDH is either 'secondary' to an underlying neurological or systemic disorder, or due to a 'primary' headache syndrome (in other words, a recognisable pattern of headache and accompanying symptoms, without underlying structural pathology). Your patient is naturally worried that she has a brain tumour. Although you must always eliminate secondary headaches from the differential diagnosis first, a brain tumour is an unlikely explanation in her case because she has no suggestive symptoms: for example, cognitive dysfunction or focal neurological symptoms. She has early morning headaches but these are not a reliable indicator of raised intracranial pressure. In the absence of symptoms indicating other causes of secondary headache (for example, head injury, infection or giant cell arteritis), this woman is most likely to have a primary headache disorder.

Primary headaches can de subdivided according to their associated symptoms, as well as the duration of pain. Cluster headaches and other rare 'trigeminal autonomic cephalgias' tend to last 90 minutes at most, whereas chronic migraine and chronic tension-type headaches tend to last for at least 4 hours. Because of the difference in treatment, it is important to distinguish between tension-type headaches, which account for almost three-quarters of chronic primary headache disorders in the population, and chronic migraine, which is the more prevalent diagnosis in hospital outpatient clinics. Nausea, photophobia, phonophobia, aggravation of pain by movement, throbbing headache and a need to lie down in a darkened room are key pointers to migraine (Box 81.1). The existence of some of these features, as well as a personal and family history of migraine, make chronic migraine the most likely diagnosis in this case.

Examination

Neurological examination, including funduscopy, is normal, but the patient looks tired and depressed. Blood pressure is 132/64 mmHg. When you palpate her cervical paraspinal muscles, they are tender. Her general practitioner performed some simple blood tests and these are shown in Box 81.2.

Have examination and initial investigations narrowed down your differential diagnosis?

Examination has provided further reassurance that there are no signs to indicate structural pathology within the central nervous system. Furthermore, neck examination has revealed another potential factor that might be contributing to this woman's chronic migraine. It was important to check her thyroid function and calcium level, given her low mood and chronic headache, but measuring the erythrocyte sedimentation rate (ESR) was unnecessary. The ESR certainly needs to be checked in anyone over the age of 50 years with a new daily persistent headache, to look for giant cell arteritis.

Further investigations

Although you might be tempted to organise a brain scan to 'rule out' a secondary cause of the headache, especially if the patient requests it, the yield of anything but incidental abnormalities on a brain scan is negligible in patients with chronic headache and a normal neurological examination. A careful drug history, including an enquiry about OTC medicines, is the crucial next step here.

Does this narrow down your differential diagnosis?

Further questioning and examination of the pill packets in the woman's handbag reveal that she has been taking at least two tablets of an OTC preparation of paracetamol and codeine on a daily basis for most of the last year. On a background of infrequent migraine with visual aura, she has developed chronic migraine, compounded by analgesic overuse and cervical muscle tension.

How will you treat this patient?

Gradual or sudden withdrawal of analgesics will eventually lead to a resolution of the headaches related to medication misuse. During drug withdrawal, a non-steroidal anti-inflammatory drug (NSAID) can safely provide some relief. Following analgesic withdrawal, the underlying headache disorder usually persists, and it is possible that this woman is suffering a perimenopausal exacerbation of migraine. Lifestyle measures can ameliorate migraine, and you should encourage a regular sleep pattern, regular meals, avoidance of over-exertion, and minimal stress; some people find that dietary exclusion of certain foodstuffs prevents some migraines. Chronic migraine can respond to amitriptyline (10–75 mg), sodium valproate (up to 1500 mg daily) or topiramate (up to 50 mg 12-hourly), the doses of which should be titrated according to their beneficial effects and/or side-effects.

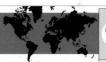

Global issues

More on migraine?

- The most prevalent neurological disorders world-wide are migraine (10% prevalence) and CDH (5% prevalence).

- Patterns of analgesic overuse depend on the regional availability of OTC analgesia.

- There are numerous potential causes of headache in patients with human immunodeficiency virus/acquired immunodeficiency syndrome (HIV/AIDS) and such individuals should be investigated thoroughly.

See Chapter 26 of
**Davidson's
Principles and
Practice of
Medicine**
(20th edn)

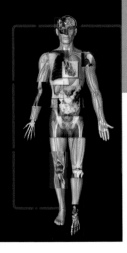

82

A young woman with numbness and sensory loss in her fingers

S. B. GUNATILAKE

Presenting problem

A 25-year-old female is seen in a neurology clinic in Colombo, Sri Lanka, with a history of numbness and loss of sensation over the left small and ring fingers. She first developed numbness about 6 months ago, and a few days prior to the clinic visit she burnt her small finger while cooking but felt no pain. The numbness has gradually worsened and now affects the whole of the two fingers, as well as part of the palm. She has also noticed that the two affected fingers tend to bend without her being aware and that it is difficult to keep them straight with the other fingers.

What would your differential diagnosis include before examining the patient?

Numbness and loss of sensation affecting the ulnar border of the hand can be due to an ulnar nerve lesion, a C8/T1 root lesion, or even a lesion within the lower cervical cord such as syringomyelia. Ulnar neuropathies at the elbow typically present with complaints of numbness and tingling of the fourth and fifth fingers.

In severe cases there is weakness and wasting of the ulnar innervated small muscles of the hand: namely, the abductor digiti minimi and the first dorsal interosseous muscle. Ulnar neuropathy can occur from excessive and repeated leaning on the elbow, entrapment of the nerve just below the elbow by the aponeurosis joining the two heads of the flexor carpi ulnaris muscle, and following fractures and dislocation of the elbow. Ulnar neuropathy can also be a presentation of a mononeuritis multiplex such as seen in vasculitides, systemic lupus erythematosus and leprosy (Box 82.1).

BOX 82.1

Vasculitides affecting peripheral nerves

- Polyarteritis nodosa
- Churg–Strauss syndrome
- Wegener's granulomatosis
- Rheumatoid arthritis
- Systemic lupus erythematosus

Examination

The patient's higher functions, speech and cranial nerves are normal. She has an ulnar claw hand on the left side and a large hypopigmented patch over the skin of the left ulnar border of the forearm (Fig. 82.1). There are burn scars on the small finger. Wasting of the first dorsal interosseous and abductor digiti minimi is present, and abduction of the second finger and

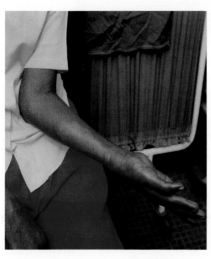

Fig. 82.1 The patient's left forearm showing the ulnar claw and the hypopigmented skin lesion.

flexion of the fourth and fifth fingers are weak. There is sensory loss to touch, pain and temperature over the ulnar nerve territory and over the hypopigmented patch. The left ulnar nerve is grossly thickened at the elbow groove. The right ulnar nerve is not thickened, but on general examination the patient has a prominent greater auricular nerve on the left side. Lower limb examination is normal, with normal tendon reflexes and plantar responses.

Has examination narrowed your differential diagnosis?

Thickened, hypertrophic nerves are seen in hereditary motor sensory demyelinating neuropathy type 1 (Charcot–Marie–Tooth type 1). However, the absence of family history and normal findings in the lower limbs make this diagnosis very unlikely. Leprosy can be diagnosed with confidence in a patient with hypopigmented anaesthetic skin lesions and thickened ulnar and greater auricular nerves from a region where leprosy is still seen or endemic (Box 82.2). Histological examination with skin biopsy or nerve biopsy is not required when all these features are present. Leprosy is a chronic granulomatous infection of the skin and peripheral nerves with the intracellular bacterium *Mycobacterium leprae*.

> **BOX 82.2**
>
> **Diagnostic signs of leprosy**
>
> - Hypopigmented or reddish patches with definite loss of sensation
> - Thickened peripheral nerves
> - Acid-fast bacilli on slit skin smears or biopsy material

Investigations

Routine blood tests are normal. The erythrocyte sedimentation rate (ESR) is 10 mm in the first hour. A vasculitis screen is negative and antinuclear antibody (ANA) is absent. Nerve conduction studies show absent sensory action potentials in the fourth and fifth digits and evidence of axonal damage in the ulnar nerve.

How will you treat this patient?

The diagnosis needs to be carefully explained to the patient and, as social stigma is still attached to the disease, counselling and reassurance are necessary. Multidrug therapy is now the standard treatment. As this patient has paucibacillary (1–5 skin lesions) or tuberculoid leprosy, she does not discharge any viable organisms and therefore is not a risk to others. Treatment is with rifampicin 600 mg once a month for 6 months and dapsone 100 mg daily for 6 months. For multibacillary or lepromatous leprosy, treatment consists of rifampicin 600 mg once a month, dapsone 100 mg daily, clofazimine 50 mg daily combined with 300 mg once a month for 1 or 2 years. For the ulnar claw hand, the patient will require a splint to keep the fingers in the neutral position and advice on proper hand care because of the sensory loss.

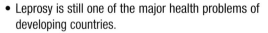

Global issues

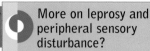

More on leprosy and peripheral sensory disturbance?

See Chapters 13 and 26
Davidson's Principles and Practice of Medicine (20th edn)

- Leprosy is still one of the major health problems of developing countries.
- When the features are typical and the patient is from a country where leprosy is still endemic (India, Brazil, Mozambique, Nepal and Madagascar) or known to occur, skin and nerve biopsies are not required.
- Leprosy should be considered in any unfamiliar skin lesion or a peripheral nerve lesion in a patient from an endemic area.

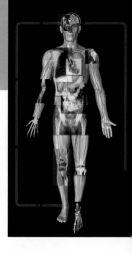

83

A 49-year-old man admitted in coma

R. J. DAVENPORT

Presenting problem

You are called to the Accident and Emergency department (A&E) to see a 49-year-old man admitted 2 hours previously. He is now unconscious and intubated, and thus unable to provide a history. The (rather vague) history is that he is a businessman who requested a doctor whilst in his hotel. He told the doctor that he felt unwell and dizzy, and had vomited once with some mild headache. Whilst the doctor was speaking to him, he developed a left-sided weakness and slurred speech, and an ambulance was called. He told the staff at the A&E when he arrived that he was usually well, and his only medication was a 'water pill'. He is a heavy smoker, and was able to request a cigarette in the A&E. His left-sided weakness improved during his transfer to hospital, but he still complained of headache and felt unwell, and also complained that his vision was not right. He then developed a rapidly evolving right-sided weakness, and whilst a brain scan was being organised, his left side became weak again. He became increasingly drowsy and proceeded to have a respiratory arrest. He was rapidly resuscitated, with no cardiac arrest, and was given short-acting sedation and paralysing agents prior to endotracheal intubation and ventilation.

What would your differential diagnosis include before examining the patient?

The differential for coma is wide and, as always, the key lies in the history. By definition, this is never directly available from a patient in coma, but you must pursue family, carers, general practitioners, ambulance crew and anyone who might be able to provide a history. Vital questions to ask are when was the patient last well, what pre-existing comorbidities are known, and what medications are being taken? In this case, you should seek to identify the patient's next of kin as soon as possible to obtain more information, and you should also speak directly to the doctors who attended to him before he lapsed into coma.

Coma is (somewhat arbitrarily) defined as a Glasgow Coma Score (GCS) of 8 or less, made up of failure to open the eyes to verbal command (E2) or less, abnormal flexion (M4) or less and making unrecognisable sounds in response to pain (V2) or less. You should always use the GCS to measure consciousness, and avoid terms like stuporose, obtunded or drowsy, which mean little. Never quote a sum score but describe the three components of the scale; to describe someone as eye opening to speech (E3), localising to pain (M5), with confused speech (V4) paints a much clearer picture than simply GCS = 12.

BOX 83.1

Clinical presentation of coma

Clinical appearance	Possible causes
Coma without focal signs or meningism	Anoxic–ischaemic, metabolic or toxic insults
Coma without focal signs with meningism*	Meningo-encephalitis, subarachnoid haemorrhage
Coma with focal signs	Intracranial haemorrhage, infarction, other structural lesions

*Meningism is not universally present in these conditions.

Coma requires either diffuse bilateral hemispheric damage, or damage to the ascending reticular activating system within the brain stem. Thus, unilateral hemispheric damage does not cause coma, unless there is associated brain-stem compression, which is why early (within 24 hours of onset of symptoms) coma due to an ischaemic hemispheric stroke is most unlikely.

It is useful to consider three clinical appearances of coma (Box 83.1), which will suggest possible underlying causes. Always consider head injury, which is usually obvious from the history but may not be, particularly in patients found unconscious with no witnesses. Beware of ascribing coma solely to alcohol. When considering 'medical' (i.e. non-traumatic) coma, stroke accounts for about 50% of all cases, with 20% due to anoxic–ischaemic injury, and metabolic and infective encephalopathies accounting for most of the rest.

In this case, the focal symptoms and signs clearly suggest a primary intracranial cause, rather than a global brain problem such as a toxic or metabolic insult. The onset is clearly abrupt, suggesting a stroke, and the alternating hemipareses and early disturbance of consciousness exclude a hemispheric ischaemic or haemorrhagic stroke, and localise the lesion to the brain stem. Thus an ischaemic brain-stem stroke is the most likely diagnosis; haemorrhage is less likely due to the fluctuating nature. The unequivocal focal signs exclude a psychogenic coma. An anoxic–ischaemic complication of this man's brief respiratory arrest is not plausible, as he clearly was developing a neurological syndrome with coma before his arrest. Rather it was a consequence of his syndrome, not the cause.

Examination and initial investigations

Prior to this man's respiratory arrest, his coma score was recorded as eye opening to pain (E2), not speaking (V1), and extending to pain (M2), a sum score of 5/15. No details relating to other neurological signs were recorded. On examination now, he is intubated with no gag response and has not received any anaesthetic drugs for about 30 minutes (and the anaesthetist tells you that the drugs she used at the time of his emergency intubation will have worn off by now). There is no rash or other skin signs, and no neck stiffness. His pulse is 90/min regular, blood pressure is 205/115 mmHg, and he is hyperventilating spontaneously. He is obese with heavy nicotine staining of his fingers.

He has no eye opening to pain (E1) and extends to painful stimuli on the left, with abnormal flexion of the right (i.e. his best motor response is M3). His pupils are 3 mm and equal, and reacting sluggishly. His oculocephalic reflexes (doll's eye response) are absent. His reflexes are uniformly brisk, and both plantar responses are extensor.

The results of initial investigations are shown in Box 83.2

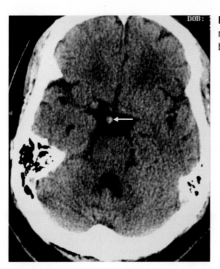

Fig. 83.1 Initial CT brain scan interpreted as normal. Closer inspection reveals a hyper-dense basilar artery (arrow), suggestive of thrombosis.

Have examination and initial investigations narrowed down your differential diagnosis?

Yes, the 'normal' computed tomography scan (CT) of the brain has excluded a haemorrhagic stroke or subarachnoid haemorrhage (although neither of these was the most likely diagnosis). The most likely diagnosis remains a brain-stem ischaemic stroke, and early CT in such cases is often normal. In fact, closer review of the CT reveals that it was not normal. There was a 'hyper-dense' basilar artery (suggesting intraluminal thrombosis) and early ischaemic change within the left occipital region; these subtle signs of early ischaemic stroke are often missed. The raised blood glucose indicates either hitherto unknown diabetes or an acute stress response.

BOX 83.2	
Initial investigations	
FBC, U&E	Normal
Blood glucose	12.1 mmol/l (218 mg/dl)
12-lead ECG	Sinus rhythm, voltage criteria for left ventricular hypertrophy, otherwise normal
Chest X-ray	Normal
CT brain	Reported as normal (Fig. 83.1)

Further investigations

The following day, the patient undergoes repeat CT imaging and CT angiography. This confirms widespread infarction of the brain stem and an occluded basilar artery (Figs 83.2 and 83.3).

Does this narrow down your differential diagnosis?

This confirms the initial clinical diagnosis of an ischaemic brain-stem stroke due to an occluded basilar artery.

How will you treat this patient?

Where available and licensed, intravenous thrombolysis within 3 hours of presentation, or randomisation into any ongoing trials would be appropriate considerations. Other more experimental techniques, such as intra-arterial thrombolysis with stenting or endovascular clot removal, might also be considered in some centres. Otherwise, standard stroke care, on an organised stroke unit, is the most appropriate management.

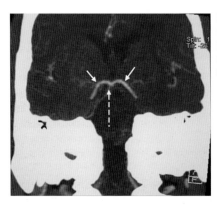

Fig. 83.2 Repeat CT brain within 24 hours. Established brain-stem and right cerebellar hemisphere infarction (arrows).

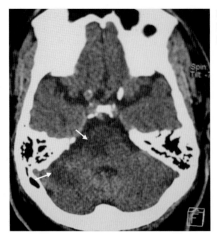

Fig. 83.3 CT angiogram revealing no flow within the basilar artery (broken arrow). The posterior cerebral arteries are filling from the anterior circulation via the circle of Willis (solid arrows).

Neurologists are sometimes asked to see such patients several days or weeks after their presentation as persisting 'coma', whereas in fact they are 'locked in' (i.e. fully conscious but paralysed, able to communicate only with eye opening and vertical eye movements). The identification of this syndrome and discriminating it from coma is essential, and the patient described above is precisely the sort of case that may recover to such a state.

Global issues

 More on coma?

- Infectious diseases account for a higher proportion of coma patients in the developing than the developed world.

- The frequency of traumatic causes of coma (i.e. traumatic brain injury) has been successfully reduced in some developed countries following the introduction of safety measures, but paradoxically is increasing in many developing countries as road traffic intensifies.

See Chapter 26 of
Davidson's Principles and Practice of Medicine
(20th edn)

84

A woman with a shaking attack

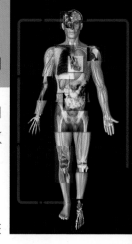

J. STONE

Presenting problem

A 30-year-old woman is admitted to hospital following an episode at home where, according to ambulance staff, she became unresponsive and apparently 'shook all over' for 'quite a long time'. There is a history of a previous episode 4 weeks before. She has a history of depression and is seeing a psychiatrist. She takes fluoxetine 20 mg once daily. By the time you see her she is feeling physically back to normal, but is upset and wants to go home.

What would your differential diagnosis include before taking a further history from the patient and a witness?

The main causes of loss of consciousness with shaking in adults are epilepsy, syncope and non-epileptic attack disorder (pseudoseizures). Separating these relies mostly on a detailed history of the attack from the patient and a witness (Box 84.1), and not on examination or investigations.

Firstly, ask the patient about any warning symptoms. In syncope there may be ringing in the ears or darkening of vision. In epilepsy there may be no warning or an indescribable 'aura'. How did she feel afterwards? Rapid recovery is more common in syncope. Patients with a long generalised seizure usually want to sleep and may have a headache. Did she bite her tongue (Fig. 84.1)? This is common in epilepsy, but rare in syncope. Urinary incontinence on the other hand happens in both epilepsy and syncope.

BOX 84.1

Features in the history that are helpful in distinguishing epilepsy from syncope

	Epilepsy	Syncope
Tongue-biting	Common	Rare
Duration of shaking, if present	60–90 seconds	5–20 seconds
Post-ictal confusion	Common	Rare
Post-ictal headache	Common	Rare
Rapid recovery	Occasional	Usual

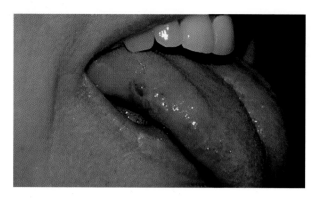

Fig. 84.1 Tongue-biting occurs commonly in generalised seizure, rarely in non-epileptic attacks and hardly ever in syncope. When the lateral tongue is visibly bitten like this, epilepsy is likely.

Secondly, spend time trying to speak to a witness. Use the telephone if you have to. This is more useful than arranging an electroencephalogram (EEG). Remember that the witness may overestimate the duration of the attack. Could the shaking have lasted less than 30 seconds? If it did, then it could easily be the kind of brief twitching that is not infrequently seen after a faint (and which is not epilepsy). In a tonic-clonic seizure there should be a tonic phase (when the patient is rigid) followed by a clonic phase (in which the patient jerks). Typically, generalised tonic-clonic seizures last around 2 minutes. If the shaking attack lasts longer than 10 minutes, then this should raise suspicion of a non-epileptic attack disorder, although you may need a specialist to make this diagnosis. Other clues to non-epileptic attacks include closed eyes, resistance to eyelid opening and flailing of limbs (rather than jerking).

In someone with suspected epilepsy, ask about a family history of epilepsy, childhood seizures, head injury or meningitis. Look hard for provoking factors, such as sleep deprivation and alcohol use (which are associated with a lowered seizure threshold the following day), as this may influence treatment. Do not let a psychiatric history put you off a diagnosis of epilepsy. However, the presence of multiple symptoms unexplained by disease would point more towards non-epileptic attack disorder. The presence of focal neurological symptoms or signs indicates the need for urgent investigations.

Further history and examination

The history obtained is that each attack occurred the day after 'binge' alcohol consumption. There was no warning, tongue-biting or incontinence, and afterwards the patient was drowsy. Although the terrified witness initially reports an attack lasting 10 minutes, after discussion he says that it was probably more like 2 minutes, but definitely longer than 30 seconds. The witness also comments that the woman's body was 'stiff' at the beginning of the attack. The previous attack was similar. Examination is normal.

Has the further history narrowed down your differential diagnosis?

The history is highly suggestive of two generalised tonic-clonic seizures provoked by alcohol abuse. Although limbs can sometimes stiffen briefly in syncope, the duration is too long for this. There are no positive features of non-epileptic attack disorder and epilepsy is more common. The use of fluoxetine may have lowered this woman's seizure threshold further, although antidepressants are not contraindicated in people with epilepsy.

Further investigations

For any adult, cerebral imaging with computed tomography (CT), and preferably magnetic resonance imaging (MRI), is usually advisable, whether or not there have been provoking factors. This is especially true for patients with focal (partial) seizures. EEG is sometimes useful in diagnosis and can be helpful in distinguishing the type of epilepsy. However, around 50% of patients with epilepsy have a normal inter-ictal EEG and there may be non-specific EEG abnormalities in patients without epilepsy. In this case, both CT of the head and EEG were normal.

Does this narrow down your differential diagnosis?

No. Usually, the diagnosis of attacks like this depends on the history.

How will you treat this patient?

The patient has had two seizures, both provoked by alcohol and perhaps partially by fluoxetine. Firstly, she needs general advice about driving and avoiding risk in day-to-day activities.

Usually, drug treatment is advised after two unprovoked generalised seizures. The decision to start anticonvulsants is a major one and should be taken collaboratively with the patient. This case is more difficult, as both seizures were provoked. The decision to treat depends on:

1. whether the patient is likely to continue to have binge drinking sessions
2. whether she will be staying on fluoxetine
3. whether she drives or not
4. how 'risk-averse' she is.

The choice of anticonvulsant depends on the type of epilepsy, age of the patient and other medical issues. The first-line drugs, sodium valproate, carbamazepine and lamotrigine, have similar efficacy.

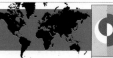

Global issues

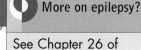

More on epilepsy?

- There are many infective causes of epilepsy to consider world-wide, including neurocysticercosis, human immunodeficiency virus (HIV), toxoplasmosis, tuberculoma and encephalitis.

- An accurate diagnosis of epilepsy should be possible in most cases on the basis of a detailed history. Investigations are there to find out the cause of epilepsy.

See Chapter 26 of
Davidson's Principles and Practice of Medicine
(20th edn)

- Phenytoin and phenobarbital have inferior pharmacokinetics and side-effect profile to newer drugs, but they are just as effective and may be more readily available in some parts of the world.

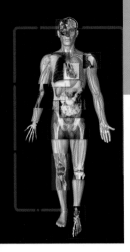

85

A young woman with progressive visual loss in her right eye

C. J. LUECK

Presenting problem

A 25-year-old woman is referred to an Accident and Emergency department with a 12-hour history of progressive visual loss in her right eye. She has been completely well until 2 days ago, when she developed a mild ache behind her right eye which was worse when she moved her eyes. The evening before presentation she thought the vision in her right eye was a bit blurred, but it was late and she went to bed hoping that it would clear up. The next morning the vision was markedly worse and it has continued to deteriorate ever since.

She has no significant past medical history. In particular, there is no history of recent infection or of any cardiovascular risk factor. There is no relevant family history and she is not taking any medication. She is still experiencing mild discomfort behind her right eye when she looks around. She can still detect movement and shapes in the periphery of her vision, but she cannot see faces. Vision out of the left eye is normal.

What would your differential diagnosis include before examining the patient?

The fact that only her right eye is involved means that the pathology must lie in the right eye, the right optic nerve or just possibly the optic chiasm. Ocular vascular disorders, such as a central retinal artery occlusion (CRAO) or anterior ischaemic optic neuropathy (AION), would be unlikely, as the evolution has been gradual. A central retinal vein occlusion (CRVO) is a possibility, as are other ocular causes such as infections or central serous retinopathy, but these should all be obvious on ophthalmic examination.

In Europe, North America or Australia, optic neuritis (ON) is the most likely diagnosis in a woman of this age with this history, but it is important to consider other possibilities. For example, nutritional optic neuropathy or optic nerve compression from an intra-orbital mass, infection, inflammation or thyroid eye disease should be considered. The history in this case is very short, making all these possibilities very unlikely.

It is also important to remember that involvement of the optic chiasm can (rarely) cause symptoms referable to only one eye. Compression of the anterior part of the chiasm where the optic nerve joins it can catch crossing fibres from the other eye and result in a small upper temporal visual field loss, of which the patient might not be aware.

Examination

General examination is normal. The patient's visual acuity is 6/60 on the right and 6/4 on the left. On confrontation, the left visual field is normal but there is an obvious right central scotoma, and this is borne out by subsequent visual field testing. Colour vision (assessed using Ishihara charts) is markedly impaired on the right. There is an obvious right relative afferent pupillary defect (Marcus Gunn pupil). Funduscopy is normal.

Has examination narrowed down your differential diagnosis?

The fact that funduscopy is normal means that ocular vascular disorders (CRAO, CRVO, AION) and macular disease are very unlikely. There is no suggestion of involvement of the left eye, making a chiasmal lesion extremely unlikely, and there is no sign of orbital disease, making thyroid disease most unlikely. It is just possible that there may be a small compressive lesion in the orbit (e.g. an optic nerve sheath meningioma), but this would be most unlikely to present so quickly.

The examination findings are those of acute ON. If the optic disc had been swollen, this would have been labelled 'papillitis'. As it is not, this is referred to as 'retrobulbar neuritis'.

Further investigations

Some practitioners would perform a magnetic resonance (MR) scan of the brain and orbits at this point. This is not essential to making the diagnosis. (Many cases of ON show no abnormality on MR imaging.) However, a great concern is whether this episode of ON might represent the first episode of what will become multiple sclerosis (MS).

MS *cannot* be diagnosed on the basis of just one episode. Thus, the MR scan will make no difference to the immediate diagnosis. A diagnosis of MS will only be made if the patient goes on to have a further episode of central nervous system inflammation or if an MR scan performed in at least 3 months' time demonstrates the development of new lesions. The MR scan is, however, useful for prognostication. If it is normal, the chance of the patient developing MS is less than 10%. If it shows abnormalities typically seen in MS (Fig. 85.1), there is at least a 50% chance that the patient will develop MS within the next 5 years.

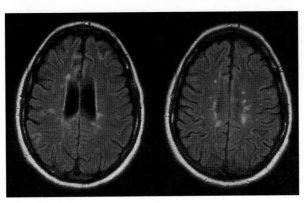

Fig. 85.1 Fluid-attenuated inversion-recovery (FLAIR) MR scan showing the typical areas of periventricular high signal seen in MS.

How will you treat this patient?

Most patients with ON recover vision over a few months, though their recovery may not be completely back to normal. The only available treatment for acute ON is corticosteroids, though these make no difference to long-term outcome and are only indicated if:

1. there is severe pain
2. vision in the other eye is already impaired, *or*
3. binocular function is crucial.

Interferon-β (IFN-β) should be considered in those patients with abnormal MR scans, as there is evidence that it delays the onset of MS after ON, and it may eventually be shown to reduce disability in MS if it is started early. However, IFN-β is not available for this indication in many countries.

Whether an MR scan is performed or not, the patient will need review in 4–6 weeks to make sure that vision is recovering, at least partially. If there is no recovery at all, the diagnosis of ON may still be correct, but other diagnoses will need consideration. Hence, a diagnosis of ON should always be seen as 'conditional' until the patient has been reviewed.

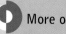

Global issues

- ON and MS are uncommon in more equatorial countries.
- Not all countries have licensed IFN-β for use after isolated ON.

More on optic neuritis

See Chapter 26 of
Davidson's Principles and Practice of Medicine
(20th edn)

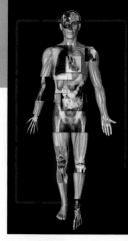

86

A man with a sudden stroke

S. KEIR

Presenting problem

A 72-year-old man presents with left-sided weakness which he noticed on waking the previous day. He is able to walk, but feels as though his leg 'might give way' and is unable to grip items with his left hand. He felt more than usually tired the evening before his symptoms started and went to bed early, but has otherwise been well. He is a smoker, takes a regular aspirin tablet and has a history of hypertension for which he also takes medication.

What would your differential diagnosis include before examining the patient?

The most common cause of this man's symptoms would be a stroke, about 90% of which are due to acute arterial occlusion (ischaemic infarct) and the remaining 10% to intracerebral haemorrhage. Contrary to popular belief, intracerebral haemorrhages can cause relatively mild symptoms. Hemispheric weakness can occur following a seizure and, in an elderly person, during acute hypoglycaemia. Other important causes to consider would be intracerebral tumour, subdural haemorrhage and intracerebral infection (e.g. abscess).

Examination

The gentleman is apyrexial and has a regular pulse rate of 84/min. His blood pressure is high at 184/106 mmHg. He is alert, orientated and able to respond to commands. His visual fields are intact. On being asked to extend his arms out in front of him, his left arm drifts down and his hand grip is noticeably weak. There is sensory inattention on the left side. Power is normal in the left leg.

Has examination narrowed down your differential diagnosis?

The history is one of the strongest pointers to the precise diagnosis; few conditions can provoke significant neurological findings without warning, in the absence of triggers such as epilepsy or hypoglycaemia. Intracranial tumours usually have a more insidious history of events that individually may seem rather inconsequential — perhaps a slight increase in the frequency of headaches, atypical clumsiness or paraesthesia. Subdural haemorrhage can also present with a prodrome of non-specific signs; families may describe the person as 'just not being themselves'. There may also be a history of fall some time previously, which may have precipitated the start of the subdural haemorrhage.

BOX 86.1

Initial investigations

Full blood count	Normal
U&E	Normal
ESR	18 mm/hr
Blood glucose	7.3 mmol/l (132 mg/dl)
Serum total cholesterol	5.8 mmol/l (224 mg/dl)
ECG	Sinus rhythm; no acute changes

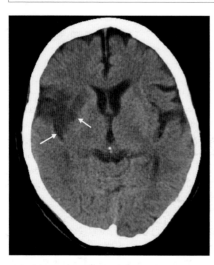

Fig. 86.1 CT scan of the brain showing an area of hypodensity in the right hemisphere consistent with an area of subacute infarction (arrows). The right lateral cerebral ventricle is distorted by the mass effect of the infarct and surrounding oedema.

There are no signs to suggest the gentleman has had a fit, such as tongue-biting or incontinence. We already know he is not a diabetic and there are no signs to suggest he drinks large amounts of alcohol, which could predispose him to hypoglycaemia. Ischaemic stroke remains the most likely diagnosis.

Investigations

Initial investigations are shown in Box 86.1. A computed tomography scan (CT) of the brain is required. This will exclude tumour and subdural haemorrhage, and will identify an intracerebral haemorrhage. CT demonstrates an area of hypodensity in the right cerebral hemisphere, consistent with a subacute, ischaemic stroke (Fig. 86.1).

Does this narrow down your differential diagnosis?

Hypoglycaemia has been ruled out. There are no signs to suggest infection. The CT has shown clear evidence of an ischaemic stroke in the area of the brain consistent with the patient's symptoms and signs. It is not possible to be certain, but the pattern of signs demonstrating involvement of the cortex (inattention), along with motor symptoms, makes the aetiology of thromboembolism a strong possibility. A normal erythrocyte sedimentation rate (ESR) makes a vasculitic cause of the stroke highly unlikely.

It is important to note that CT of the brain may be normal in some patients with ischaemic stroke, particularly if performed very early on after the onset of symptoms. Abnormalities may be demonstrable with magnetic resonance imaging (MRI), but even if this is not available, it is still possible to make a positive diagnosis of ischaemic stroke if the other differential diagnoses have been confidently excluded.

How will you treat this patient?

This gentleman has presented too late for thrombolysis (with tissue plasminogen activator) to be considered. This has to be given within 3 hours of onset of symptoms and intracerebral haemorrhage has to be excluded as the cause of the stroke. Blood pressure should be monitored closely, but unless very high, early aggressive lowering should be avoided, as this can provoke neurological deterioration. However, if the blood pressure remains high after the first week, his antihypertensive medication should be adjusted until his blood pressure is well under 140/80 mmHg. A statin should be commenced to reduce cholesterol and further stroke risk. The gentleman is already taking aspirin. A further antiplatelet drug, modified-release dipyridamole 200 mg 12-hourly, should be added.

Doppler ultrasound of the internal carotid arteries should be performed, as carotid artery stenosis represents an important source of thromboembolism. If carotid Dopplers demonstrate a stenosis of greater than 70% in the internal carotid on the same side as the hemisphere responsible for the symptoms, consideration should be given for carotid endarterectomy. This can markedly reduce the risk of further stroke, but does carry with it a chance of provoking a stroke at the time of operation. Whether this is considered should be determined locally and depends on when the operation could be performed in relation to onset of symptoms and on the local vascular surgeon's peri-operative stroke rate.

Transthoracic echocardiography should also be considered to investigate cardiac sources of embolism (if carotid Doppler studies do not identify a causative lesion); if normal, however, this does not necessarily exclude a cardiac source. If clinical suspicion remains high, transoesophageal echocardiography should be performed.

Global issues   More on stroke?

- Stroke is the third most common cause of death world-wide after heart disease and all cancers combined.

- Stroke is one of the leading causes of adult disability.

- Takayasu's arteritis in young females is an uncommon but important cause of stroke, especially in Asia.

See Chapter 26 of
Davidson's
Principles and
Practice of
Medicine
(20th edn)

- Vasculitis secondary to tuberculosis meningitis is an important cause of stroke in those countries where tuberculosis and human immunodeficiency virus (HIV) are common.

- Moyamoya syndrome is a rare cause of stroke characterised by occlusion of one or both internal carotid arteries with accompanying new vessel formation. (Moyamoya is Japanese for 'puff of smoke'; the new vessels are said to resemble this on cerebral angiography.) It has a number of causes, including clotting and endothelial abnormalities. It can cause ischaemic and haemorrhagic strokes. It was originally noted in Japan and is more common in the Asian population, but it can be seen in any population group.

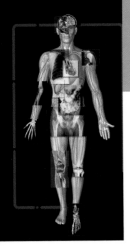

A young girl with a changing mole

J. A. A. HUNTER

Presenting problem

A 16-year-old white girl is referred urgently by her general practitioner to the dermatology clinic. She says that a black mole on her right calf appeared 3 months ago. It is enlarging, becoming more prominent and began to itch about 2 weeks ago. It bled, just once and a tiny amount, a week ago. On closer questioning she thinks that there might have been a small flat brown mark near the same spot previously, but is not certain. Her general health is good and she does not take any regular medication. Although dark-haired, she has a fair skin and says that she usually burns with even short sun exposure and tans poorly (skin type II). Nevertheless, she does sunbathe and holidays in the sun every year. She has never used a sunbed. Nobody in her family has ever had a skin tumour.

What would your differential diagnosis include before examining the patient?

Her GP is obviously concerned or she would not have been referred urgently to the clinic. The sudden appearance of a black lesion on a white female's leg, together with itch and bleeding, is indeed a major CHANGE and should sound a loud alarm bell. First and foremost, malignant melanoma must be excluded; this diagnosis would fit in with her history of sunbathing. However, if she is lucky, this might be due to a benign pigmented lesion such as a melanocytic naevus; but why has it enlarged so much recently? A Spitz naevus (previously called juvenile melanoma) is another benign lesion; although it usually presents as a pink or red nodule, it is a possibility in this case. Dermatofibromas are common at this site and occur in this age group, but they are usually skin-coloured or just lightly pigmented. Seborrhoeic warts are most common on the trunk in older age groups, but are occasionally seen on the leg in the young. Pigmented basal cell carcinomas are almost never seen at this site in this age group. Acquired haemangiomas, including the misnamed pyogenic granuloma, are sometimes very dark and, if thrombosed, black; they should be borne in mind. A rare pigmented adnexal (from a sweat gland or hair follicle) tumour would also be at the end of the differential diagnosis list of most smart dermatologists.

Examination

The girl looks anxious but otherwise well. There is a dark brown-black nodule, measuring 1cm in diameter, on the right calf (Fig. 87.1). On the surface of the nodule there is a tiny area of crusting. There are no hairs. The

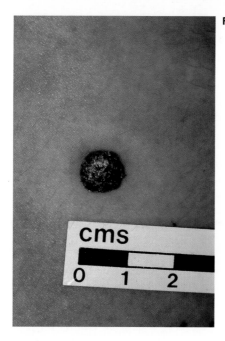

Fig. 87.1 A nodule on the right calf

nodule is symmetrical, the border sharply demarcated, the colour uniform and the elevation regular. There is a narrow (1–2 mm) rim of erythema around most of the nodule. She has a sprinkling (about 20–30 in all) of unexceptional-looking melanocytic naevi on her trunk and legs. There is no significant local or distal lymphadenopathy. The liver is not palpable.

Investigations

Examination of the lesion with a hand-held dermatoscope indicates that it is of melanocytic origin and that there are many microscopic features suggestive of malignant melanoma; the appearance rules out a heavily pigmented seborrhoeic wart and a haemangioma.

Dermatoscopy is a relatively recent diagnostic aid, additional to clinical examination. Helpful in expert hands, it in no way replaces careful observation with the help of a hand lens.

Has examination narrowed down your differential diagnosis?

It seems all but certain that this is a malignant melanoma. Multiple benign melanocytic naevi (as this girl has) are a risk factor, as well as her skin type. The examination, confirmed by the dermatoscopic appearance, has ruled out most of the alternatives mentioned above, with the exception of a Spitz naevus. But, as already mentioned, these naevi are usually pink or red and seldom heavily pigmented.

The useful ABCDE (**A**symmetry, irregular **B**order, irregular **C**olour, **D**iameter greater than 5 mm, irregular **E**levation) rule, relating to examination of the tumour, was not helpful here — a reminder that no rules are sacrosanct and that common sense must always prevail. In this case, the warning light was the history of sudden and undoubted change in a pigmented skin lesion.

Histological confirmation is required and the lesion should be excised straight away, under local anaesthetic, with a 5 mm margin of normal skin around (including deep to) the tumour.

Further investigations

The pathology report concludes, 'This is a nodular malignant melanoma, with incipient ulceration. Tumour thickness (Breslow): 2.5 mm.' A standard chest X-ray is reported as normal.

Does this narrow down your differential diagnosis?

Yes; the diagnosis of an intermediate-thickness, nodular malignant melanoma is confirmed.

How will you treat this patient?

Wider excision of the area is indicated. For tumours of this thickness the margin of excision around the excision biopsy site should be 2 cm. Radical surgery (4–6 cm excision margins) provides no greater benefit, in terms of local recurrence or survival, than more conservative (1–2 cm) excision.

Some surgeons in specialist centres will examine a sentinel node (the first and often nearest local node in the lymphatic drainage of the tumour) at the time of wider excision, if the tumour already removed was thicker than 1.5 mm. If metastatic tumour is found in the sentinel node, then block dissection of the regional nodes (the ilio-femoral group in this case) should be performed.

If there are no facilities for sentinel node biopsy and if the local nodes are not clinically enlarged, then no further treatment is required. Prophylactic lymph node dissection is no longer advised in this group but, should clinically enlarged local nodes be noted at follow-up, then the entire lymph node basin should be removed.

The patient should be followed up regularly. Many advise lifetime follow-up but, in busy hospitals, a common regimen for a patient with an invasive melanoma is at 3-month intervals for the first 3 years and then, if all is well, yearly for a total follow-up time of 5 years. At these appointments, advice about avoiding excessive sun exposure and using appropriate sunblocks should be continually reinforced. Assessment should also include a whole-body examination to

---

BOX 87.1

Prognostic indicators in malignant melanoma

Indicator	Significance
Depth of primary tumour (Breslow)	< 0.75 mm, 5-year survival 95%
	0.76–1.5 mm, 5-year survival 85%
	1.51–3.5 mm, 5-year survival 75%
	> 3.5 mm, 5-year survival 50%
Sex	Females do better than males
Age	Prognosis worsens after 50 years of age, especially in males
Site	Prognosis is poorer for tumours on trunk, upper arms, neck and scalp
Ulceration	Signifies a poor prognosis
Sentinel node	Prognosis worsens with tumour-positive sentinel node
Clinical stage	Prognosis worsens with advancing stage

check for second primary melanomas (risk about 2%). Further investigations at follow-up clinics are not routine unless there are specific clinical indications.

This patient has a clinical stage 1 malignant melanoma (primary lesion only with no nodal or distant metastases). The thickness of the tumour, measured microscopically by Breslow's method, gives a very good estimate of the prognosis. This girl has around an 80% chance of being alive and tumour-free in 5 years' time (Box 87.1). At present there is no compelling evidence that any adjunctive chemotherapy will improve her prognosis.

Global issues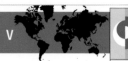

- Episodic exposure of fair-skinned individuals to intense sunlight is thought to be the main cause of the steadily increasing incidence of melanoma world-wide.

- There is a higher incidence of malignant melanoma in white people living near the equator than in temperate zones.

- The highest incidence, more than 40 per 100 000 per year, is seen in white people living in Australia and New Zealand.

- The tumour is rare before puberty and in black people, Asians and Orientals; when it does occur in these races, it is most often on the palms, soles or mucous membranes.

 More on the changing mole?

See Chapter 27 of
Davidson's Principles and Practice of Medicine (20th edn)

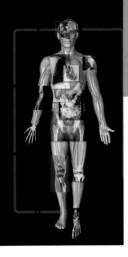

88

A baby with
incessant scratching

J. D. BOS

Presenting problem

A baby boy, aged 4 months, is brought to the clinic with a 3-week history of scratching, intermittent initially, but almost continuous in the last few days. Scratching has been followed by an ever-increasing number of skin lesions all over the body, especially on the face and hands. There is a family history of atopy, with childhood flexural eczema in the mother and some relatives with allergic asthma. The boy is an only child and otherwise healthy. The parents have no itch, eczema or asthma.

What would your differential diagnosis include before examining the patient?

The history fits most obviously with infantile atopic eczema, which often starts on the cheeks and is notorious for being associated with severe itch. Other itchy skin diseases with prominent facial involvement in this age group include atopiform dermatitis (where there is no atopy, as allergen-specific immunoglobulin (Ig) E cannot be detected), seborrhoeic dermatitis and scabies. Erythema infectiosum (fifth disease) and other viral exanthems may affect the face, but are not very itchy.

Examination

A number of papules, vesicles and serous crusts are visible on both cheeks, more or less symmetrically, on a background of ill-bordered erythema (Fig. 88.1). Similar lesions are present (but not as grouped) elsewhere, especially on the trunk, arms, and palmar and plantar skin. There are a few excoriations. No burrows can be seen. There are no hives (urticaria). The child is almost continuously scratching and rubbing his skin.

Has examination narrowed down your differential diagnosis?

Yes; if it were not for the involvement of the palms and soles, the appearance would fit nicely with a diagnosis of infantile atopic (or atopiform) eczema. Acute atopic eczema is characterised by papulation, vesiculation and the appearance of serous crusts. The absence of lichenification (a common sign in chronic cases) fits in with the short history of the lesions. In the infantile type of atopic eczema, the lesions are mainly on the face but can be found in patches elsewhere, not necessarily in skin folds such as elbows and knees. The flexural type of atopic eczema is characteristic for childhood atopic eczema, but palmar and plantar lesions are unusual in both infantile and childhood eczema.

Seborrhoeic eczema of infants is a misnomer. It has nothing to do with seborrhoea, involves the face, axillae and groin and does not appear to be very itchy, as judged by the relative lack of scratching. Again the palms and soles are seldom involved.

Scabies still sounds a real possibility. It would be well worth-while going back to the baby with a magnifying glass and checking more carefully for burrows, especially on the palms, soles and genitals. Burrows — grey-white, slightly scaly, tortuous lines of up to 1 cm in length — are easily missed (Fig. 88.2). They are caused by the scabies mite, which may be seen through a magnifying glass as

Fig. 88.1 An itchy rash on both cheeks.

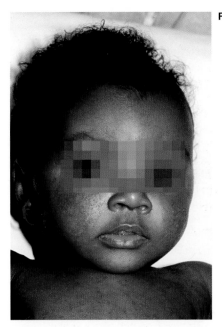

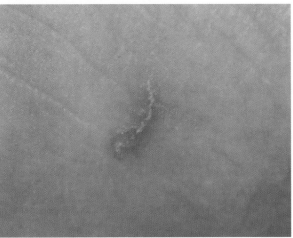

Fig. 88.2 A burrow on the palm of a Caucasian adult

a small dark dot at the most recent, least scaly end of the burrow. With experience it can be removed with a needle for microscopic confirmation.

It is only by inference from the incessant scratching that we deduce that the baby is itchy, for he is much too young to tell us! Be that as it may, we do not have to consider the numerous systemic causes of generalised pruritus in an adult when considering this baby.

Further investigations
It would be unfair and unnecessary to carry out skin-prick or blood tests to detect allergen-specific IgE in so young a child. However, a further direct examination of scales taken from a palmar lesion duly reveals the mite, *Sarcoptes scabiei*.

How will you treat this patient?
Treatment of scabies depends on the local availability of antiparasitic preparations. Contacts and other household members of the patient should be identified and treated. In this case, the parents do not seem to be infected but they should be treated as well. Further history-taking reveals that the contact from whom the baby has acquired the disease is a nanny. She is invited to the clinic and identified as having scabies.

All personal clothing and bed linen should be washed or air-dried for at least 4 hours. The safest preparation with which to treat a baby of this age is 6% precipitated sulphur in petrolatum applied to the whole body each night for 3 days. If this fails, 5% permethrin cream should be tried. Permethrin is the first choice when treating adults; the cream should be applied to the whole body and washed off 8 hours later. The application should be repeated in 1 week. Economic considerations may favour the traditional 25% benzyl benzoate emulsion for the treatment of adults in low-resource settings. In a few countries, oral ivermectin is being used more and more for the treatment of adult scabies. A single oral intake of 200 μg/kg is generally sufficient. As ivermectin comes in tablets of 3 mg, 1 tablet is given for each 15 kg of body weight.

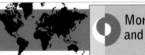

Global issues

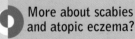

More about scabies and atopic eczema?

- Scabies is mainly a childhood dermatosis in the tropics and subtropics and mainly a sexually transmitted disease in countries with a cold climate.

- Treatment differs, depending on availability of antiparasitic drugs. Permethrin cream is the most commonly used treatment in developed countries; topical benzyl benzoate is a classic; systemic ivermectin may become one.

See Chapter 27 of
Davidson's Principles and Practice of Medicine (20th edn)

- Norwegian scabies occurs in hosts with compromised immune system and may be more relevant in regions with increased prevalence of HIV. The skin manifestations include thick hyperkeratotic crusts. Pruritus may not be severe.

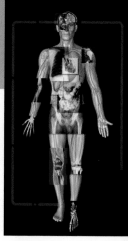

89

A young woman with a widespread scaly rash

J. D. BOS

Presenting problem

A 28-year-old woman presents with a 2-week history of a widespread rash. It erupted over a few days, starting on the face and then spreading to most of the body. She complains of a deep and severe burning sensation that prevents her from sleeping. Itch is a less troubling feature. During the night, she walks around her apartment, taking cold showers and trying ointments and creams, including lotions containing menthol, without effect. She is otherwise healthy but has been treated for moderate acne with topical and systemic agents, including topical benzoyl peroxide, occasional use of topical erythromycin lotion and systemic antibiotics. There is no history of atopy. She is a hairdresser and beautician, and has never had hand eczema. Her skin is not easily irritated and she denies any allergies to cosmetics. She knows that she is allergic to nickel and avoids wearing jewellery that contains nickel.

What would your differential diagnosis include before examining the patient?

We have a patient with an eruptive and widespread red, scaly rash. Box 89.1 lists the most common causes of this presentation. Examination should help to narrow down the differential diagnosis.

Examination

On full examination of the skin, a widespread, symmetrical and somewhat violet, erythematous rash is apparent (Fig. 89.1). The eruption involves the face, trunk and extremities. There is an obvious photosensitive distribution of the rash with relative sparing of the skin unexposed to sun. The rash comprises confluent plaques which are oedematous and indurated in places. There are scattered papules between the plaques and a few tiny vesicles, some of which are haemorrhagic. There is a little scaling and no excoriations. The buccal mucosa and the nails appear normal.

BOX 89.1

Sudden widespread red, scaly rashes

- Eczema
- Psoriasis
- Pityriasis rosea
- Lichen planus
- Drug eruption
- Fungal infection

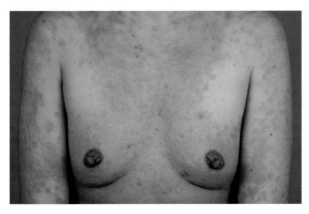

Fig. 89.1 A widespread
erythematous rash.

Has examination narrowed down your differential diagnosis?

Yes; we can now exclude most of the conditions in Box 89.1, but we have also to explain the photosensitive distribution. Psoriasis and eczema seem non-starters. Other than her known nickel sensitivity, the patient has no history of either condition in the past. The appearance of the rash, with minimal scaling, absent scalp involvement and nail changes, rules out psoriasis. Burning rather than itch, together with a paucity of vesicles and absence of weeping or crusting, does not point to a diagnosis of eczema.

There is a violet hue to the rash and acute lichen planus should be considered. This seems unlikely, however, because there is no involvement of the buccal mucosa and the classic flat shiny papules (showing Wickham's striae and the Köbner effect) are not seen. It is not pityriasis rosea. There was no 'herald plaque' preceding the generalised eruption and the typical small, oval, pink plaques with collarette scaling are not evident. The rash is too symmetrical for a fungal infection and there are no signs of peripheral scaling, vesicles or pustules at an advancing edge of the large plaques. A drug eruption is the only other common cause left in Box 89.1 and this must be a distinct possibility.

The photosensitive distribution would fit in with a reaction to a photosensitising drug, though there are some dermatoses that are initiated or exacerbated by exposure to ultraviolet radiation. These include lupus erythematosus and even photosensitive variants of psoriasis and atopic eczema. The patient is too well generally to have systemic lupus erythematosus (SLE) and there are no other systemic features of this condition, such as joint, kidney or haematological disorders. But some further investigations would exclude the possibility of this and of subacute cutaneous lupus erythematosus. The rash is not scaly enough, and is too widespread and too acute for chronic discoid erythematosus.

A phototoxic drug eruption now seems to be the most obvious diagnosis. Further enquiry about the precise use of systemic antibiotics reveals that the patient had taken oral minocycline for her acne for 2 weeks preceding the onset of skin problems.

Investigations

Urine examination reveals no proteinuria. A full blood count and erythrocyte sedimentation rate (ESR) are normal. The antinuclear antibody (ANA) test is negative and no antibodies to Ro (SSA) and La (SSB) antigens are detected.

Has the diagnosis been clinched?

All forms of lupus erythematosus are excluded and a confident diagnosis of minocycline-induced phototoxic rash can be made.

Photosensitivity-induced drug eruptions come in two forms. Certain compounds, when given systemically, may induce subsequent photoallergic reactions. Others are known to be phototoxic, without immunological mechanisms (Box 89.2).

How will you treat this patient?

Oral minocycline should be stopped immediately and prohibited for the rest of her life. The rash may be treated symptomatically with topical glucocorticoids of moderate strength, applied once daily in the evening. Avoidance of sun exposure is advised and a broad (ultra-violet (UV) A and UVB) sunscreen also prescribed. Acne therapy could be adjusted by advising the use of an androgen-inhibiting oral contraceptive (e.g. Dianette) in combination with a topical vitamin A derivative, applied once daily in the morning.

BOX 89.2

Systemic drugs inducing photosensitivity

Phototoxic

- Amiodarone
- Retinoids
- Non-steroidal anti-inflammatory drugs (NSAIDs)
- Diuretics (chlorothiazides)
- Phenothiazines

Photoallergic

- Thiazides
- Enalapril
- NSAIDs
- Hydroxychloroquine
- Phenothiazines

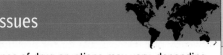 Global issues

 More on sudden widespread scaly rashes and drug eruptions?

- The incidence of drug eruptions may vary, depending on regional patterns of drug use.
- Photosensitive drug reactions are more common in the tropics and subtropics than in temperate climates.

See Chapter 27 of

Davidson's Principles and Practice of Medicine
(20th edn)

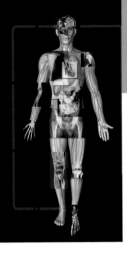

90

Palpable purpura in an elderly woman with psoriasis

O. M. SCHOFIELD

Presenting problem

A 65-year-old lady who has a long history of psoriasis and psoriatic arthritis presents with a 4-day history of a rash on her lower limbs, lethargy and fever. The rash is quite different to her psoriasis. Rather than being red and scaly, it is purplish and in some areas almost black. She says that these lesions started off as small papules, some of which blistered. The affected area has extended and now there are large purplish lesions which are beginning to 'break down'. Besides psoriasis, this lady has a history of hypertension and type 2 diabetes mellitus. She has had bilateral knee replacements in the past. Her current medication includes diclofenac, aspirin, omeprazole, metformin, lisinopril, amlodipine and tramadol. She is being treated with weekly oral methotrexate for her psoriasis and she has been treated with myocrisin and etanercept unsuccessfully for her psoriatic arthritis in the past.

BOX 90.1
Causes of vasculitis
• Drugs
• Infection
• Connective tissue disease
• Malignancy
• Idiopathic (Henoch–Schönlein purpura)

What would your differential diagnosis include before examining the patient?

The differential diagnosis of a purple-coloured skin eruption would include purpura and vasculitis. Purpura does not blanch on pressure and can be traumatic in origin, related to a low platelet count or abnormal clotting, or secondary to a Gram-negative coccal septicaemia. Clinically, vasculitis is characterised by palpable purpura and can be due to a wide variety of causes: in particular, a drug eruption, infections, connective tissue disease or an underlying malignancy (Box 90.1).

Examination

The lady is pale, apyrexial and in some pain from her rash. She has significant signs of chronic arthritis with ulnar deviation of her fingers and reduced grip strength. She has reduced range of movement of several large joints but no evidence of active synovitis of any joints. General examination shows no features to cause concern: in particular, no breast lumps or lymphadenopathy. She has evidence of ongoing chronic plaque psoriasis on her back, extensor surfaces and scalp. She has nail changes of pitting and onycholysis consistent with this condition. On her legs she has an eruption that consists of individual scattered lesions which are palpable and purpuric, ranging from a few millimetres to 5 cm in size.

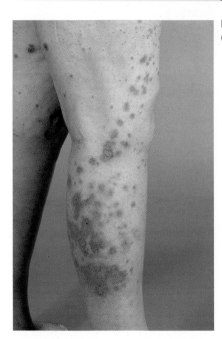

Fig. 90.1 The rash of cutaneous vasculitis (palpable purpura).

Some of the lesions have vesicles within them and larger areas are beginning to show necrosis of the superficial portion of skin (the epidermis) (Fig. 90.1).

Has examination narrowed down your differential diagnosis?

This lady has a florid vasculitis evident in the skin of her legs. Her medication has not changed recently and so it is unlikely that a drug is causative. Further investigations are needed to determine the cause of the patient's vasculitis.

Further investigations

Initially and most importantly, urinalysis is performed to look for haematuria, which might indicate renal involvement. A full 'vasculitis screen' is performed, including a full blood count, erythrocyte sedimentation rate (ESR) and C-reactive protein (CRP), urea and electrolytes, liver function tests, serum immunoglobulins, antinuclear factor and anti-double-stranded DNA antibody, rheumatoid factor, antineutrophil cytoplasmic antibodies (ANCA), viral and hepatitis serology, cryoglobulins, a throat swab and chest X-ray. The results of her investigations are shown in Box 90.2. A skin biopsy is taken from one of the lesions on her leg and confirms the diagnosis of a small-vessel vasculitis with leucocytoclasis. A section of the biopsy is sent for immunofluorescence examination and shows deposition of immunoglobulin (Ig) A, IgM and C3 within small vessels.

Does this narrow down your differential diagnosis?

The histology confirms the diagnosis of vasculitis. This is a leucocytoclastic vasculitis with the presence of large numbers of neutrophils. Taken together with the direct immunofluorescence results and elevated serum IgA, this is typical of the idiopathic form of vasculitis, Henoch–Schönlein purpura. This condition can be seen at all ages and has no clear precipitating cause. It can occur as one attack or become more chronic with repeated attacks. As with all causes of vasculitis, it can affect several organs.

BOX 90.2

Further investigations

Urinalysis	Negative for blood and protein
Haemoglobin	102 g/l (10.2 g/dl)
ESR	99 mm/hr
CRP	154 mg/l
ANF	1:40
Anti-dsDNA	Negative
ANCA	Negative
RF	Negative
Cryoglobulins	Negative
Serum immunoglobulins	IgG normal, IgM normal, IgA elevated
Hepatitis serology	Negative
Viral serology	Negative
Chest X-ray	Mild cardiomegaly, lung fields clear

How will you treat this patient?

In view of the severity of this lady's rash and the localised areas of ulceration, she is treated with oral prednisolone starting at a dose of 40 mg daily. The effect of prednisolone on her diabetes makes it likely that she will need insulin temporarily. Topically, she has a very potent topical corticosteroid (clobetasol propionate 0.05%) applied 12-hourly to the lesions on her legs and a topical antibacterial cream (silver sulfadiazine 1% cream) under a Jelonet dressing applied to any ulcerated areas. For her psoriasis she just has simple emollients applied. As the rash improves, her treatment with oral steroids is slowly reduced. In the case of severe recurrent attacks, treatment with an alternative form of immunosuppressant, such as azathioprine, should be considered. The systemic steroids are phased out over several months to avoid a significant flare-up of her psoriasis.

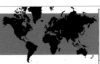

Global issues

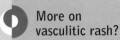

More on vasculitic rash?

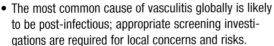

- The most common cause of vasculitis globally is likely to be post-infectious; appropriate screening investigations are required for local concerns and risks.

- Malignancy, when suspected, should be investigated by appropriate directed tests.

- Renal involvement is the most serious complication of vasculitis; involvement of the kidneys should be carefully monitored and investigated early if suspected.

- Although leucocytoclastic vasculitis is more common in a younger age group, there is a significant incidence in older people. In the elderly there is a significant risk of gastrointestinal involvement in Henoch–Schönlein purpura.

See Chapter 27 of
Davidson's Principles and Practice of Medicine
(20th edn)

91

A non-healing leg ulcer in an elderly man

M. J. TIDMAN

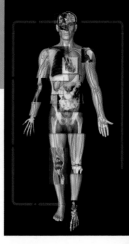

Presenting problem

A 73-year-old man presents with an uncomfortable enlarging ulcer over his left calf of 6 weeks duration. He is known to have type 2 diabetes mellitus, controlled with dietary measures, and after complaining to his general practitioner of being tired, he has recently been found to have anaemia (Box 91.1).

What would your differential diagnosis include before examining the patient?

The most common cause of leg ulceration in the UK is venous hypertension, but varicose/venous ulcers typically occur over the malleolar regions. An arterial (ischaemic) ulcer is a possibility, for which this man's diabetes would be a risk factor, as it is for neuropathic ulcers. However, these are usually painless and situated over pressure points. Necrobiosis lipoidica, a cutaneous manifestation of diabetes that usually involves the shins, may ulcerate. Cutaneous malignancy, particularly basal cell and squamous cell carcinomas, should always be considered in chronic leg ulceration, especially if there is background actinic damage. Remember that, very occasionally, chronic venous ulcers may undergo malignant change to a squamous cell carcinoma ('Marjolin ulcer').

Leg ulcers may be the result of an underlying vasculitis, either confined to the skin or as part of a systemic condition such as rheumatoid arthritis. Hypertension is said to predispose to painful leg ulceration (Martorell's ulcer), typically situated more proximally than a venous ulcer. Infections of bacterial (including mycobacterial), fungal, parasitic or treponemal aetiology have also to be considered, especially in tropical regions. Pyoderma gangrenosum, a necrotising inflammatory disorder, may also be confined to the legs. Haemoglobinopathies, such as

BOX 91.1	
Initial investigations	
Haemoglobin	96 g/l (9.6 g/dl)
MCV	101 fl
WCC	3.7×10^9/l (10^3/mm^3)
Platelets	86×10^9/l (10^3/mm^3)

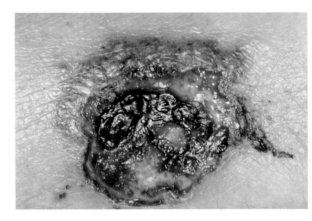

Fig. 91.1 Typical clinical presentation of pyoderma gangrenosum, showing an ulcer with an undermined inflamed margin.

sickle-cell disease and spherocytosis, and genetic predisposition, such as prolidase deficiency, would probably have been diagnosed earlier in life, and thrombophilic disorders, such as antiphospholipid syndrome and platelet aggregability, may need to be excluded. Certain drugs, such as hydroxyurea and methotrexate, may cause leg ulcers. Finally, leg ulcers may be self-inflicted (dermatitis artefacta), but this is usually a diagnosis made by excluding other causes.

Examination

The ulcer measures several centimetres in diameter. The margin is duskily erythematous and somewhat undermined, and the base is covered with a purulent slough (Fig. 91.1). The absence of bolstering of the ulcer edge is reassuring that this is not a malignant ulcer, and there are no signs of venous hypertension (such as pinpoint purpura, pigmentation, atrophie blanche and venular dilatation) or arterial insufficiency (pallor, mottled skin, poor capillary filling and dystrophic nails). The patient's pedal pulses are easily palpable and there are no objective signs of peripheral sensory loss. The absence of palpable purpura elsewhere on his legs militates against a vasculitic aetiology.

Has examination narrowed down your differential diagnosis?

The appearance of the margin suggests that this ulcer is pyoderma gangrenosum. This condition is diagnosed principally on its clinical features; the histology is not specific, although characterised by a neutrophil-abundant inflammatory process. Although the clinical signs may be typical of pyoderma gangrenosum, a biopsy from the ulcer edge is always advisable for definite exclusion of infection, malignancy and vasculitis.

An important aspect of pyoderma gangrenosum is that, in up to 80% of cases, it is associated with an underlying disease, most commonly inflammatory bowel disease, rheumatoid arthritis, plasma cell dyscrasias (monoclonal gammopathy and myeloma) and myeloproliferative disorders (leukaemia and myelofibrosis). When associated with haematological malignancy, pyoderma gangrenosum may present as a haemorrhagic blister.

Further investigations

Histological examination of a skin biopsy from the lesion shows the features of an abscess with haemorrhage, tissue necrosis and vascular thrombosis. Bacterial and fungal culture of a sample of skin reveals no organisms.

The full blood count, as well as showing mild anaemia, also demonstrates low white cell and platelet counts, i.e. a pancytopenia. Vitamin B_{12} and folate levels are within the normal range and a subsequent bone marrow examination shows features consistent with myelofibrosis.

Does this narrow down your differential diagnosis?

The association of a chronic ulcer, characterised by a bluish, undermined margin and a neutrophil-rich histology, and a myeloproliferative disorder makes the diagnosis of pyoderma gangrenosum very likely. A note of caution, however, is that the absence of an objective diagnostic test means that pyoderma gangrenosum is, perhaps, too freely diagnosed. This clinical scenario is an example of how changes in the skin can, quite frequently, act as a window for the diagnosis of internal disorders.

How will you treat this patient?

The management of pyoderma gangrenosum depends on the extent and degree of inflammation. If there is an underlying medical problem, this will require appropriate treatment. In this particular case of a single lesion, the combination of the daily application of a topical antiseptic, such as potassium permanganate (1:10 000 dilution), with the 12-hourly application of a very potent topical corticosteroid, such as clobetasol propionate, under polythene occlusion is a reasonable initial therapeutic option. However, if this is not quickly effective in settling the inflammation, a tapering course of prednisolone, commencing with a dose of 1–3 mg/kg body weight daily, is indicated. Other systemic therapeutic options include minocycline and ciclosporin. Surgical excision is contraindicated, as this may precipitate aggressive recurrence because of the phenomenon of pathergy (hyper-reactivity of the skin) that characterises pyoderma gangrenosum.

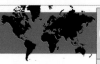

Global issues

More on leg ulcers?

- Yaws, leishmaniasis, leprosy, syphilis, tuberculosis and atypical mycobacterial infections can all cause indolent leg ulcers; although rare in Western Europe, they should be considered in other ethnicities.

- A Buruli ulcer is caused by *Mycobacterium ulcerans* and occurs in rural African areas. It is the third most common mycobacterial infection world-wide after tuberculosis and leprosy. Surgery is the treatment of choice.

- Cutaneous amoebiasis, blastomycosis, cryptococcosis and tropical ulcer may mimic pyoderma gangrenosum.

See Chapter 27 of
Davidson's Principles and Practice of Medicine (20th edn)

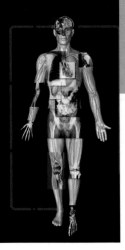

92

A man with a blistering disorder

J. A. A. HUNTER

Presenting problem

A 70-year-old white man presents at a skin clinic with numerous, discrete, large, tense blisters on his trunk. These developed over 10 days, appearing within red and irritable patches. The patient does not feel ill. His general health has been good in the past and he is not taking any form of medication.

What would your differential diagnosis include before examining the patient?

Not many conditions need to be considered with such a concise history. The inherited forms of epidermolysis bullosa would have presented early in life. Lack of pain, the large size of the blisters and lack of systemic symptoms rule out widespread herpes simplex and herpes zoster (also excluded, as unilateral blisters are not described). Dermatitis herpetiformis would have declared itself earlier in life; characteristically its lesions are itchy and vesicular (a few millimetres in diameter) rather than bullous and appear mostly on the elbows, shoulders and buttocks. Toxic epidermal necrolysis is a non-starter; although this may appear initially as widespread blistering, the blisters soon coalesce and the blister roofs peel off, leaving large, painful, moist denuded areas like a scald. It cannot be a bullous drug eruption because the patient is not taking any drugs. Bullous pemphigoid must be at the top of the list of possibilities, but pemphigus, bullous erythema multiforme, acquired epidermolysis bullosa, cicatricial pemphigoid and even bullous impetigo need to be excluded. Examination should help here.

Examination

The patient is apyrexial and remarkably unperturbed by the extensive blisters. The eruption is bullous (blisters over 0.5 cm in diameter) rather than vesicular (blisters less 0.5 cm in diameter) and predominantly involves the trunk (especially flexures) and limbs (Fig. 92.1). The bullae are tense and filled with clear fluid; many have an erythematous rim and there are discrete urticarial-like plaques with small blisters developing within them. There are scattered erosions at the site of some previous blisters. Shearing stress on normal-looking skin between the blisters does not cause an erosion (negative Nikolsky sign). There are no blisters in the mouth. Physical examination is otherwise unremarkable.

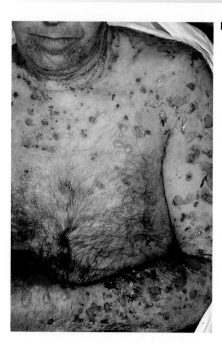

Fig 92.1 Bullous pemphigoid.

Has examination narrowed down your differential diagnosis?

The appearance of many skin diseases is diagnostic, providing the whole skin is examined carefully and under optimal conditions. The history and clinical findings here are so typical of bullous pemphigoid that subsequent investigations will only be necessary for confirmation. Patients with pemphigus vulgaris invariably feel ill, the mouth is usually involved, the blisters are flaccid, numerous erosions are seen and the Nikolsky sign may be positive. There are no purple target-like lesions with an acral distribution to give rise to suspicion of bullous erythema multiforme, and in this condition the mucous membranes of the mouth, conjunctivae and genitalia are frequently involved. The blisters of porphyria cutanea tarda are induced by minor trauma, occur only on exposed skin and leave milia in their wake. Acquired epidermolysis bullosa can be excluded because there is no history of blisters developing as a result of trauma, and there are no milia at the site of previous blisters. In this condition the blisters appear on normal skin rather than within urticarial-like plaques. Cicatricial pemphigoid differs from pemphigoid in that its blisters occur mainly on mucous membranes such as the conjunctivae, mouth and genital tract. As the name suggests, these lesions heal with scarring. Bullous impetigo is more common in children but may be seen in the elderly, especially those immunosuppressed. The bullae are flaccid, often contain pus and are frequently grouped or located in body folds.

Has the diagnosis been clinched?

The clinical picture is all but diagnostic, but histology of a small fresh blister with immunofluorescence will confirm it.

Further investigations

Histology reveals a subepidermal blister filled with eosinophils. Direct immunofluorescence shows a linear band of immunoglobulin (Ig) G and C3 along the basement membrane zone.

Circulating IgG antibodies, reacting with the basement membrane zone of skin, are found in 70% of patients. The test is simple and (stored) serum from the patient, acquired before starting treatment, may easily be sent to a laboratory offering this service. Tzanck smears remain popular in some countries. A blister roof is removed and cells taken from the base of the blister with a surgical blade. These cells are smeared on to a glass slide, fixed with methanol and then stained with Giemsa, toluidine blue or Wright's stain. Distinctive cells are seen in pemphigus (acantholytic cells) and herpes simplex/zoster infections (multinucleate giant cells). A fresh blister swab would reveal no bacterial growth in bullous pemphigoid (compare *Staphylococcus aureus* in bullous impetigo).

How will you treat this patient?

Systemic corticosteroids (provided there are no contraindications) should be given straight away, without waiting for the results of confirmatory diagnostic tests. In the acute phase prednisolone at a dosage of 40–60 mg/day should control the eruption, but immunosuppressive agents (e.g. azathioprine) may also be required. The patient should be followed up regularly, with urine and blood screening standard for a patient taking a prolonged course of corticosteroids. The dosage is reduced as soon as fresh blisters stop appearing and, within a month or two, the patient should end up on a low-maintenance regimen (e.g. prednisolone 5–10 mg on alternate days) of systemic corticosteroids, until stopped. Bullous pemphigoid is usually self-limiting and treatment can often be stopped after 1–2 years.

Global issues

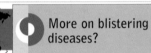

More on blistering diseases?

- Bullous pemphigoid is relatively common in the West but uncommon in the East. Pemphigus vulgaris is more common than bullous pemphigoid in India and Pakistan.

- Dermatitis herpetiformis appears to be less common in Asia and the USA, compared with Europe.

- In a case as typical as this, it could be argued that further investigations in a developing country would be an expensive luxury that would simply confirm a very sound clinical diagnosis. However, in developed countries confirmation would be required with a biopsy of a small recent blister and immunofluorescent investigation.

See Chapter 27 of **Davidson's Principles and Practice of Medicine** (20th edn)

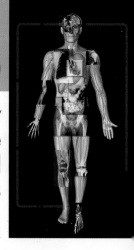

93

A young boy with multiple hypopigmented lesions

B. KUMAR

Presenting problem

A 14-year-old Indian boy presents with multiple hypopigmented lesions over the trunk and extremities. Three years ago, he noticed a hypopigmented dry patch over his right forearm. Since then he has noted an increase in the size of this lesion and has developed similar patches over his trunk and limbs. He has not bothered to seek medical attention because the lesions were almost asymptomatic. Over the last 6 months he has developed numbness and weakness of the right hand, which are now interfering with his daily activities. The use of some indigenous local medication has produced no improvement. There has been no significant medical or dermatological illness in the past and he has no systemic complaints.

What would your differential diagnosis include before examining the patient?

Hypopigmented lesions are a common finding in practice. There are several conditions which can produce them. A careful history regarding the evolution of the lesions and a thorough systematic examination greatly help to limit the differential diagnoses. In this boy the absence of systemic features, at present or in the past, makes malignant, metabolic and endocrine causes of hypopigmentation most unlikely. Most stable lesions are likely to be congenital and progressive lesions are usually inflammatory or immunological.

Causes of hypopigmented patches include pityriasis alba, pityriasis versicolor, post-inflammatory hypopigmentation and leprosy (Box 93.1). Pityriasis alba is especially common in children. A few hypopigmented, minimally scaly patches with ill-defined margins usually appear on the face, but may also involve the trunk and limbs. They take weeks to months to subside. Pityriasis versicolor is a common superficial fungal infection of the skin caused by *Malassezia furfur*. These lesions are

> **BOX 93.1**
>
> **Causes of hypopigmented lesions**
>
> **Common**
> - Pityriasis alba
> - Pityriasis versicolor
> - Post-inflammatory hypopigmentation
> - Vitiligo
> - Leprosy
>
> **Rare**
> - Sarcoidosis
> - Idiopathic guttate hypomelanosis
> - Progressive macular hypopigmentation
> - Tuberous sclerosis
> - Naevus anaemicus
> - Naevus depigmentosus
> - Hypomelanosis of Ito
> - Mycosis fungoides
> - Hypopigmented malignant melanoma

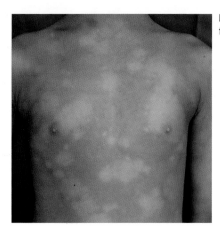

Fig. 93.1 Multiple hypopigmented patches over the trunk.

seen in young adults with dark skin as multiple small hypopigmented macules with powdery scales, and are generally distributed over the chest and upper back. In those with white skin, the initial lesions appear as fawn areas standing out against the light background. The lesions are often asymptomatic but may occasionally be itchy. Patches of hypopigmentation with raised margins, covering large parts of the body, may be seen on patients in the tropics. Post-inflammatory hypopigmentation is another common cause of such a presentation. It may follow a variety of inflammatory dermatoses, including psoriasis, pityriasis rosea, adverse cutaneous drug reactions, trauma and contact dermatitis. Vitiligo, also known as leucoderma, is characterised by milky white or depigmented lesions, sometimes with a hyperpigmented border. However, evolving lesions may sometimes be hypopigmented. The sharply defined lesions of the generalised type are especially common on the backs of the hands, the wrists, the fronts of knees and the neck, and around body orifices.

Leprosy is undoubtedly the most important cause of hypopigmented lesions and often, for months or even years, these are the only manifestation of the disease before a neurological deficit develops. For those practising in a non-endemic country who are not familiar with this disease, the diagnosis may be missed and subsequent neurological symptoms may be attributed to some other disease. An insidious onset and slow progression of these often asymptomatic or anaesthetic hypopigmented lesions in a patient living in an endemic country, or in an immigrant from such a part of the world, should raise a high index of suspicion. Further clinical examination of the lesions and peripheral nerves will help to confirm the diagnosis.

Some rarer causes of hypopigmented skin lesions are also listed in Box 93.1.

Examination

The patient is apparently healthy and remarkably unperturbed by the skin lesions, more than 30, distributed over his body. The hypopigmented and slightly indurated lesions are of varying sizes, measuring up to 10 cm (Fig. 93.1). The lesions have sparse hair and, within them, there is partial loss of sensation, including temperature. The boy's right ulnar nerve (above the elbow) is thickened and non-tender, with associated sensory impairment and weakness of small muscles of the hand on the ulnar side (ulnar claw hand). His greater auricular nerves, radial cutaneous nerves and left lateral popliteal nerve are also thickened.

Has examination narrowed down your differential diagnosis?

Often in dermatology, there is not always an easy spot diagnosis (as the morphology of many dermatoses is so similar), and astute observation, with correlation of the findings, helps the physician to arrive at the final diagnosis. But the combination of typical skin and neurological signs in this case positively proclaim a diagnosis of leprosy! The diagnosis and classification of leprosy are based on the clinical features and skin smears when facilities are available. The clinical diagnosis of leprosy is based on patients having one or more of the three cardinal signs (Box 93.2).

> **BOX 93.2**
>
> **Cardinal signs of leprosy**
>
> - Hypopigmented or erythematous skin lesion(s) with definite loss or impairment of sensation
> - Involvement of the peripheral nerves, as demonstrated by definite thickening with sensory impairment
> - Slit skin smear positive for acid-fast bacilli

Further investigations

A slit skin smear (SSS) is performed and is positive for acid-fast bacilli with a bacteriological index (BI) of 2+ and a morphological index (MI) of 1%. A skin biopsy reveals perivascular, peri-appendageal and perineural lymphocytic infiltrates, granulomas in the dermis and foam cells filled with lepra bacilli. These findings are consistent with a diagnosis of borderline lepromatous (BL) leprosy.

How will you treat this patient?

The treatment of leprosy is based on the type of disease. Patients with paucibacillary leprosy ($\leq$ 5 skin lesions or negative SSS) are treated with the World Health Organization (WHO) recommended multidrug therapy (MDT) paucibacillary (PB) regimen. Patients with multibacillary (MB) leprosy (> 5 skin lesions or positive SSS) are treated with the WHO MDT multibacillary (MB) regimen. This young man has multibacillary disease and should be treated with the WHO-MDT-MB regimen (Box 93.3). A course of systemic corticosteroids (prednisolone) for 4–6 months will be required for the recent neurological deficit involving the right hand. Physiotherapy, counselling for compliance with the treatment, advice for care of hands and feet, and examination of close household contacts are important components of total treatment.

> **BOX 93.3**
>
> **MDT-MB regimen for multibacillary leprosy (12 months) in a child of 10–14 years**
>
> **Dapsone**
> - 50 mg given daily
>
> **Rifampicin**
> - 450 mg given once a month under supervision
>
> **Clofazimine**
> - 50 mg given daily *and*
> - 150 mg given once a month under supervision

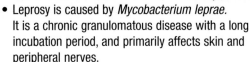

Global issues

- Leprosy is caused by *Mycobacterium leprae.* It is a chronic granulomatous disease with a long incubation period, and primarily affects skin and peripheral nerves.

- Leprosy is the most common cause of peripheral nerve thickening.

 More on leprosy?

See Chapter 13 of
Davidson's Principles and Practice of Medicine
(20th edn)

- Leprosy still remains a huge public health problem in some thickly populated countries of the world. About 70% of the world's leprosy patients live in India, with Brazil, Indonesia, Mozambique, Madagascar, Tanzania and Nepal being the next most endemic countries.

- Slit skin smears are useful for confirming the diagnosis and monitoring response to treatment.

- MDT, recommended by the WHO in 1982, has rapidly become the standard treatment of leprosy. It consists of three drugs: dapsone, rifampicin and clofazimine. PB patients are treated with an MDT-PB (rifampicin + dapsone) regimen for 6 months, and MB patients are treated with an MDT-MB (rifampicin + dapsone + clofazimine) regimen for 12 months.

- In countries where this disease is uncommon, a high index of suspicion is required to diagnose, treat early and prevent the transmission of infection and development of deformities.

- With increased migration, leprosy will occur globally until the disease is eradicated.

Appendix

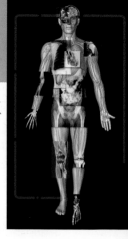

S. W. WALKER

Biochemical and haematological values

A.1		
Urea and electrolytes in venous blood		
	Reference range	
Analyte	**SI units**	**Non-SI units**
Sodium	135–145 mmol/l	135–145 meq/l
Potassium (plasma)	3.3–4.7 mmol/l	3.3–4.7 meq/l
Potassium (serum)	3.6–5.1 mmol/l	3.6–5.1 meq/l
Chloride	95–107 mmol/l	95–107 meq/l
Urea	2.5–6.6 mmol/l	15–40 mg/dl
Creatinine	60–120 µmol/l	0.68–1.36 mg/dl

A.2		
Arterial blood analysis		
	Reference range	
Analyte	**SI units**	**Non-SI units**
Bicarbonate	21–29 mmol/l	21–29 meq/l
Hydrogen ion	37–45 nmol/l	pH 7.35–7.43
$PaCO_2$	4.5–6.0 kPa	34–45 mmHg
PaO_2	12–15 kPa	90–113 mmHg
Oxygen saturation	> 97%	

A.3

Hormones in venous blood

Hormone	Reference range SI units	Non-SI units
Adrenocorticotrophic hormone (ACTH) (plasma)	1.5–11.2 pmol/l (0700–1000 hrs)	7–51 pg/ml
Aldosterone		
Supine	45–440 pmol/l	1.63–15.9 ng/dl
Erect	110–860 pmol/l	3.97–31.0 ng/dl
Cortisol	Dynamic tests are required	
Follicle-stimulating hormone (FSH)		
Male	1.5–9.0 U/l	0.3–2.0 ng/ml
Female	3.0–15 U/l (early follicular, luteal)	0.7–3.3 ng/ml
	< 20 U/l (mid-cycle)	< 4.4 ng/ml
	> 30 U/l (post-menopausal)	> 6.7 ng/ml
Gastrin (plasma, fasting)	< 57 pmol/l	< 120 pg/ml
Growth hormone (GH)	< 2 mU/l excludes acromegaly	Conversion to mass units depends on assay
	> 20 mU/l excludes GH deficiency	
	Dynamic tests are usually required	
Insulin	Highly variable and interpretable only in relation to plasma glucose and body habitus	–
Luteinising hormone (LH)		
Male	1.5–9.0 U/l	0.17–1.0 µg/l
Female	2.5–9.0 U/l (early follicular, luteal)	0.3–1.0 µg/l
	Up to 90 U/l (mid-cycle)	Up to 10 µg/l
	> 20 U/l (post-menopausal)	> 2.2 µg/l
17β-Oestradiol		
Male	< 200 pmol/l	< 54 pg/ml
Female	110–180 pmol/l (early follicular)	30–49 pg/ml
	550–1650 pmol/l (mid-cycle)	150–449 pg/ml
	370–770 pmol/l (luteal)	101–209 pg/ml
	< 150 pmol/l (post-menopausal)	< 41 pg/ml
Parathyroid hormone (PTH)	1.0–6.5 pmol/l	10–65 pg/ml
Progesterone		
Male	< 2.0 nmol/l	< 0.63 ng/ml
Female	< 2.0 nmol/l (follicular)	< 0.63 ng/ml
	> 15 nmol/l (mid-luteal)	> 4.7 ng/ml
	< 2.0 nmol/l (post-menopausal)	< 0.63 ng/ml
Prolactin (PRL)	60–500 mU/l	–
Renin activity		
Erect	0.6–2.8 ng/ml/h	–
Supine	< 1.5 ng/ml/h	–
Testosterone		
Male	10–30 nmol/l	2.88–8.64 ng/ml
Female	0.4–2.8 nmol/l	0.12–0.81 ng/ml

A.3		
Hormones in venous blood		

	Reference range	
Hormone	**SI units**	**Non-SI units**
Thyroid-stimulating hormone (TSH)	0.15–3.5 mU/l	–
Thyroxine (free) (free T_4)	8–27 pmol/l	622–2098 pg/dl
Triiodothyronine (T_3)	1.0–2.6 nmol/l	65–169 ng/dl

Notes

1. A number of hormones are unstable and collection details are critical to obtaining a meaningful result. Refer to local laboratory handbook.
2. Values in the table are only a guideline; hormone levels can often only be meaningfully understood in relation to factors such as sex (e.g. testosterone), age (e.g. FSH in women), time of day (e.g. cortisol) or regulatory factors (e.g. insulin and glucose, PTH and $[Ca^{2+}]$).
3. Reference ranges may be critically method-dependent.

A.4

Other common analytes in venous blood in adults

Analyte	Reference range SI units	Non-SI units
α_1-antitrypsin	1.1–2.1 g/l	110–210 mg/dl
Alanine amino-transferase (ALT)	10–50 U/l	–
Albumin	35–50 g/l	3.5–5.0 g/dl
Alkaline phosphatase	40–125 U/l	–
Amylase	< 100 U/l	–
Aspartate amino-transferase (AST)	10–45 U/l	–
Bilirubin (total)	2–17 μmol/l	0.12–1.0 mg/dl
Calcium (total)	2.12–2.62 mmol/l	4.24–5.24 meq/l or 8.50–10.50 mg/dl
Carboxy-haemoglobin	< 1.5% in non-smokers	–
Caeruloplasmin	150–600 mg/l	15–60 mg/dl
Cholesterol (total)	Ideal level varies according to cardiovascular risk (see cardiovascular risk chart, p. 328) so reference ranges can be misleading. The following values were described by the European Atherosclerosis Society:	
	Mild increase 5.2–6.5 mmol/l	200–250 mg/dl
	Moderate increase 6.5–7.8 mmol/l	250–300 mg/dl
	Severe increase > 7.8 mmol/l	> 300 mg/dl
HDL-cholesterol	Ideal level varies according to cardiovascular risk so reference ranges can be misleading. According to the National Cholesterol Education Programme Adult Treatment Panel III (ATPIII), a low HDL-cholesterol is:	
	< 1.0 mmol/l	< 40 mg/dl
Copper	13–24 μmol/l	85–153 μg/dl
C-reactive protein	< 5 mg/l	
	Highly sensitive CRP assays also exist which measure lower values and may be useful in estimating cardiovascular risk	
Creatine kinase (total)		
Male	55–170 U/l	–
Female	30–135 U/l	–
Creatine kinase MB isoenzyme	< 6% of total CK	–
Ethanol	Not normally detectable	
	Marked intoxication 65–87 mmol/l	300–400 mg/dl
	Stupor 87–109 mmol/l	400–500 mg/dl
	Coma > 109 mmol/l	> 500 mg/dl
Gamma-glutamyl transferase (GGT)		
Male	5–55 U/l	–
Female	5–35 U/l	–
Glucose (fasting)	3.6–5.8 mmol/l	65–104 mg/dl
Glycated haemoglobin (HbA$_{1c}$)	5.0–6.5%	–

A.4

Other common analytes in venous blood in adults

Analyte	Reference range	
	SI units	Non-SI units
Immunoglobulin A	0.8–4.5 g/l	80–450 mg/dl
Immunoglobulin G	6.0–15.0 g/l	600–1500 mg/dl
Immunoglobulin M	0.35–2.90 g/l	35–290 mg/dl
Lactate	0.6–2.4 mmol/l	5.40–21.6 mg/dl
Lactate dehydrogenase (total)	208–460 U/l	–
Lead	< 1.0 µmol/l	< 21 µg/dl
Magnesium	0.75–1.0 mmol/l	1.5–2.0 meq/l or 1.82–2.43 mg/dl
Osmolality	280–290 mmol/kg	–
Osmolarity	280–290 mosm/l	–
Phosphate (fasting)	0.8–1.4 mmol/l	2.48–4.34 mg/dl
Protein (total)	60–80 g/l	6–8 g/dl
Triglycerides (fasting)	0.6–1.7 mmol/l	53–150 mg/dl
Troponins	Values consistent with 'myocyte necrosis' or myocardial infarction are crucially dependent upon which troponin is measured (I or T) and on the method employed	
Urate		
Male	0.12–0.42 mmol/l	2.0–7.0 mg/dl
Female	0.12–0.36 mmol/l	2.0–6.0 mg/dl
Vitamin D		
25(OH)D		
Winter	15–50 nmol/l	6–20 ng/ml
Summer	15–100 nmol/l	6–40 ng/ml
1,25(OH)$_2$D	20–120 pmol/l	7.7–46 pg/ml
Zinc	11–22 µmol/l	72–144 µg/dl

A.5

Haematological values

Analyte	Reference range	
	SI units	**Non-SI units**
Bleeding time (Ivy)	< 8 min	–
Blood volume		
Male	75 ± 10 ml/kg	–
Female	70 ± 10 ml/kg	–
Coagulation screen		
Prothrombin time	12–15 sec	–
Activated partial thromboplastin time	26–37 sec	–
D-dimer		
Routine	< 0.2 mg/l	
Sensitive (for venous thromboembolism)	Variable threshold (dependent on method)	–
Erythrocyte sedimentation rate	Higher values in older patients are not necessarily abnormal	
Adult male	0–10 mm/hr	–
Adult female	3–15 mm/hr	–
Ferritin		
Male	17–300 µg/l	17–300 ng/ml
Pre-menopausal female	7–280 µg/l	7–280 ng/ml
Post-menopausal female	4–233 µg/l	4–233 ng/ml
Fibrinogen	1.5–4.0 g/l	0.15–0.4 g/dl
Folate		
Serum	2.0–13.5 µg/l	2.0–13.5 ng/ml
Red cell	95–570 µg/l	95–570 ng/ml
Haemoglobin		
Male	130–180 g/l	13–18 g/dl
Female	115–165 g/l	11.5–16.5 g/dl
Haptoglobin	0.4–2.4 g/l	0.04–0.24 g/dl
Iron		
Male	14–32 µmol/l	78–178 µg/dl
Female	10–28 µmol/l	56–156 µg/dl
Leucocytes (adults)	$4.0–11.0 \times 10^9/l$	$4.0–11.0 \times 10^3/mm^3$
Differential white cell count		
Neutrophil granulocytes	$2.0–7.5 \times 10^9/l$	$2.0–7.5 \times 10^3/mm^3$
Lymphocytes	$1.5–4.0 \times 10^9/l$	$1.5–4.0 \times 10^3/mm^3$
Monocytes	$0.2–0.8 \times 10^9/l$	$0.2–0.8 \times 10^3/mm^3$
Eosinophil granulocytes	$0.04–0.4 \times 10^9/l$	$0.04–0.4 \times 10^3/mm^3$
Basophil granulocytes	$0.01–0.1 \times 10^9/l$	$0.01–0.1 \times 10^3/mm^3$
Mean corpuscular haemoglobin (MCH)	27–32 pg	–
Mean corpuscular volume (MCV)	78–98 fl	–

A.5

Haematological values

Analyte	Reference range	
	SI units	Non-SI units
Packed cell volume (PCV) or haematocrit		
Male	0.40–0.54	–
Female	0.37–0.47	–
Platelets	$150–350 \times 10^9/l$	$150–350 \times 10^3/mm^3$
Red cell count		
Male	$4.5–6.5 \times 10^{12}/l$	$4.5–6.5 \times 10^6/mm^3$
Female	$3.8–5.8 \times 10^{12}/l$	$3.8–5.8 \times 10^6/mm^3$
Red cell lifespan		
Mean	120 days	–
Half-life (^{51}Cr)	25–35 days	–
Reticulocytes (adults)	$25–85 \times 10^9/l$	$25–85 \times 10^3/mm^3$
Transferrin	2.0–4.0 g/l	0.2–0.4 g/dl
Transferrin saturation		
Male	25–56%	–
Female	14–51%	–
Vitamin B$_{12}$	130–770 pg/ml	–

A.6

Cerebrospinal fluid analysis

Analyte	Reference range	
	SI units	Non-SI units
Cells	$<5 \times 10^6$ cells/l (all mononuclear)	<5 cells/mm^3
Glucose	2.3–4.0 mmol/l	41–72 mg/dl
IgG index*	<0.65	–
Total protein	140–450 mg/l	0.014–0.045 g/dl

*A crude index of increase in IgG attributable to intrathecal synthesis.

Cardiovascular risk prediction charts

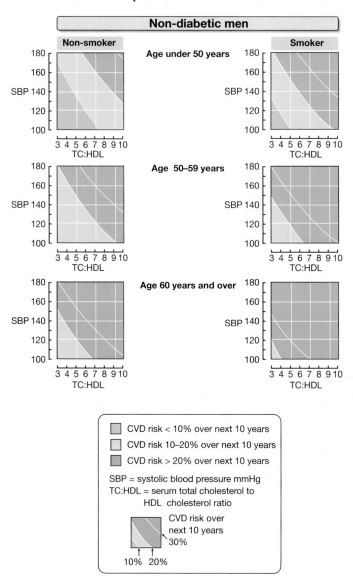

Non-diabetic men

Non-smoker		Smoker

Age under 50 years

Age 50–59 years

Age 60 years and over

SBP 180 160 140 120 100

TC:HDL 3 4 5 6 7 8 9 10

□ CVD risk < 10% over next 10 years
□ CVD risk 10–20% over next 10 years
■ CVD risk > 20% over next 10 years

SBP = systolic blood pressure mmHg
TC:HDL = serum total cholesterol to
HDL cholesterol ratio

CVD risk over
next 10 years
30%

10% 20%

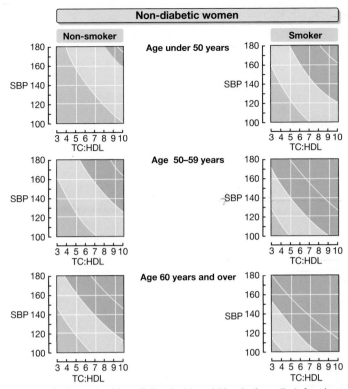

Fig. 94.1 Cardiovascular risk prediction chart to assist in selecting patients for primary prevention therapy.

- To estimate an individual's absolute 10-year risk of developing cardiovascular disease (CVD), choose the panel for the gender, smoking status and age. Within this, define the level of risk from the point where the coordinates for SBP and ratio of the total to high-density lipoprotein (HDL)-cholesterol cross. If no HDL-cholesterol result is available, assume it is 1.0 mmol/l and use the lipid scale as total serum cholesterol.
- Highest-risk individuals (red areas) are those whose 10-year CVD risk exceeds 20%, which is approximately equivalent to a 10-year coronary heart disease risk of > 15%. As a minimum, those with CVD risk > 30% (shown by the line within the red area) should be targeted and treated now. When resources allow, others with a CVD risk > 20% should be targeted progressively.
- The chart also assists in identification of individuals with a moderately high 10-year CVD risk—in the range of 10–20% (orange area) and those in whom it is lower than 10% (green area).
- Smoking status should reflect lifetime exposure to tobacco.

Index

Note: Entries in cases have been referenced by case number rather than page number. References have been given to the more possible or likely differential diagnoses in addition to the correct diagnoses. Where possible countries of the case (patient's) location or origin in the Asian subcontinent have been indexed as these are often of diagnostic relevance. Numbers preceded by an 'A' are to the Appendix. Numbers in red indicate the major presenting symptom of a case; numbers in bold indicate page numbers of cardiovascular risk prediction charts.

rash *see* rash
tumors, 87
sleepiness and snoring, obese man, 45
smoking
cardiovascular risk prediction and, **328, 329**
lung cancer and, 44
snake bite, 8, 31
snoring and sleepiness, obese man, 45
sodium disturbances, 25
somatoform disorder, 12
South Asia *see* Asian subcontinent
spinal cord compression, 14
spinal disease, back pain, 14, 78
splenohepatomegaly, 68, 71
splenomegaly and fever, 71
spondylitis, ankylosing, 78
squamous cell carcinoma
bronchogenic, 44
oesophageal, 58
Sri Lanka
numbness and sensory loss in fingers, 82
snake bite, 8
Staphylococcus aureus infective
endocarditis, 38
steroid replacement therapy, 53
stings, scorpion, 9
Streptococcus infection
endocarditis, 38, 39
glomerulonephritis, 29
group A, 29, 39
rheumatic fever, 39
S. viridans, 38
stroke (cerebrovascular accident)
elderly, 6, 86
young person, 79
subarachnoid haemorrhage, 80
suicide attempt, drug overdose, 10, 11
supraventricular tachycardia, 37
swallowing difficulty, 58
syncope vs seizure, 36, 84
syndrome of inappropriate ADH secretion, 25
syndrome X (metabolic syndrome), 55
syphilis, 21
systemic lupus erythematosus, 13, 89

tachycardia, supraventricular, 37
thrombocytopenia after hip surgery, 73
thrombocytosis, 74
thromboembolic disease, antiphospholipid
syndrome, 79
thrombosis
basilar artery, 83
deep venous, 42
thrombotic thrombocytopenic purpura, 73
thyroid disease, 47, 48
thyrotoxicosis, 47
tiredness *see* fatigue
TNF-α inhibitors/antagonists, 77
tonic–clonic seizure, generalised, 84
toxins (venoms), 8
transfusion reactions, 75

purpura, 73
transplantation, renal, 32
traveller's diarrhoea, 18
tropical disorders
infections, 16, 17, 19, 71
pulmonary eosinophilia, 19
tuberculosis, 15
arthritis, 76
cryptic miliary, 7
elderly, 5, 7, 76
haemoptysis and previous history of, 43
hepatosplenic, 71
HIV and, 20
intestinal, 62
odynophagia, 58
spinal, 14
vasculitis, 86
tumour(s) (neoplasms)
benign/in general
adrenal cortisol-producing, 52
lung, 44
pancreatic insulin-producing, 54
parathyroid, 50
pituitary, 49
skin, 87
malignant *see* cancer
tumour necrosis factor-α inhibitors/
antagonists, 77

ulcer, foot, 57
ulnar neuropathy, 82
unconsciousness *see* coma; consciousness, loss
urea, venous blood values, A.1
urethral discharge, 22
urination pain and vulval pain, 21
urine
blood in, 29
retention, 14
urticaria and eyelid swelling, 2

vaginal discharge, 24
valvular heart disease, 12, 39
vascular disease, peripheral, type 2 diabetes, 57
vasculitis, 90
tuberculous, 86
vasovagal syncope, 36
venoms (bites and stings), 8, 9, 31
veno-occlusive disease, 65
venous blood values
hormones, A.3
urea and electrolytes, A.1
other common analytes, A.4
venous leg ulcer, 91
venous thrombosis, deep, 42
ventricular septal defect, 38
vertebrae
osteoporosis, 78
tuberculosis, 14
viper bites, 8
visceral leishmaniasis, 71
vision, progressive monocular loss, 85